The Ethics of Personalised Medicine

Critical Perspectives

Edited by

JOCHEN VOLLMANN, VERENA SANDOW,
SEBASTIAN WÄSCHER AND JAN SCHILDMANN
*Institute for Medical Ethics and History of Medicine,
Ruhr-University Bochum, Germany*

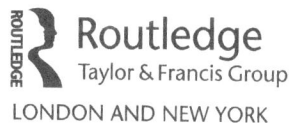

LONDON AND NEW YORK

First published 2015 by Ashgate Publishing

2 Park Square, Milton Park, Abingdon, Oxfordshire OX14 4RN
52 Vanderbilt Avenue, New York, NY 10017

Routledge is an imprint of the Taylor & Francis Group, an informa business

First issued in paperback 2020

British Library Cataloguing in Publication Data
A catalogue record for this book is available from the British Library.

The Library of Congress has cataloged the printed edition as follows:
The ethics of personalised medicine : critical perspectives / [edited] by Jochen Vollmann, Verena Sandow, Sebastian Wäscher and Jan Schildmann.
    p. ; cm.
Includes bibliographical references and index.
ISBN 978-1-4724-4796-8 (hardback)
    I. Vollmann, Jochen, editor. II. Sandow, Verena, editor. III. Wäscher, Sebastian, editor.
IV. Schildmann, Jan, 1974– , editor.
    [DNLM: 1. Ethics, Clinical. 2. Individualized Medicine—ethics. WB 60]
    R724
    174.2–dc23

2014042996

ISBN 978-1-4724-4796-8 (hbk)
ISBN 978-0-367-59909-6 (pbk)

THE ETHICS OF PERSONALISED MEDICINE

This volume is a landmark for demythologising the buzzword 'personalised medicine', critically differentiating between hype and false hopes on the one hand and realistic approaches and outlooks on the other. By comprehensively comprising a wide range of excellent normative and empirical studies, it empowers anyone interested in better understanding the presuppositions and consequences of the term 'personalised medicine' to form a well-informed judgement on one of the most augured ideas in cutting-edge medicine.

Peter Dabrock, University of Erlangen, Germany, and Vice Chair of the German Ethics Council and member of the European Group on Ethics in Science and New Technologies (EGE)

The concept 'personalised medicine' has become a buzz word in contemporary medicine. However, it is not at all clear what the concept entails. The suggestion is that treatment will be adapted to the individual patient. Yet, the basis is not knowledge of the individual patient, but statistical analysis of characteristics of patient groups. Moreover, individual patient wishes and preferences may become less relevant, if treatment options are seen in terms of chances of patient groups. This book contains critical discussions of the concept of 'personalised medicine', both from an empirical and a normative perspective. It provides a timely and needed contribution to the debate.

Guy Widdershoven, VU University Medical Center, Netherlands

Gathering together a broad range of academics working in this important area, this book considers comprehensively the conceptual, ethical and practical issues associated with the ethics of personalised medicine. The editors are to be congratulated on this volume and for the way in which it carefully reflects on the issues involved in personalised medicine and its application in practice.

Mark Sheehan, University of Oxford, UK

Contents

CONTENTS

PART IV: PERSONALISED MEDICINE IN ONCOLOGY: RECOMMENDATIONS FOR FUTURE DEVELOPMENT

List of Figures

List of Tables

Notes on Contributors

Teresa Bertram is a medical student at the Technical University Munich and works as a student research assistant at the Institute of Ethics, History and Theory of Medicine at the Ludwig-Maximilians-University Munich. She also studies at the Munich School of Philosophy and holds a scholarship from the German National Merit Foundation (Studienstiftung des deutschen Volkes).

Miriam Böttcher is a medical student in the tenth semester at the Hannover Medical School (since 2009). In the context of the research association 'Personalised medicine in Oncology' supported by the Bundesministerium für Bildung und Forschung (BMBF) she works on her medical dissertation in the medical subproject. After her general higher education entrance qualification (Abitur) in 2005 at the Caecilienschule Oldenburg she passed her final examination at the end of her training of nurses in 2009 at the Evangelisches Krankenhaus Oldenburg.

Caroline Brall holds a Master's degree in Public Health and is currently working on her dissertation in public health ethics at Maastricht University, Netherlands. During her studies, she conducted one semester at the University of Buenos Aires, Argentina and worked in a project – launched and supported by the Association of Schools of Public Health in the European Region (ASPHER) in Brussels, Belgium – exploring how ethics is taught in European Schools of Public Health. After graduating, she worked as a research assistant at the Institute of Medical Ethics and History of Medicine, Ruhr-University-Bochum, Germany. Caroline Brall obtained an Honours degree from the Faculty of Health, Medicine and Life Sciences, Maastricht University and was awarded with the Young Scholar Award of the European Association of Centres of Medical Ethics (EACME). Her main research interests focus on ethics within public health, including ethics education, priority-setting in health care, personalised medicine and ethical issues of governing innovations in health care.

George P. Browman is a cancer physician with a special interest in health services research and evidence-based decision making at the clinical and policy levels. He has contributed to tools development to facilitate ethical resource allocation decisions related to funding of new cancer drugs. Currently a healthcare consultant, Dr Browman has served as an academic leader and health-care manager in the cancer field. His past appointments include Professor and Chair of the academic Department of Clinical Epidemiology & Biostatistics at McMaster University in Hamilton Ontario (1989–97) and the Department of Oncology at the University of Calgary (2004–7). As a health-care manager he served as President of the Juravinski Cancer Centre and Vice President, Hamilton Health Sciences in Hamilton Ontario as well as Vice President, Cancer Care Ontario (1997–2004). He served as Director of the Tom Baker Cancer Centre and Vice President of the Alberta Cancer Board (2003–7). Dr Browman is the Founding Director of Cancer Care Ontario's Program in Evidence-based Care. Dr Browman retains an Adjunct appointment as Professor in the Department of Clinical Epidemiology & Biostatistics at McMaster and is Clinical Professor at the School of Population and Public Health at the University of British Columbia. Most recently, Dr Browman served as Chair of the Research Ethics Board for the University of British Columbia, BC Cancer Agency (2007–14) and as medical oncologist at the BC Cancer Agency, Vancouver Island Centre. In 2000 he was awarded the O. Harold Warwick Prize from the National Cancer Institute of Canada/ Canadian Cancer Society for 'career contributions to cancer control in Canada'. He lives and works in Victoria, British Columbia, Canada.

Marcus Dörr is a cardiologist and holds a Professorship for Cardiovascular Epidemiology and Prevention. He is a senior physician at the Department of Internal Medicine B, University Medicine Greifswald, Germany. Moreover, he is a principle investigator of the DZHK (German Centre for Cardiovascular Research) and a co-ordinator of the individualised medicine project GANI_MED (Greifswald Approach to Individualised Medicine). Professor Dörr's research interests include cardiovascular epidemiology, individualised medicine, novel heart failure therapies and exercise in cardiovascular diseases.

Tobias Fischer is a philosopher and ethicist. He is a Lecturer for Bioethics, Scientific Co-ordinator of the Department of Ethics, Theory and History of Life Sciences at the University Medicine Greifswald, Germany and member of the GANI_MED consortium. In addition, Dr Fischer is subdivision head of the BMBF-funded project MENON, which deals with ethical and economic implications of systems medicine. His research interest includes the theory and ethics of personalised medicine, reproductive medicine and the application of ethics in clinical practice.

Maria Gabriel entered Hannover Medical School in 2007 as a medical student after her general higher education entrance qualification (Abitur) in 2007 at the secondary school Hermannsburg. In the context of the research association 'Personalised medicine in Oncology' supported by the German Federal Ministry of Education and Research (Bundesministerium für Bildung und Forschung – BMBF) she works on her medical dissertation in the medical subproject.

Arnold Ganser has been chief of the Department of Hematology, Hemostasis, Oncology, and Stem Cell Transplantation within the Center of Internal Medicine at Hannover Medical School in Hannover, Germany, since 1995. He is an internationally recognised expert in the acute leukaemias and the myelodysplastic syndromes, both clinically and in translational research, with special emphasis on molecular genetics and individualised treatment strategies. In recent years his research interests have included the ethical and economic impact of individualised therapy. His scientific work has been published in more than 650 original publications in the *New England Journal of Medicine*, *Cancer Cell*, *Lancet*, *Blood*, *Journal of Clinical Oncology*, *Leukemia*, and others. He is co-chair of the German-Austrian Acute Myeloid Leukemia Study Group (AMLSG), speaker of the German MDS Study Group, and member of the executive committee of the German Network of Competence for Acute and Chronic Leukemias. He has been editor-in-chief of the *Annals of Hematology* since 2003. He also served as chair of the International Members Committee of the American Society of Hematology 2008–11, and is at present a member of the ASH Nominating Committee. His work has been honoured with the Artur Pappenheim Prize of the German Society of Hematology and Oncology, the Cancer Award of Hessen, the Dr. Paul and Cilli Weil Prize of the Johann Wolfgang Goethe University Frankfurt am Main, and the Cooperation Prize of the State of Lower Saxony.

Hanno Glimm has been section head of Applied Stem Cell Biology since 2006 and is Senior Attending Physician at the Department of Translational Oncology at the National Centre for Tumour Diseases (NCT) Heidelberg. He received his MD and Medical PhD degree from the University of Köln and worked at the University of Köln and Freiburg and at the Terry Fox Lab in Vancouver followed by his habilitation in 2005. At the NCT, Prof. Glimm co-ordinates the Personalised Oncology Programme (NCT-POP) providing individual patient treatment based on in-depth molecular analysis. He has a specific interest in normal and malignant stem cell biology, gene therapy approaches of the haematopoietic system and in developing molecular targeting approaches against solid tumour-initiating cells in solid cancers and leukaemia. Prof. Glimm serves on the ASH Scientific Committee Stem Cells and Regenerative Medicine and is a member of several scientific associations, including the German Society for Haematology and Oncology (DGHO), the American Society of Hematology (ASH), the American Association of Cancer Research (AACR), and the International Society of Stem Cell Research (ISSCR).

Sina Gottwald studied Law at the Ruhr-University Bochum and passed her first state law examination in 2008. After a two-year stage of practical legal training, she passed the second state law examination in 2011. From 2011 to 2014, she was a research assistant at the Institute for Social Law and Medical Law, Ruhr-University Bochum. She has been in practice as a lawyer since 2011.

Scott D. Grosse is a public health economist and health services researcher and works at the US Centers for Disease Control and Prevention (CDC), Atlanta, Georgia. Dr Grosse has authored and co-authored more than 150 journal articles and book chapters. His research interests include policy and cost-effectiveness analyses of strategies such as newborn screening and genetic testing, assessments of the economic burden of congenital disorders, and health economic measures and methods.

Robin Haring graduated as Demographer (Diploma) from the University of Rostock, Germany, in 2006, and was awarded a PhD in Epidemiology with distinction from the University of Greifswald, Germany, in 2010. He was awarded with the Dissertation of the Year Prize from the University of Greifswald and granted a scholarship from the Alfried Krupp von Bohlen und Halbach Foundation for a postdoc research fellowship in the Framingham Heart Study, Boston University, in 2010/11. Given his strong interest in endocrine and cardiovascular epidemiology, he successfully completed his habilitation about 'Low total testosterone concentrations as a biomarker of increased cardiometabolic risk factor burden in men' in 2013, with an overall number of 55 publications in international peer-reviewed journals and a cumulative Impact Factor of 275. He is currently head of the Biobanking Core Unit at the University Medicine Greifswald, Germany.

Franz Hessel is a physician and holds a Master's degree in Public Health. He has served as Professor for Health-Care Management at the SRH University Berlin as programme head of the Executive MBA Health-Care Management course since July 2011. He was research fellow and senior researcher at the University of Greifswald and the University of Essen, Germany, participating in and leading numerous research projects in economic evaluation, medical decision-making, health technology assessment and health services research. From 2006 to 2011, he was head of HEOR (Health Economics Outcomes Research) of Sanofi Germany and Abbott Diagnostics. Professor Hessel's current research interests include the medical and economic evaluation of biomarker tests and personalised medicine strategies in oncology, infectious diseases, diabetes and other disease areas, the health-care patterns in addiction treatments and aspects of hospital management, such as risk management and human resources management. He has been working as a consultant for market access and HEOR for industry and non-commercial health-care institutions for over 15 years.

Peter Heusser is a physician and has a Master's of Medical Education. He serves as Professor and Director of the Institute of Integrative Medicine and as chair holder of the Gerhard Kienle Chair for Theory of Medicine, Integrative and Anthroposophic Medicine at Witten/Herdecke University, Germany. He is co-chairman of the Centre for Medical Research and Education at the Community Hospital in Herdecke, Germany. Professor Heusser's research interests include integrative medicine, person-centred medicine, anthroposophic medicine, medical anthropology and medical education.

Irene Hirschberg, MD, MPH, born in 1977, is a Research Associate at the Institute for History, Ethics and Philosophy of Medicine at the Centre for Public Health and Health-care, Hannover Medical School (Germany) and member of CELLS – Centre of Ethics and Law in the Life Sciences (Hannover). She studied Medicine and Public Health (both in Hannover). After a short period as a clinician in paediatrics, she undertook a traineeship in project management and editing at a German medical publishing company. She has worked in the fields of public health ethics, clinical ethics and research ethics since 2007. Her current research interests include informed consent evaluation, research ethics and public involvement activities.

Stefan Huster studied Law and Philosophy at the universities of Bielefeld and Frankfurt/Main. From 1990 to 2002, he was a research assistant at Heidelberg University, where he received his PhD and *venia docendi* in Public Law, European Law, Legal Philosophy and Social Law. From 2002 to 2004, he was Professor of German and European Constitutional and Administrative Law at FernUniversität in Hagen. In 2004, he joined the Ruhr-University Bochum (Germany) as Professor of Public Law and Social Law and Director of the Institute of Social Law and Health Law. He was awarded a fellowship at the Institute of Advanced Studies, Berlin, for the academic year 2010/11. His research areas are public law, social law, health law and philosophy of law.

Rebecca Jahn is a senior researcher and has been head of the research unit 'Health Systems, Health Policy and Pharmaceutical Regulation' at the Institute for Health Care Management and Research, University of Duisburg-Essen, Germany, since 2007. She studied Nutritional Sciences at the University of Gießen, Germany, and completed her doctorate at the University of Duisburg-Essen. Dr Jahn mainly analyses health policy in Western welfare states and the regulation of the pharmaceutical industry.

Hannes Kahrass, MPH, born in 1983, has a degree in Physiotherapy and Public Health. Since 2010, he has worked as a research associate at the Institute for History, Ethics & Philosophy of Medicine at the Centre for Public Health and Healthcare, Hannover Medical School (Germany) and CELLS – Centre for Ethics and Law in the Life Sciences (Hannover). He passed the state examination in Physiotherapy in 2008 (University Medical Centre Göttingen) and completed his Bachelor of Science in Physiotherapy in 2009 (HAWK Hildesheim). He successfully completed his Master of Public Health in 2011 (Hannover Medical School). His current research interests include informed consent evaluation, research ethics, knowledge translation and health policy analysis.

Corinna Klingler is a research associate and PhD student at the Institute of Ethics, History and Theory of Medicine at the Ludwig Maximilians-University Munich. She received her BA in Philosophy and Economics from the University of Bayreuth and her MSc in International Health Policy from the London School of Economics and Political Science. Currently, she has a scholarship from the German National Merit Foundation (Studienstiftung des deutschen Volkes) for her doctoral research, which is concerned with the difficulties faced by immigrant physicians practising in German hospitals and questions of responsibility distribution. In addition, she is engaged in other projects at the institute and has worked on definitions of personalised medicine and economic implications of advance care planning. She developed an ethical framework for evaluating health-care programmes for chronically ill patients. Her main research interests are normative health services research, public health ethics and rationing/prioritising scarce health-care resources.

Martin Langanke is a philosopher and ethicist. Dr Langanke serves as a lecturer for ethics at the Faculty of Theology, Ernst-Moritz-Arndt-University Greifswald, Germany. He is a member of the GANI_MED consortium at Greifswald University and general co-ordinator of the BMBF-funded project MENON, which deals with ethical and economic implications of systems medicine. Dr Langanke's research interests include the foundations of ethics, philosophical anthropology, theory and ethics of personalised medicine, medical research ethics and animal ethics.

Stefan Lange completed his medical studies at the Heinrich-Heine-University in Düsseldorf in 1989 and received his MD in 1994. From 1989–93 he was initially in practical training at the Ferdinand-Sauerbruch-Clinic in Wuppertal, then assumed the position of intern/resident physician. In 1993 he joined the department of medical computer sciences, biometrics and epidemiology at the Ruhr-University in Bochum and was appointed to the position of research assistant in 1995. He was awarded the certificate of Biometrics in Medicine with the title of 'Qualified Statistician' by the German Association for Medical Computer Sciences, Biometry and Epidemiology (GMDS) in 1999. In 2003 he received his PhD (second thesis, the *Habilitationsschrift*) at the Ruhr University and received the venia legendi (right to teach) in Medical Biometry and Clinical Epidemiology. He joined the Institute for Quality and Efficiency in Health Care in 2004 and headed the department of Non-Medical Interventions until 2007. Since 2005 he has held the position of Deputy Director of the Institute.

Georg Marckmann studied medicine and philosophy at the University of Tübingen (Germany) and received a Master's degree in Public Health from the Harvard School of Public Health (Boston, MA). He was a scholar in the Postgraduate College 'Ethics in the Sciences and Humanities' in Tübingen from 1992 to 1995. He received a doctoral degree in medicine in 1997. From 1998 to 2010, he was Assistant Professor at the Institute of Ethics and History of Medicine at the University of Tübingen and has been Vice Director of the institute since 2003. He has been a full Professor of Medical Ethics and Director of the Institute of Ethics, History, and Theory of Medicine at Ludwig-Maximilians-University of Munich since 2010. His main research interests include ethical issues of end-of-life care, clinical ethics consultation, distributive justice in health care, ethical issues in organ transplantation and public health ethics.

Anja Neumann, MD, PhD in Economics, is a Research Assistant at the Institute of Health-Care Management and Research at the University of Duisburg-Essen in Essen, Germany. She is head of the working group 'Health Economic Evaluation and Outcomes Research'. Her research interests include health economic evaluation and outcomes research, personalised medicine, systematic reviews and decision-analytic modelling.

Michael Noweski is a political scientist. He has been a research associate at the Institute for Health-Care Management and Research, University of Duisburg-Essen, Germany, since 2012. After completing his doctorate at the Free University of Berlin in 2007, he was a research associate at the WZB Berlin Social Science Centre. Dr Noweski analyses the regulation of health-care markets and the structure and developmental dynamics of policy subsystems.

Julia Perry is a Master's student in Sociology with a minor in Gender Studies at the University of Göttingen, Germany. She completed her undergraduate studies in Sociology at the University of Bremen. She has been a student Research Assistant to Prof. S. Schicktanz at the Department of Medical Ethics and History of Medicine at the University Medical Centre Göttingen since 2012. She also worked there within the DFG-funded project of the clinical research unit

(KFO 179/2) 'Ethical aspects in individualized rectal cancer therapy: patients' expectations and attitudes toward prognostic tests using biomarkers – a socio-empirical and medical-ethical analysis'. Currently, she is finalising her Master's thesis: 'The complexity of medical information in cancer treatment: needs and uncertainties regarding information on treatment procedure, side effects, risks, and genetic testing – a qualitative study of 10 rectal carcinoma patients in longitudinal section' (working title) which is linked to data of the KFO project.

Matthias Port is a physician specialising in haematology, oncology, palliative care and radiobiology. He serves as a scientist and Director of the Bundeswehr Institute of Radiobiology affiliated to the University of Ulm, Munich, Germany. His fellowship included training at the Federal Armed Forces Hospitals in Koblenz and Ulm/Germany and Hannover Medical School (MHH), Hannover, Germany. While working as consultant at the MHH, he was responsible for the academic teaching in palliative care. Dr Port's research interests include tumourbiology, radiobiology and personalised medicine.

Laura Pouryamout, MA, is a research assistant at the Institute of Health-Care Management and Research at University of Duisburg-Essen in Essen, Germany. She is part of the working group 'Health Economic Evaluation and Outcomes Research'. She finished her bachelor studies in Health Communication at the Faculty of Health Science at the University of Bielefeld and then continued her education with a Master's degree in Medical Management at the Institute of Health-Care Management and Research at University of Duisburg-Essen. Her research interests include health economic evaluation and outcomes research, personalised medicine, systematic reviews and decision-analytic modelling.

Barbara Prainsack is a professor at the Department of Social Science, Health and Medicine at King's College London. A political scientist by background, Prof. Prainsack is interested in the regulatory, social and ethical dimensions of bioscience and biomedicine. She has published widely on these topics, in particular, on DNA testing in forensics and medicine. Her recent book publications include: *Genetics as Social Practice* (Ashgate, 2014; ed. with Silke Schicktanz and Gabriele Werner-Felmayer); *Solidarity: Reflections on an Emerging Concept in Bioethics* (Nuffield Council on Bioethics, 2011; with Alena Buyx); and *Genetic Suspects: Global Governance of Forensic DNA Profiling and Databasing* (Cambridge University Press, 2010; ed. with R. Hindmarsh). Professor Prainsack is a member of the Austrian Bioethics Commission advising the government in Vienna, the National DNA Database Ethics Board in England and Wales, and she is the British representative in the Domain Committee Individuals, Societies, Cultures, and Health (ISCH) at COST (cost.eu). She led the European Science Foundation's (ESF) Forward Look on 'Personalised Medicine for the European

Citizen' from 2011–13, alongside Aarno Palotie and Stephen Holgate. She is also a senior editor of the second *Encyclopedia of Social and Behavioral Sciences* (Elsevier, publication date 2015).

Wolf H. Rogowski is a health economist at the Helmholtz Centre Munich, Institute of Health Economics and Health-Care Management, in Germany. He has headed the institute's research unit 'Translational Health Economics' since August 2009. He holds a PhD from Ludwig-Maximilians-University Munich and has held visiting fellowships at the Centre of Health Economics at the University of York (UK), the Hastings Center in Garrison, New York (USA) and the Harvard School of Public Health, Boston (USA). Dr Rogowski explores the process of translational medicine from a health economics perspective. This includes the application of cost-effectiveness and value of information analysis to new health technologies; the empirical and theoretical assessment of methods and procedures applied in decision-making; and the development of instruments for decision support. He has a particular interest in the intersection of ethics and economics in the evaluation of medical innovations. Focusing on genetic testing and personalised medicine, Dr Rogowski serves as a member of the European Society for Human Genetics' Professional and Public Policy Committee and the scientific advisory board of the *Journal of Community Genetics*. He holds a *venia legendi* in Health Economics and Health-Care Management and teaches at the Ludwig-Maximilians-University Munich, Germany, at the LMU Entrepreneurship Centre and in the Master of Public Health programme, among others.

Verena Sandow, MA, is a researcher in Medical Ethics and Applied Ethics at the Institute for Medical Ethics and History of Medicine, Ruhr-University Bochum, Germany. Following her studies in Philosophy, Media Studies and Economic History at the Heinrich-Heine-University Düsseldorf, she was a member of the research training group 'Bioethics' at the International Centre in Science and Humanities, Eberhard-Karls-University Tübingen. She works in the field of human medical research, research ethics and has co-organised several conferences in the field of medical ethics.

Silke Schicktanz has been full Professor of Cultural and Ethical Studies of Biomedicine at the Department of Medical Ethics and History of Medicine at the University Medical Centre Göttingen, Germany, since 2010. She studied Biology and Philosophy at the University of Tübingen and finalised her PhD in the field of Ethics of Life Sciences in 2002. She was Junior Professor of History, Ethics and Theory of Medicine at the University of Göttingen from 2006 to 2010. She relies on her established international research collaborations with the Ben-Gurion University (Israel), JNU Delhi

(India), Uppsala University (Sweden), University of California, Berkeley and San Francisco State University (USA) and CESAGEN Lancaster (UK) for her cross-cultural research interest. Most recently, she led a research project funded by the Deutsche Forschungsgemeinschaft (DFG) investigating patients' views on individualised medicine in rectum cancer treatment (2011–14, KFO 179/2). Professor Schicktanz is also a PI in the European Joint Programme 'Mind the risk' funded by the Swedish Riksbankens Jubileumsfond (2013–18) in which she is investigating the ethical and cultural implications of individualised genetic medical information for treatment and prevention. Her other research fields include ethics of organ transplantation and ageing medicine, cultural differences in bioethics and biopolitics, the intersection of professional views and patients' perspectives, and new methodological approaches in empirical-ethical research.

Jan Schildmann, MD MA, studied medicine at the Charité Medical School, Berlin, and received an MA in Medical Law and Ethics from King's College, University of London. He has qualified as a specialist in internal medicine and is currently head of the North Rhine-Westphalia Junior Research Group 'Medical Ethics at the End of Life: Norm and Empiricism' at the Institute of Medical Ethics and History of Medicine, Ruhr-University Bochum, Germany. His research focuses on clinical ethics (i.e. end-of-life decisions, ethics support services), research ethics (i.e. personalised medicine, conflict of interest) and methodological aspects of empirical medical ethics. His work has been published in more than 70 contributions in peer-reviewed journals and awarded with research prizes by the European Society for Philosophy of Medicine and Healthcare, and the German Society for Palliative Medicine.

Sebastian Schleidgen is a philosopher and ethicist. He works as Research Fellow at the National Center for Tumor Diseases (NCT), Ruprecht-Karls-University Heidelberg, Germany. He was trained in Philosophy and Sociology at the University of Constance, Germany (2000–7). He was a PhD student at the research training group 'Bioethics' at the International Centre for Ethics in the Sciences and Humanities (IZEW), Eberhard-Karls-University Tübingen, Germany (2007–10) and a Fellow in Philosophy at the Department of Philosophy, Harvard University, Cambridge, MA, USA (2009/10). He worked as Research Fellow at the Institute of Ethics, History and Theory of Medicine, Ludwig-Maximilians-University Munich, Germany (2011–14). His research interests are mainly in ethics, medical ethics, metaethics and political philosophy.

Jörg Schmidtke is a clinical geneticist. He studied medicine in Freiburg and Basel. He obtained his doctoral degree in 1974 at the University of Freiburg, and has held postdoctoral positions in Freiburg and Göttingen. He was a visiting scientist at the MRC Mammalian Genome Unit, Edinburgh, 1981–2, the Gesellschaft für Biotechnologische Forschung, Braunschweig, Dept. Genetics, 1982, and Johns Hopkins University, Baltimore, 1995. He obtained a Professorship for Human Genetics at the Free University of Berlin in 1988 and was Director of the Institute of Human Genetics at Hannover Medical School from 1990 to 2014. He was Chairman of the German Board of Medical Genetics 1993–7, President of the German Society of Human Genetics 1998–2000, Member of the Ethics Council, Federal Ministry of Health, Germany, 1999–2002, coordinator of ORPHANET Germany, since 2002, appointed member and elected chair of the 'Gendiagnostik-Kommission' at the Robert-Koch-Institut, Berlin since 2009, and President of the European Society of Human Genetics 2011–12. He was honoured with Scientific Prizes of the German Society of Human Genetics and the German Cystic Fibrosis Society in 1987, habilitation and Heisenberg fellowships of the Deutsche Forschungsgemeinschaft. He is currently Editor-in-Chief of the *Journal of Community Genetics* and Clinical Utility Gene Cards Section Editor of the *European Journal of Human Genetics*. His current research interests include community genetics and translational medicine.

Daniel Strech, MD, PhD, born 1975, is Assistant Professor at the Institute for History, Ethics and Philosophy of Medicine at the Centre for Public Health and Healthcare, Hannover Medical School (Germany) and co-director of CELLS – Centre of Ethics and Law in the Life Sciences (Hannover). He studied Medicine and Philosophy and worked for two years as a clinician and researcher in the field of Psychiatry. He has worked full-time in the fields of Public Health Ethics, Research Ethics and Health Policy Analysis. He is a board member of the German Network for Evidence-based Medicine (DNEbM). He served as Interim Director at the Institute of Biomedical Ethics, University of Zurich (Switzerland), from January 2012 to June 2013.

Klaus Tanner (born 1953) has been the Professor of Systematic Theology and Ethics at the Faculty of Theology at the Ruprecht-Karls-University Heidelberg since 2008. He taught at the Martin Luther University Halle-Wittenberg (2000–8), at the Philosophical Faculty of the Technical University Dresden (1993–8) and at the Theological Faculty at Ludwig-Maximilians-University in Munich. He is an ordained pastor of the Lutheran Church in Bavaria. He was a member of the German Parliament's Study Commission on 'Law and Ethics in Modern Medicine' (2000–2). He has been a member of the federal government's 'Central Ethics Committee for Stem Cell Research' (ZES at the Robert-Koch-Institute) since 2002 and the German Research Foundation's 'Senate Commission on Genetic Research'. He is an elected member of the German Academy of Sciences Leopoldina (National Academy). He is on the board of directors of the Centre for Medicine- Ethics-Law (MER) at the Martin-Luther-Universität Halle-Wittenberg. He is on the Advisory Commission of the Evangelical Church in Germany (EKD) regarding Social Responsibility. Professor Tanner's research fields are Protestantism and political culture in Germany, bioethics, history of ethics and hermeneutics. He has written on Protestantism and democracy, the natural law traditions, bioethics, law and culture.

Felicitas Thol is a physician and researcher in the field of hematology. She serves as an attending physician at the Department of Hematology, Hemostasis, Oncology, and Stem Cell Transplantation at Hannover Medical School, Hannover, Germany. She completed her residence in internal medicine at Dartmouth Hitchcock Medical Center (USA). She is additionally board certified in internal medicine as well as in hematology/oncology in Germany. Her clinical as well as research interest are in the field of hematological malignancies, especially acute myeloid leukemia and myelodysplastic syndromes. She is co-leader of the AML-SG reference lab in Hannover. Prices for her work on molecular markers in myeloid malignancies include the Rudolf Schoen-price of the TUI-Stiftung, the MHH Cancer Center Research Fellowship, the ASH Abstract Achievement Award as well as the EHA ASH Translational Research Training in Hematology Award.

Nicole Trachte, Dipl.-Kffr., is a consultant in the consulting agency CURATIS GmbH in Bremen, Germany. She is part of the working group which specialises in the secondary and tertiary facilities in the health-care system, primarily in hospitals. She finished her degree in business administration at the Faculty of Business and Economics at University of Duisburg-Essen, Campus Essen.

Jochen Vollmann is a physician and medical ethicist. He serves as Professor and Director of the Institute for Medical Ethics and History of Medicine and President of the Centre for Medical Ethics, Ruhr-University Bochum, Germany. Professor Vollmann was Visiting Fellow at the Kennedy Institute of Ethics, Georgetown University, Washington, DC (1994/5), Visiting Professor at the San Francisco School of Medicine, University of California and at the Mount Sinai School of Medicine, New York (1999/2000), at the Institute for the Medical Humanities UTMB, Texas (2001) and at the Centre for Values, Ethics and the Law in Medicine at the University of Sydney (2004, 2008, 2009, 2010, 2012, 2013 and 2014). He was honoured with the Prize for Brain Research in Geriatrics of the University of Witten/Herdecke, the Stehr-Boldt-Prize for Medical Ethics of the University of Zurich, the Research Award of the German Association of Palliative Medicine, as well as the University Teaching Award *lehrreich* of the Ruhr-University Bochum and the Gaudium docendi Teaching Award of the Society of Friends and Sponsors of the Ruhr-University Bochum. Professor Vollmann's research interests include informed consent and capacity assessment, mental health ethics, end-of-life decision-making, advance directives, personalised medicine, medical professionalism, clinical ethics committees and clinical ethics consultation.

Christof von Kalle has been Director of the Department of Translational Oncology at NCT and DKFZ since July 2005, chairing the NCT Board of Directors. As a physician scientist, with a clinical background in haematology/oncology, Prof. von Kalle is an internationally renowned scientific leader in stem-cell research, mutation analysis and gene transfer, with >150 high-impact publications. He is an elected member of the European Academy of Cancer Sciences and serves as chair of the CCC Network of German Cancer Aid. Professor von Kalle co-ordinates overall NCT activities, with the primary goal of facilitating excellence in translational and clinical research. The department is home to internationally renowned research groups for stem-cell research, applied functional genomics, lymphoma research, molecular diagnostics and gene therapy. Physician scientists are involved in clinical activities, patient care and innovative clinical trials. The department oversees NCT POP, providing individual patient treatment based on in-depth molecular analysis.

Thomas Wabel is Professor of Protestant Theology (with a focus on Systematic Theology) at the University of Bamberg. Following his studies in Heidelberg, Bonn and Oxford, and after a research year at Harvard University in 1994, Wabel received his PhD in Systematic Theology from Heidelberg University in 1996. He has taught Systematic Theology at Frankfurt University, Humboldt University of Berlin, Justus-Liebig-University, Gießen, and Hamburg University, and he is a pastor in the Protestant Church of Hessen and Nassau (Germany). Professor Wabel held the Ernst Cassirer Fellowship at the Swedish Collegium for Advanced Study (SCAS) in Uppsala (Sweden) in 2008. He is author of *Sprache als Grenze in Luthers theologischer Hermeneutik und Wittgensteins Sprachphilosophie* (Berlin and New York: de Gruyter, 1998) and of *Die nahe ferne Kirche. Studien zu einer protestantischen Ekklesiologie in kulturhermeneutischer Perspektive* (Tübingen: Mohr Siebeck, 2010). Furthermore, his publications include books (both as editor and co-editor) on bioethics and medical ethics (2004, 2007), on neurophysiology, legal responsibility and free will (2005), and on commentary as a practice of liberal arts (2011). His articles in journals and books cover such topics as the role of intuition in moral reasoning (2005), religion and aesthetics (2006, 2007), the hiddenness of God (2010) and medical ethics (2012, 2013).

Anke Walendzik studied Economics at the Universities of Cologne and Warsaw and completed her doctorate at the University of Duisburg-Essen. She was working as a research associate from 2005 and has been working as head of the research unit 'Health Systems, Health Policy and Pharmaceutical Regulation' at the Institute for Health-Care Management and Research,

University of Duisburg-Essen, Germany, since 2009. Dr Walendzik mainly analyses the remuneration of health services and economic incentives in healthcare markets.

Sebastian Wäscher, MA, is a researcher in Medical Ethics, with a focus on social science aspects. He has a background in Communication, Sociology and Philosophy. Sebastian has been a Research Assistant at the Institute for Medical Ethics and History of Medicine, Ruhr-University Bochum, Germany, and a member of the NRW-Junior Research Group 'Medical Ethics at the End of Life: Norm and Empiricism' since 2011. His research interests are questions at the end of life, empirical ethics, personalised medicine and qualitative research methodology.

Jürgen Wasem is an economist and public health researcher by training. He has served as a full Professor and Director of the Alfried Krupp von Bohlen und Halbach Endowed Chair for Health-Care Management and Research, University Duisburg-Essen, since 2003. Professor Wasem is a member of the medical faculty as well as of the faculty for Business and Economics at the University. Among former positions he was full Professor for Health-Care Management at the Department for Law and Economics of the Ernst Moritz Arndt University Greifswald, Professor for Health Economics in the School of Public Health of the Ludwig-Maximilans-University Munich, a senior researcher at the Max Planck Institute for the Study of Societies, Cologne, and consultant at the Department for Health Care and Health Insurance of the Federal Ministry of Labour and Social Policy. He is a member of the board of directors of the German Health Economics Association (dggoe), where he was chairman in 2013/14. He was the president of the German Association for Disease Management (DGDM), and is a member of the board of directors of the Federal Association for Managed Care (BMC). He is chairperson of the Academic Advisory Board on Risk Adjustment which is affiliated to the Federal Insurance Office.

Jürgen Windeler is a physician and the current Director of the Institute for Quality and Efficiency in Health Care (IQWiG) in Cologne, Germany. Between 1985 and 1993, Professor Windeler worked as an assistant physician, was a fellowship holder of the German Research Foundation, and worked as a research associate at various universities and hospitals, including the Department of Medical Informatics and Biomathematics at the Ruhr University of Bochum. Between 1993 and 1999, he was a university lecturer and Deputy Head of the Department of Medical Biometry at the Ruprecht Karls University of Heidelberg. He then joined the Medical Advisory Service of the German Social Health Insurance (MDS) in Essen, initially as the Head of the

Department of Evidence-based Medicine (1999–2004) and then as the Deputy Chief Executive and Chief Physician (2004–10). In September 2010 he took up the position of Director of IQWiG. Besides evidence-based medicine (EbM) in general, Professor Windeler's research interests include the application of EbM principles to medical devices, screening programmes, and personalised medicine. He has held an extraordinary professorship in Medical Biometry and Clinical Epidemiology at the Ruhr University of Bochum since 2001.

Eva C. Winkler is a physician ethicist at the National Centre for Tumour Diseases (NCT) in Heidelberg. She holds a PhD in cancer research from the University of Heidelberg as well as in Medical and Health-Care Ethics from the University of Basel (*summa cum laude*). Before she entered the PhD programme in Basel, she did research and training in Medical Ethics at the Harvard Medical School, Division of Medical Ethics (ethics fellowship) and as a Faculty Fellow at the Center for Ethics and the Professions, Harvard University, Kennedy School of Government. She is a board-certified internist who has been working in oncology both with in- and outpatient care for 15 years and as a consultant for many years. Dr Winkler works as a consultant at the Centre for Oncology at the NCT Heidelberg and is a group leader of the research programme Ethics and Patient-Oriented Care in Oncology (NCT-EPOC). She is co-directing the 'Ethics and Medicine' Working Group of the German Association for Haematology and Oncology. She is a fellow of the Marsilius Kolleg and project speaker for the interdisciplinary project 'Ethical and Legal Aspects of Whole Genome Sequencing (EURAT)' of the Marsilius Kolleg in Heidelberg.

Mathias Wirth is a theologian and ethicist who studied both Catholic and Protestant Theology with Philosophy. He holds the position of Lecturer and Research Associate at the Department of History and Ethics at the University Medical Centre Hamburg-Eppendorf, Germany. His research and teaching interests encompass Anthropology and Ethics, with a particular focus on Hebrew-Christian tradition in dialogue with current ethical debates on medicine, freedom and vulnerability. Examples of his work include *Can One Murder Out of Compassion? Ethics of Compassion according to Emmanuel Lévinas's Concept of Alteration* (2012), *The (In)Visible Human in Life Sciences: How Accurate is Karl Rahner's Enigmatic Human after Genome Sequencing and Brain Imaging?* (2012), and *Regula Tactus: The Actuality of an Ecclesiastical Norm as Prevention of and a Plea against Sexual Violence* (2013).

Sabine Wöhlke completed her studies in Cultural Anthropology and Gender Studies at the University of Göttingen, Germany. She has been a research assistant for Prof. S. Schicktanz at the Department of Medical Ethics and History of Medicine at the University Medical Centre, Göttingen, since 2006.

Her main interests include ethical aspects of genetic testing and predictive genetic testing, qualitative social-empirical research, and ethical and medical anthropological research on organ transplantation. She was scientific co-ordinator of the project 'Ethical aspects in individualized rectal cancer therapy: patients' expectations and attitudes toward prognostic tests using biomarkers – a socio-empirical and medical-ethical analysis' (funded by the DFG, KFO 179/2) from 2011 to 2014. She has been a member of the European working group 'Mind the risk' – ethical, psychological and social implications of provision of risk information from genetic and related technologies (funded by the Swedish Riksbankens Jubileumsfond), since 2014.

In 2014, Dr Wöhlke finalised her PhD with the title: 'Medical anthropological perspectives towards decisions and motivations of living kidney donations, with a special focus on gender differences'.

Introduction

Jochen Vollmann, Verena Sandow, Sebastian Wäscher and Jan Schildmann

'Personalised medicine' is commonly understood as the application of biological (for example, genomic) data to improve the diagnosis, therapy and prevention of diseases. Over the last few years, this phrase has become the symbol of medical progress and a label for better health care in the future. However, a controversial debate has developed whether these promises of better, more personal and more cost-efficient medicine are realistic. Therefore, the book assembles contributions of leading experts from normative and empirical disciplines with a focus on a critical reflection about 'personalised medicine' – a topic which is often dealt with in a rather uncritical way in current literature.

One important source for the research comprised in this volume is the four-year collaborative research project *Personalised Medicine in Oncology: An Interdisciplinary Study on Ethical, Medical, Economical and Legal Aspects* funded by the German Federal Ministry for Education and Research (Bundesministerium für Bildung und Forschung – BMBF). Experts from the fields of medical ethics, oncology, health-economics and law present findings from this joint research collaboration. The second source for contributions is a selection of presentations from the 2013 conference of the European Association of Centres of Medical Ethics (EACME) *'Personalised Medicine' – Medicine for the Person? Ethical Challenges for Medical Research and Practice.* The conference attracted leading researchers from Europe, North America and other continents which provided a forum for a multidisciplinary debate on the current state of research on the ethical, legal and social implications of personalised medicine.

The book is structured in three main parts which cover important topics in the field of personalised medicine beginning with the clarification of the vague concept of personalised medicine, through the presentation and reflection of clinical application, to a discussion on structural aspects of personalised medicine. A fourth part completes the book with recommendations for future development in personalised medicine.

Part I: Personalised Medicine – Medicine for the Person? Concepts and Contextual Aspects

The first part of the book reflects on the general concepts of personalised medicine. Therefore, questions on the meaning of the term 'personalised medicine' and related topics are discussed. The contributions stretch from definitions (Schleidgen and colleagues) and possible paradigm shifts (Fischer and colleagues; Browman) to the question of personhood (Wabel; Wirth; Heusser).

Sebastian Schleidgen and his colleagues argue that the lack of a clear definition of personalised medicine is problematic for both conceptual and empirical research. The aim of their chapter, 'What is Personalised Medicine? Sharpening a Vague Term Based on a Systematic Literature Review', is to develop a definition of personalised medicine to solve the problems arising from the vague use of the term. The authors conduct a systematic review in order to derive a definition of the term 'personalised medicine'.

Tobias Fischer and his colleagues locate the discussion on personalised medicine between hypes, hopes and risks. The authors state that aspects of personalised medicine are situated in the realm of hypothetical ethics. With their chapter, 'Alarming Symptoms of a Paradigm Shift? An Approach to Bridge the Gap between Hypothetical Ethics and the Current Status of Individualised Medicine Research', they present an approach to bridge the gap between hypothetical ethics and the current status of research on personalised medicine.

Thinking of personalised medicine in terms of a paradigm shift, George P. Browman illuminates in his chapter, 'Personalised Medicine: Getting Past the Controversies', how new ways of thinking often begin with controversial discussions and then, slowly, arrive at more fruitful conversations. The aim of his chapter is to contribute to the discussion on personalised medicine in order to change the way of speaking from controversy to consensus. He sets up a framework for the future accessibility of personalised medicine and differentiates between two conceptual packages with unsolved and rising problems.

While these three chapters discuss very foundational questions of personalised medicine, the following three chapters focus on aspects of personhood and autonomy in personalised medicine.

Thomas Wabel argues in favour of a concept of 'embodied autonomy' in his chapter, 'Patient as Person in Personalised Medicine: Autonomy, Responsibility and the Body'. This concept avoids a dualism of body and mind and is driven by the idea that 'mind is essentially embodied'. To strengthen his argumentation, he uses empirical results from interview studies on personalised medicine as an example of how to conceptualise 'embodied autonomy'.

Matthias Wirth analyses the term 'personalised' from a phenomenological theoretical perspective. In his chapter, 'The Authority of Corporeality and Emotions: The New Phenomenology and its Relevance to the German Debate on Personalised Medicine', he shows how a concept of corporeality broadens our view of a personalised medical treatment. He argues that neither the immaterial nor the material aspect of human existence refers exclusively to the phrase 'personalised'.

In line with Wabel and Wirth, Peter Heusser analyses the term 'person' in personalised medicine and agrees that a person is more than a mere genetic set-up. In his chapter, 'Towards Integration of "Personalised" and "Person-centred" Medicine: The Concept of "Integrative and Personalised Health Care"', he shows a friction between the scientific concept of personalised medicine as molecular medicine and the understanding of the term by lay people.

Part II: Personalised Medicine in Clinical and Practical Research

The second part of the book shifts from the theoretical perspective to the application of personalised medicine and draws a line from critical conceptual contributions on biobanking (Winkler and colleagues; Hirschberg and colleagues), through clinical research on new genetic biomarkers (Port and colleagues) to a general reflection from a social science perspective (Wöhlke and colleagues; Wäscher and colleagues; Prainsack).

The first two chapters discuss aspects of biobank research in the context of informed consent. Both chapters present various problems of biobank research and concentrate on informed consent procedures, but choose different ways of coping with the complex issue of consent in biobank research.

Eva C. Winkler and her colleagues argue from a clinical perspective and develop an ethical framework on this basis. They point out several ethical issues connected to genomic data use in medicine in their chapter, 'Ethical Considerations for Developing a Best-Practice Guideline for Next Generation Sequencing in Oncology'. The main aim of the chapter is to give an overview of ethical and clinical questions concerned with the patient information process and consent in biobank-based genomic research.

Closely connected with Winkler, Irene Hirschberg and colleagues analyse guidelines on consent in biomedical research in order to develop a tool to distinguish relevant aspects of informed consent in biobank research in their chapter, 'Practice Variation across Consent Templates for Biobank Research: A Survey of German Biobanks'.

On the basis of a meta-analysis of publications dealing with acute myeloid leukemia (AML), Matthias Port and his colleagues provide an account of the current evidence on the role of biomarkers for treatment and prognosis of this disease. In the chapter 'Individualised Medicine in the Diagnosis and Prognosis of Patients Younger Than 65 Years with Normal Karyotype Acute Myeloid Leukemia: A Systematic Review and Meta-Analysis of the Impact of Fms-Related

Tyrosine Kinase 3 Internal Tandem Duplication (FLT3-ITD)', the authors identify the FLT3-ITD mutation as an important prognostic parameter in AML therapy and also discuss the challenges to critically appraise the relevance of biomarkers.

Three chapters take a social science perspective on clinical research in personalised medicine.

Sabine Wöhlke and colleagues analyse patients' perspectives on personalised medicine with a qualitative research design (observations and interviews). In their chapter, 'Taking it Personally: Patients' Perspectives on Personalised Medicine and its Ethical Relevance', they concentrate on ethical aspects of information and decision-making within the context of stratified treatment of rectal carcinoma.

Sebastian Wäscher and his colleagues give insights into the clinical social reality with their chapter, '"Personalised Medicine" in Oncology: Physicians' Perspectives on Contributions to and Challenges for Clinical Practice'. They use qualitative interviews to illuminate the attitudes and values of oncologists who are confronted with the development of personalised medicine in their daily practice. The physicians draw a differentiated picture of personalised medicine in which they stress the advantages of stratifying therapies as well as the practical problems resulting from such a development.

Barbara Prainsack links the discussion on biobanking and the application of specific genomic data to a larger discussion on the clinical use of personalised medicine in her chapter, 'Through Thick and Big: Data-Rich Medicine in the Era of Personalisation'. She critically asks questions on the use of data and points out several challenges, such as the clinical utility of 'big data'.

Part III: Personalised Medicine in Health-Care Systems

The third part of the book assembles contributions on methodological and normative aspects relevant to the implementation of personalised medicine in health-care systems. This includes research on methodological characteristics of drug assessment (Windeler and Lange), aspects of reimbursement decision-making (Hessel; Noweski and colleagues), questions on the fair allocation of genetic testing (Rogowski and colleagues), legal aspects of orphanisation (Gottwald and Huster) and a critical analysis of priority setting and opportunity costs in European public health-care systems (Vollmann).

Jürgen Windeler and Stefan Lange argue in their chapter, 'Benefit Assessment of Personalised Interventions: Methodological Challenges and Approaches to a Solution', that, from a methodological point of view, no new concepts of quality assessment for personalised medicine are needed. Personalised medicine can be judged under the stance of evidence-based medicine, which usually means prospective controlled intervention trials.

The chapter 'The Relevance of the Analytic Validity of Genetic Biomarker Tests in Personalised Medicine in Oncology' by Franz Hessel discusses the validity of genetic testing and the resulting therapy decisions. The author clarifies that genetic testing alone does not lead to causal inferences on therapy decisions. However, these tests are more often one piece of a complex diagnostic puzzle.

The following chapter on 'Approval and Reimbursement of Personalised Drugs: Interim Results of the Adjustment Process' also focuses on economic topics. Michael Noweski and his colleagues examine the system of drug approval and reimbursement in the United States and in Europe and take a closer look at the reimbursement system in Germany. They especially discuss the problem of how to deal with genetic tests within the reimbursement process.

Wolf H. Rogowski and his colleagues analyse criteria for prioritising genetic tests from an economic point of view in their chapter, 'Criteria for Fairly Allocating Scarce Health-Care Resources to Genetic Tests: Which Matter Most?'. They ask what a fair allocation of health-care costs related to genetic testing should look like. They are aware of the complex mixture of criteria which have to be ethically firm, sufficiently specific and able to be operationalised.

'Personalised Medicine as Orphan Drugs? Legal and Ethical Questions' sheds a light onto the German legislative handling of personalised medicine. After discussing general considerations on the reimbursement in the German pharmaceutical market, Sina Gottwald and Stefan Huster analyse the possibility of classifying personalised medicine therapies into an orphan drugs status. With this, they round off the discussion on the German process of reimbursement and early benefit assessment which was also touched on previously by Windeler and Lange, Hessel, and Noweski et al.

In the final chapter of this section, Jochen Vollmann provides a critical analysis on 'Personalised Medicine: Priority Setting and Opportunity Costs in European Public Health-Care Systems'. In this chapter, many issues previously addressed are brought together, for example, aspects of personhood, research progress, actual clinical benefit to patients, and opportunity costs and priority setting in solidarity-based health-care systems. Vollmann argues strongly in favour of a public discussion and democratically legitimised priority setting and provides a complex understanding of medical developments.

Part IV: Personalised Medicine in Oncology: Recommendations for Future Development

The last part of the book is an interdisciplinary collaboration of all researchers involved in the collaborative research project *'Personalised Medicine' in Oncology: An Interdisciplinary Study on Ethical, Medical, Economical and Legal Aspects* funded by the German Federal Ministry for Education and Research (Bundesministerium für Bildung und Forschung – BMBF). Jan Schildmann and his colleagues provide an account of the state of research reached as part of the work within and across the disciplines of medical ethics, oncology, health-economy and law. Following an introduction, this chapter summarises important aspects as viewed from the perspectives of the various disciplines, including a case study on the benefits and costs of personalised medicine in acute myeloid leukaemia. The chapter concludes with jointly developed *recommendations for future development of research and practice of 'personalised medicine'*.

With this book, the editors provide an interdisciplinary and critical contribution to the growing field of so-called 'personalised medicine', which is often discussed too optimistically and interest-driven. Therefore, we believe that this volume is not only relevant to biomedical researchers and clinicians, but also to the fields of social science, psychology, economics, law, health-care administration, education, politics and media.

The editors thank all the authors for their chapters and their willingness to contribute to this volume. We also thank the German Federal Ministry of Education and Research for the funding of the collaborative research project *Personalised Medicine in Oncology: An Interdisciplinary Study on Ethical, Medical, Economical and Legal Aspects* (01 GP 1001A-C), including the funding of this publication. We thank Philip Saunders for proof reading and formatting the papers. Furthermore, we thank Ashgate Publishing for all the professional co-operation.

PART I
Personalised Medicine – Medicine for the Person? Concepts and Contextual Aspects

Chapter 1

What is Personalised Medicine? Sharpening a Vague Term Based on a Systematic Literature Review[1]

Sebastian Schleidgen, Corinna Klingler, Teresa Bertram,
Wolf H. Rogowski and Georg Marckmann

Background

In recent years, individualised or personalised medicine (IM/PM)[2] has become a buzzword in the academic as well as public debate surrounding health care. Promising to make health care more effective and efficient by tailored medical interventions it has become one of the core areas of public research funding and pharmaceutical research investment (Vollmann, 2013). However, PM lacks a clear definition and is open to interpretation (Schleidgen and Marckmann, 2013). Consequently, a whole continuum of PM understandings exists, in which three main positions can be identified: (a) PM is not a new concept as medicine has always been individualised; (b) PM is holistic health care centred on the needs of the individual patient; and (c) PM is treatment targeted at stratified subgroups (for example, pharmacogenetics) (Müller, 2012).

The prevailing vagueness of the term poses several problems. First and foremost, it unduly complicates public discourse on the chances, risks and limits of PM: if the meaning of a term like PM is not clearly defined, it is impossible to debate questions of its matter as well as its (future) handling. As a consequence, it is difficult to develop regulatory mechanisms that ensure effectiveness as well as ethical acceptability of research on and provision of PM. Furthermore, stakeholders might utilise the term's vagueness to further their respective,

---

1   Abridged reprint from BMC Medical Ethics 2013, 14:55: doi:10.1186/1472–6939–14–55 (http://www.biomedcentral.com/1472–6939/14/55) © 2013 Schleidgen et al.; licensee BioMed Central Ltd. This is an Open Access article distributed under the terms of the Creative Commons Attribution License (http://creativecommons.org/licenses/by/2.0), which permits unrestricted use, distribution, and reproduction in any medium, provided the original work is properly cited.

2   For pragmatic reasons we will use the acronym PM in the following to refer to both individualised and personalised medicine.

especially economic, interests and preferences. In the medical context, however, this seems to be morally unacceptable; on the contrary, medical actions ultimately must be directed towards the patients' needs. Finally, PM's underspecification may lead to unwarranted fears of patients as well as unfounded hopes like a perfectly tailored or patient-centred medicine (Bondio and Michl, 2010; Dabrock, 2011). Against this background, the goal of this chapter is to help structure the debate over PM's meaning by developing a *sufficiently* precise definition, which is formally adequate while at the same time reflecting the actual scientific possibilities as well as limitations of medical measures labelled as PM.

A definition declares that a term (the *definiendum*) is equivalent with another set of terms whose meaning is well-established (the *definiens*) (Whitehead and Russel, 1910; Brown, 1998). Hurley (2007) differentiates, among others, between stipulative, lexical and precising definitions. While a lexical definition simply tries to capture the way a word is commonly used, a stipulative definition arbitrarily assigns a meaning to a certain expression, whereas a precising definition tries to reduce the vagueness of a term used in practice:

> [A precising definition] differs from a stipulative definition because its definiendum is not a new term, but one whose usage is established, although vague. The makers of a precising definition, therefore, are not free to assign any meaning they choose to the definiendum. They must remain true to established usage as far as that is possible. The aim is to make a known term more precise. At the same time they must go beyond established usage if the vagueness of the definiendum is to be reduced. (Copi and Cohen, 1990)

As the term PM is already established in public discourse, however vaguely defined, the goal of this chapter can only be to derive a precising definition. For this purpose, we first have to describe the current usage of the term. As one central goal of our chapter consists in clarifying the actual possibilities and limitations of PM, we decided to analyse its current usage in the sciences. This decision followed the assumption that the scientific debate on PM centres on its actual state-of-the-art. Analysing the stakeholders' discourse, on the other hand, would potentially have captured the respective hopes and interests instead of the actual development labelled as PM. Accordingly, we conducted a systematic review of definitions appearing in the academic literature. Based on those findings, in a second step, we developed a precising definition of PM which is formally adequate as well as sufficiently precise and hence can be regarded as an adequate basis for public discourse on PM.

Methods

For our systematic review, PubMed was searched using the keywords 'individualized medicine', 'individualised medicine', 'personalized medicine' and 'personalised medicine' connected by the Boolean operator OR. We refrained from including MeSH-terms in the search strategy as the term 'individualized medicine' specified in the thesaurus of PubMed already contains a specific definition. Including MeSH-terms would therefore have pre-selected certain articles according to this understanding of PM. Excluding MeSH-terms, on the contrary, allowed us to stay open to alternative understandings of PM. We only searched titles and abstracts to identify those articles in which PM is the main focus. We assumed that those articles were more likely to contain a definition of PM. We did not restrict the date of publication; our last research was conducted on 15 August 2012. Furthermore, we included only English articles as our goal was to capture the international debate. Subsequently, we checked full-text availability of the articles identified via the Bavarian State Library. Where full-texts were not available, we contacted the authors where contact details were provided.

A data extraction tabloid was developed which puts forward a means/ends division. This decision is based on the assumption that medical interventions are defined by the means they employ to reach certain ends. A stethoscope, for instance, is not defined by its form or colour or technical details – they may vary – but rather that it allows listening to internal sounds (means) to detect pathologies of the lung, heart or abdomen (ends).

Articles available were screened for definitions by SS and TB; definitions were extracted using the extraction tabloid by TB. This resulted in a list of ends and means constitutive for PM.

We did not interpret the data, but followed the authors' understanding of what constitutes ends and means. To reduce complexity of the resulting list, summary categories were developed inductively from the data using thematic analysis adapted to the research aim (Thomas and Harden, 2008). Two researchers, SS and CK, independently derived categories from the data. In case their assessments differed, discrepancies were discussed and resolved consensually (thereby ensuring inter-coder reliability). Where technical details were not clear, a medical expert was consulted for clarification.

Results

We identified 2457 articles containing the term PM in the title or abstract. Full-texts were available for 1443 papers. Of those articles 683 contained a definition of PM and were thus included in our review.[3]

---

3   See   http://www.biomedcentral.com/1472–6939/14/55/additional   for   an overview of all the papers identified (including information on whether they were scanned and included in our analysis).

The data proves that there is no consensus on the meaning of PM. After extracting and analyzing the definitions of PM, we found 1459 different ends and 1025 different means. A shortened version of the resulting category system is depicted in Tables 1.1 and 1.2.[4]

Table 1.1   Ends of PM in the literature

Ends in (1459)

1 Research (156)

  A. Basic research (43)
    On causes and processes of diseases (9)
    On risk factors for diseases (3)

    On disease classification (18)
    To further the development of new treatment measures (13)

  B. Research on new diagnostic and prognostic/predictive measures (30)
    Unspecified (10)
    Regarding tailoring (2)
    Regarding stratification (4)
    Regarding improved diagnostic/prognostic/ predictive measures (9)
      unspecified (2)
      effectiveness (6)
      efficiency (1)
    Regarding companion diagnostics (5)

  C. Research on new therapeutic measures (83)
    Unspecified (15)
    Regarding tailoring (15)
    Regarding stratification (40)
    Regarding improved treatment measures (13)
      unspecified (5)
      safety (3)
      effectiveness (3)
      efficiency (2)

2 Drug approval (14)

  A. Improved validation processes (1)

  B. Improved clinical trials (11)
    Unspecified (4)
    Efficiency (7)

  C. Improved approval processes (2)

---

4   See http://www.biomedcentral.com/1472–6939/14/55/additional for the complete tables containing the original definitions' components.

3 Health care (1202)

A. Health care in general (69)
 Unspecified (1)
 Decision making in health care(3)
 Tailoring health care (37)
 Improved health care (28)
  unspecified (17)
  effectiveness/efficacy (1)
  efficiency (2)
  safety (2)
  choices in health care (1)
  tailoring health care (5)
B. Prevention (158)
 Risk prognosis/prediction (82)
  unspecified (52)
  at the individual level (26)
  at the population level (3)
  improved risk prognosis/prediction (1)
 Primary prevention (76)
  unspecified (34)
  tailoring preventive measures (22)
  stratified preventive measures (1)
  improved prevention/preventive strategies (19)
   unspecified (16)
   effectiveness (1)
   timing (2)
C. Therapy (975)
 Diagnosis (68)
  unspecified (18)
  tailored diagnosis/diagnostics (28)
  improved diagnosis/diagnostic measures (22)
   unspecified (10)
   effectiveness/efficacy (5)
   timing (6)
   tailored diagnostics (1)
 Prognosis/Prediction (158)
  unspecified (4)
  prediction of disease progression/recurrence (5)
  predictive information guiding clinical decision making (21)
  prediction of treatment effects/effectiveness (60)
  tailoring prognosis/prediction (39)
  stratification by predicted treatment effects (25)
  improvement of prognostic/predictive measures (4)
   unspecified (2)
   safety (1)
   effectiveness/efficacy (1)
 Treatment (749)
  unspecified (27)

choice of therapeutic measure (104)
regarding treatment monitoring (12)
effectiveness/efficacy of treatment (16)
efficiency of treatment (2)
safety of treatment (6)
treatment outcomes (2)
tailoring therapy/therapeutic measures (269)
stratified therapeutic measure (18)
improvement of therapy/therapeutic measures (293)
   unspecified (41)
   choice of treatment (32)
   effectiveness/efficacy (92)
   efficiency (2)
   timing (4)
   safety (83)
   tailoring treatment measures (39)

4 Improved health (10)

5 Further ends (77)

Unspecified (11)
(Tailored) patient management (3)
Stratification (1)
Reduce/control costs (30)
Improved effectiveness/efficacy (24)
Improved timing (1)
Improved safety (3)
Improved quality of life (4)

Table 1.2   Means of PM in the literature

Means in (1025)

1 Research (97)

A. On individual differences (4)
B. On genetics/genomics (39)
   Unspecified (11)
   Regarding the influence of genes on disease development/progression (5)
   Regarding the influence of genes on drug response (22)
   Regarding the interaction of genes with other factors that influence disease development/
   progression (1)
C. On further factors that influence disease progression/development (8)
D. On further factors that influence drug response (4)
E. On biomarkers (40)
F. On new technologies (2)

2 Application in patient care (928)

A. Usage of clinical information/clinical indicators (718)
    Unspecified (11)
    Using information on medical history (12)
        unspecified (6)
        regarding family history (6)
    Using biological information/biomarkers (689)
        unspecified (81)
        of the individual (21)
        of the disease (13)
        on the molecular level (574)
            unspecified (101)
            information on disease pathways (7)
            genetic information (417)
                unspecified (19)
                regarding knowledge of genes/genetic variation (215)
                regarding gene expression (13)
                regarding genomics/genomic variation (98)
                regarding the transcriptome (4)
                regarding DNA/RNA (6)
                regarding epigenetics (8)
                regarding gene-environment interaction (4)
                regarding pharmacogenetics/pharmacogenomics (41)
                regarding further points (9)
            information on proteomics (35)
            information on metabolomics (14)
        Further points mentioned (6)
B. Usage of environmental factors/information (33)
C. Usage of further individual factors/information (126)
    Unspecified (77)
    Age-related information (4)
    Phenotypic factors/information (19)
        unspecified (5)
        referring to gender (4)
        referring to weight (3)
        referring to membership of a certain (ethnic) group (7)
    Personal preferences (4)
    Behaviour (22)
        unspecified (8)
        referring to nutrition (5)
        referring to lifestyle (6)
        referring to toxins (3)
D. Usage of (specific) technology (51)
    Unspecified (17)
    (New) technology for genetic analysis (30)
    Information technology (4)

Deriving a Precising Definition

Six Criteria for Adequate Definitions

As stated above, a precising definition intends to reduce the vagueness of terms *used in practice*. Hence, we have to start with the empirical information about the scientific usage of PM and search for a combination of ends and means which satisfies certain criteria. This raises the problem of adequately balancing the two main demands of a precising definition: staying close to the actual usage of a term while at the same time focusing its meaning for the sake of precision. One possible way to approach this problem would be to include definitional elements only if they occur with a certain frequency in the literature. This, however, requires establishing thresholds above which an element is to be included in our definition. As such thresholds necessarily are arbitrary, we chose an analytical approach instead. Accordingly, we used six criteria of adequate definitions which allowed us to filter the various components encountered in the literature. These criteria provide an analytical way to deal adequately with the two demands: sticking to the established usage of PM and reducing its vagueness. The criteria are:

1. A definition must be necessary, that is, there must not exist any well-established term equivalent with its *definiens*.
2. A definition must be neither too broad nor too narrow, that is, it must be adequately distinctive (for instance, the definition 'antibiotics are drugs used to treat infectious diseases' is too broad as antifungal agents – amongst others – are also used to treat infectious diseases. The definition 'antibiotics are drugs used to treat streptococcal infections', on the other hand, is too narrow as other bacterial infections can also be treated with antibiotics).
3. A definition must not be circular, that is, the *definiendum* must not appear in the *definiens*.
4. A definition must not be redundant, that is, it must not contain any components which are implied by any other of its components.
5. A definition must not be inconsistent, that is, it must not include any logical contradictions.
6. A definition must not be ambiguous, that is, the *definiens* must be clearly described (Copi and Cohen, 1990; Hurley, 2007).

Obviously, many definitions we found in the literature do not meet these criteria. For instance, most of the mentioned ends and means are far too broad to specify PM adequately: defining PM as pursuing the *end* of 'treating diseases' is not adequately distinctive (criterion 2), as any therapeutic measure's end consists in treating diseases. The same holds for a definition of PM that refers to the *means* of 'using clinical information'.

Adequate Ends of Personalised Medicine

When taking a closer look at the ends of PM encountered in the literature (Table 1.1), the first main category listed is research. Basic research as well as research on new diagnostic and therapeutic measures is to be excluded from the ends of PM as it violates criterion 5: in the medical context,[5] research is always a means to a given end, but never an end in itself. Usually – although not always – the end consists in improving medical measures or to generate medical knowledge. Therefore it would not be consistent to include research as an end in a definition of PM.

The second main category is 'drug approval' which neither is an adequate end for defining PM. After all, we search for a definition of individualised/personalised *medicine*. Accordingly, medicine is the *genus* of PM that denotes a main category to which a certain term belongs and which thereby specifies the limits of a term's meaning. For instance, 'hammer' belongs to the genus 'tools' whereas 'rose' belongs to the genus 'flowers'. The genus 'medicine', however, does not imply the term 'drug approval'. Rather, drug approval belongs to the genus 'health policy'. Consequently, including drug approval in a definition of PM violates criterion 2 as it would imply an understanding of PM that transcends the *genus* 'medicine'.

The category 'further ends' is also inadequate for defining PM as the terms listed here are either too broad or too narrow. For instance, the ends of 'decision making' or 'reduce/control costs' do not even (necessarily) belong to the genus 'medicine', but rather to the genus 'human action' or 'business administration', respectively.[6] As such they are far too broad to define PM adequately. Somewhat narrower, yet still too broad, are ends like 'patient management' or 'use stratification': it seems to be an end of almost every medical intervention to manage patients and use stratification. On the other hand, some of the findings categorised as further ends like 'tailored wellness plan for individuals' are too narrow to define PM adequately: medicine necessarily transcends wellness as it ultimately refers to the health of patients while the term wellness targets only

---

5 By medical context we refer to medicine as in medical *care*. This results from the insight that PM is generally discussed as a means to improve medical care.

6 Of course, '*medical* decision making' would belong to the genus 'medicine'. The rather general reference to 'decision making', however, does not necessarily belong to the genus 'medicine'. Therefore, we refrained from including 'decision making' in our definition.

one aspect of health (if it counts as health related at all). For many diseases, increases in wellness will not result in improvements in *health*.

The remaining categories 'health care'[7] and 'improved health' are plausible candidates for inclusion. Before taking a closer look at their subcategories, we can generally exclude the subcategories 'unspecified' from a definition of PM. To cut the argument short: all ends contained here are too broad to define PM adequately. Having said this, we will first turn to the subcategories 'prevention' and 'therapy'. To explain the argumentation underlying our decisions for exclusion, we have to take a closer look at the criterion of necessity (1): we assume that a new term becomes necessary only if changes occur or new discoveries are made that cannot be described by an already well-established term (for example, it was necessary to introduce the term 'laptop' because the established term 'personal computer' did not imply the mobility that the new device exhibits). Consequently, in the medical context, a new term is necessary if the ends and means of medical interventions change in a way that is not captured by any well-established term. Accordingly, the question is whether any of the subcategories of 'prevention' and 'treatment' necessitate the introduction of a new term? We argue that only categories speaking of *improvements* fulfil the necessity criterion. The other subcategories, for example, 'risk prognosis/ prediction' or 'primary prevention', are already well-established terms which do not justify introducing a novel term. This holds for both the subcategories of 'prevention' and of 'therapy'. Accordingly, we excluded all subcategories except the ones that refer to an improvement.

Across the categories included thus far we find subcategories that describe different dimensions of improvement: 'effectiveness/efficacy', 'timing', 'tailoring', 'choice of treatment', 'efficiency' and 'safety'. Some of these specifications can be regarded as inadequate ends for defining PM because they violate the criterion of non-redundancy (4). In health care we are confronted with a hierarchy of ends. Certain ends (for example, better timing of treatment) are not pursued for their own sake, but rather for the sake of certain higher-order ends (for example, more effective treatment). To put it differently: effectiveness, efficiency and safety of an intervention are the dimensions that define improvements in health care. For instance, a medication is considered better as an alternative medication if it either results in a more effective treatment measured on some health-related indicator, has less side effects (safety) or is more efficient (that is, costs less while producing the same health effect or has a bigger effect at the same cost). Improvements of treatment choices as well as of timing and tailoring always imply improvements on one or all of the dimensions 'effectiveness', 'efficiency' and 'safety'. Of course,

---

7   By 'health care' we understand medical care both on the population and on the individual level.

improving treatment choices, tailoring and timing does not necessarily reach all of those higher-order ends. Nevertheless, they are the ultimate ends of any improvement in health care. Therefore, 'effectiveness', 'efficiency' and 'safety' are to be understood as a triad of ultimate ends of health care innovations that are implied in any adequate lower-order end. In accordance with criterion (4) we therefore excluded improvements in 'effectiveness', 'efficiency' and 'safety' from our definition as they are necessarily implied by any medical improvement.

Additionally, improvements in choices of treatment are themselves implied by improved tailoring of treatment. To be able to choose a treatment – or the *right* treatment, respectively – one needs to tailor the treatment to the specific (sub-)type of disease. An improvement in tailoring diagnostic, prognostic, or treatment measures therefore necessarily leads to an improvement in treatment choices which is therefore redundant and can be excluded. Left are improvements of tailoring and timing of preventive and therapeutic measures as ends of PM. Those ends, however, imply improvements in *health* as the ultimate end of any improvement in *health care*. The category 'improved health' can therefore be excluded from our definition in accordance with criterion of non-redundancy (4) following the same line of argument.

Consequently, only 'improvement in tailoring and timing of health care' are plausible ends of PM. They satisfy criterion (4) and can be considered adequately distinctive (2), are neither circular (3) nor inconsistent (5) nor ambiguous (6).

Adequate Means of Personalised Medicine

However, we did not show so far that criterion (1) is ultimately satisfied: an improvement *could* potentially render a new term necessary, but it does not necessarily. Ultimately, many changes introduced to the health care system aim at improving timing and tailoring of prevention or therapy. However, not all of them require the introduction of a new term (for example, new screening interventions to improve timing of cancer treatment). However, as stated above, a new term becomes necessary if the ends *and* the means of medical measures change in a way that is not captured by any well-established term. Consequently, we have to examine whether we can find means mentioned in the literature which satisfy criteria 1–6 and thereby specify the ends in a way that criterion 1 is satisfied.

First, the subcategories 'unspecified' are excluded based on a similar argument as brought forward above: all means contained here are too broad to define PM adequately. Furthermore, only the means 'utilizing biological information and biomarkers on the level of molecular disease pathways, genetics, proteomics as well as metabolomics' satisfy criterion 2. All other means in the category 'application in the health care system' – excluding the category 'usage of (specific) technology'[8] – are not adequately distinctive as they are means employed in any medical measure (for example, questions concerning gender and weight should be part of any routine anamnesis). Those means – usage of information on the genetic, proteomic, metabolomic and molecular pathway level – are adequately distinctive and can, furthermore, be considered new in the sense requested by criterion 1: they indicate the necessity of a novel term that emphasises their use in contrast to using standard information like medical history or other non-genetic biomarkers (for example, blood pressure). One could criticise that we call the use of genetic information new and adequately distinctive as it has long been informing medical decision-making, especially in the context of prenatal diagnostics. However, recent technological developments have rendered it possible to extend the informational base to genomic information, epigenetic information or pharmacogenetic information and also further information on the influence of single genes. The genetic information relevant in our context is of a new quality. We therefore did not exclude genetic information on the basis of criteria 1 and 2. It furthermore satisfies criteria 3–6.

Combining Ends and Means: An Adequate Definition of Personalised Medicine

Accordingly, we can now derive an adequate precising definition of PM:

> PM seeks to improve tailoring and timing of preventive and therapeutic measures by utilising biological information and biomarkers on the level of molecular disease pathways, genetics, proteomics as well as metabolomics.

Although it is not clear whether improvement of tailoring and timing as ends satisfies criterion 1, tailoring and timing based on genetic/proteomic/metabolomic/molecular pathway-related information is conceptually new and therefore justifies a new term. Moreover, the definition satisfies criteria 2–6.

Several further remarks are important: first, it might not be clear why we have not included 'research' as a means in our definition. As stated above, in the medical context, research is always a means for a given end where the end usually consists in improving medical measures or possibilities. In analogy to the argumentation concerning higher- and lower-order ends, whenever medical measures, for example, diagnostic tools, are applied, there usage is necessarily grounded on research. Hence, research is implied in any medical intervention or means – in the case of PM the use of information on molecular pathways, genetics, proteomics and metabolomics – and therefore has to be excluded from our definition in order to satisfy criterion 4.

---

8 We will return to that category later.

Second, a similar point applies to the subcategory 'usage of (specific) technology': like any medical intervention, measures considered to be personalised utilise certain (specific) technologies. Our definition therefore analytically implies the utilisation of specific technologies that allow for the measurement and evaluation of the respective biological information and biomarkers. 'Usage of (specific) technology' must accordingly not be included in the definition.

Third, our definition contains 'improving tailoring of prevention and therapy' as one end of PM. If this is understood on the individual level, tailoring becomes impossible and the definition would be useless: it is impossible to find the drug that works perfectly for a single individual. The processes we employ to test medical devices and pharmaceuticals are clinical trials involving patient *groups* and not individual patients. Accordingly, tailoring means no more than stratification. In turn, stratification means the detection of subgroups of patients that benefit from a certain measure. Tailoring treatment to a patient can therefore only mean assigning the patient to a certain subgroup of patients that appear to respond particularly well to a specific intervention.

A final remark regards the part of the definition that refers to 'improved preventive and therapeutic measures'. 'Improved health care' is equivalent to 'improved preventive and therapeutic measures' as prevention and therapy are what constitutes health care. To put it differently, improved preventive and therapeutic measures are implied in improved health care and vice versa. According to criterion 4, we can replace the former with the latter in the definition, but should not include both formulations. Against the background of these considerations, we can slightly adapt our definition:

> PM seeks to improve stratification and timing of health care by utilising biological information and biomarkers on the level of molecular disease pathways, genetics, proteomics as well as metabolomics.

Discussion

We have now derived a precising definition. Four issues still need to be addressed: first, we only included the usage of information on the genetic, proteomic, metabolomic and molecular pathway level as means of PM. In medical practice, however, we will rarely witness a medical encounter where decisions are based exclusively on information of such biomarkers. Rather, in the majority of cases information from both standard biomarkers (like blood pressure) and new molecular biomarkers (for instance, the existence of a specific genetic variant) will be combined to come to a reasonable treatment decision. Therefore, we realise that PM can only be understood as an add-on to standard medical care. Consequently, the aspired improvements can only be realised by combining both approaches.

Second, regarding our empirical analysis a potential limitation is that we only screened 1443 full-texts for definitions of PM, although we found 2312 papers that included the term PM in the title or abstract. This problem is, however, commonly encountered in systematic reviews. It can also be criticised that we only searched PubMed for definitions. Seemingly, this poses the risk of introducing a bias as it is unclear whether the papers not scanned by us contained further definitional elements. However, analysing our sample of 1443 papers led to conceptual saturation meaning no new themes emerged after analysing a certain amount of articles (Thomas and Harden, 2008). Furthermore, we had no reason to suspect that our sample was significantly different from the general population of papers.

Third, one may criticise our exclusion decisions. To derive a precising definition we had to interpret terms like 'tailored', 'health care' or 'adequately distinctive'. For example, we define health care as being constituted by preventive and therapeutic measures. Naturally, those assumptions can be discussed critically as most terms are not as clearly delineated as would be desirable for the construction of a definition. However, as these terms are well-established in scientific discourse and interpretation only becomes necessary at the margin, this should not weaken our analysis in any significant way. Our definition can therefore help to re-focus the discourse on PM by reducing its conceptual vagueness.

Fourth, as mentioned above, people debating PM hold understandings that diverge from what PM technology actually can achieve. As our results show, PM is *not* medicine with a special focus on the interests and preferences of the individual patient. For instance, PM does not include any reference to an adequate doctor–patient relationship. Hence, PM as such is not related to the term patient-centred medicine. Moving towards a more patient-centred medicine may be desirable, but cannot be achieved by solely furthering PM technology. To forestall false hopes attached to the concept and accordingly wrong decisions regarding investments, it might be reasonable to adapt terminology. Stratifying medicine, for example, would be a more appropriate term than personalised medicine to describe the developments currently labelled as PM.

Conclusion

Above we have shown that the literature exhibits a huge variety of definitions of PM. A shared understanding that could facilitate the discourse on limits and chances of PM and preselect reasonable arguments is lacking. At the same time the relative amount of PM definitions given in the literature has been decreasing over the last years which we might carefully interpret as a trend: it gives cause to worry that people conceive PM as a well-described concept. This is especially worrisome because interpretations like 'tailored wellness plan for individuals' (ends) or 'consider belief of patients' (means) demonstrate that PM can be misused as a flexible void with a positive connotation that stakeholders fill with divergent meanings according to their interests and preferences.

To forestall such developments, we tried to supply the discourse with a precising definition. The starting point was our empirical data. Based on these findings, we analytically derived a *sufficiently* precise definition of PM that satisfies well-established criteria of adequate definitions:[9]

> PM seeks to improve stratification and timing of health care by utilising biological information and biomarkers on the level of molecular disease pathways, genetics, proteomics as well as metabolomics.

Hence, an adequate definition of PM is one of type (c) mentioned in the beginning as it refers to treatment targeted at stratified subgroups (for example, pharmacogenetics). Interestingly, our definition is also supported by a quantitative analysis of PM definitions in the literature. The number of occurrences of definitional elements suggests that PM should be understood as the use of genetic information (417 occurrences) – for example, knowing of a specific genetic variation – to improve the treatment of patients by better tailoring their treatment (308) – for example, by choosing a drug that does not exhibit severe side effects in the patient subgroup showing a specific genetic variation. The fact that our definition converges with the understanding of the majority suggests that it is widely *acceptable*.

This, of course, does not entail that it actually *will be accepted*. We hope, however, to stimulate a discussion on the understanding of PM that might help clarifying conceptual differences between stakeholders concerned with PM as well as avoiding unrealistic over- and underestimations in the public discourse on PM mentioned in the beginning.

---

9 Langanke et al. (2012) developed an alternative purely analytically derived definition of PM. By characterising our definition as sufficiently precise, we want to point out that it obviously cannot be perfectly precise. The construction of a perfectly precise definition would demand defining every element of the definiendum, for example the terms 'biomarker', 'proteomics' or 'metabolomics'. It is sufficiently precise in the sense that it can decrease the chances of misusing the term PM. For this purpose, it is not necessary to provide an exact definition of terms like proteomics or metabolomics. Rather, it is sufficient to point out that certain biological sub-disciplines are decisive for PM's development and implementation.

References

Bondio, M.G. and Michl, S., 2010. Individualisierte Medizin: Die neue Medizin und ihre Versprechen. *Deutsches Ärzteblatt*, 107, pp.A1062–A1064.

Brown, J.R., 1998. What is a Definition? *Foundations of Science*, 1, pp.111–132.

Copi, I.M. and Cohen, C., 1990. *Introduction to Logic*. New York and London: Macmillan.

Dabrock, P., 2011. Die konstruierte Realität der sog. individualisierten Medizin. Sozialethische und theologische Anmerkungen. In: V. Schumpelick and B. Vogel, eds. *Medizin nach Maß: Individualisierte Medizin – Wunsch und Wirklichkeit*. Freiburg: Herder. Ch.18.

Hurley, P.J., 2007. *A Concise Introduction to Logic*. Belmont, CA: Wadsworth Publishing.

Langanke, M., Lieb, W., Erdmann, P., Dörr, M., Fischer, T., Kroemer, H., Flessa, S. and Assel, H., 2012. Was ist Individualisierte Medizin? Zur terminologischen Justierung eines schillernden Begriffs. *Zeitschrift für medizinische Ethik*, 58, pp.295–314.

Müller, H., 2012. Chancen und Risiken der 'individualisierten' Medizin für das Gesundheitssystem. *Welt der Krankenversicherung*, 2, pp.40–41.

Schleidgen, S. and Marckmann, G., 2013. Alter Wein in neuen Schläuchen? Ethische Implikationen der Individualisierten Medizin. *Ethik in der Medizin*, 25, pp.223–231.

Thomas, J. and Harden, A., 2008. Methods for the Thematic Synthesis of Qualitative Research in Systematic Reviews. *BMC Medical Research Methodology*, 8, p.45.

Vollmann, J., 2013. Persönlicher – besser – kostengünstiger? Kritische medizinethische Anfragen an die 'personalisierte Medizin'. *Ethik in der Medizin*, 25, pp.233–241.

Whitehead, A.N. and Russel, B., 1910. *Principia Mathematica*. Cambridge: Cambridge University Press.

Chapter 2

Alarming Symptoms of a Paradigm Shift? An Approach to Bridge the Gap between Hypothetical Ethics and the Current Status of Individualised Medicine Research

Tobias Fischer, Marcus Dörr, Robin Haring and Martin Langanke[1]

The bioethical discourse about the projected 'shifts' that individualised medicine (IM) is going to bring to all levels of the health-care system is based on the hypothesis that IM is capable of significantly contributing to the field of medicine, health economics and public health despite the current infancy of its state. However, making bioethical reflections about IM means reflecting on a rapidly changing area because, in spite of definitional efforts (Langanke et al., 2012; Chapter 1, this volume) and concise statements such as -omics,[2] knowledge plus prevention equals 'IM', and there is still no common idea of what is involved in IM and of what IM could bring to medicine. Moreover, much of what is being researched and developed under the heading of IM could have been researched and developed under any other heading as well. The main reason for this is probably that individual conceptual moments have always

1   This work is part of the research project Greifswald Approach to Individualized Medicine (GANI_MED). The GANI_MED consortium is funded by the Federal Ministry of Education and Research and the Ministry of Cultural Affairs of the Federal State of Mecklenburg-West Pomerania (support codes: 03IS2061A & 03IS2061E).

    Gratitude is expressed to James Wells for proofreading and Sally Werner for support of the compilation of the footnotes.

2   The suffix '-omics' refers to certain research areas in biomedicine ending in -omics (for example, metabolomics, proteomics or genomics) that aim at characterising molecules that translate into the structure, function and dynamics of an organism.

been traditional concepts and goals of any progress in medicine (Gadebusch Bondio and Michl, 2010).

Hype, Hope and Risks versus the Current Status of IM Research

Due to the reason stated above, the framing of bioethical discussions also has a broad range. Whether it is a mere hype or a profound change that will really shake the basis of medicine is controversial and seriously discussed (Grill and Hackenbroch, 2011). The views extend across a wide spectrum between 'old wine in new bottles' (Schleidgen and Marckmann, 2013) to a 'great transformation of medicine' (Snyderman and Langheier, 2006). It remains unclear, even within the professional disciplines, where the main discourse is to be situated (*Nature Biotechnology*, 2012). However, it is probably situated somewhere between the following three points: (1) the turning away from the 'one size fits all' (Mancinelli et al., 2000; Hudson, 2009) approach, (2) the more health-policy question of what type of medicine is needed for an (aging) society in general (*Ärzte Zeitung*, 2013), and (3) it is only a public relations strategy of the pharmaceutical industry and interested scientists on their way to claim research funds (Bartens, 2011). Therefore, instead of a common idea, the discussion is led by a lot of proclaimed 'hypes', 'hopes' and 'risks' instead of the mere medical progress or biomedical research. One of the more often proclaimed goals of IM is that of transforming medicine towards new borders in a revolutionary approach, as Francis Collins (2010) pointed out: 'We are on the leading edge of a true revolution in medicine, one that promises to transform the traditional "one-size-fits-all" approach into a much more powerful strategy that considers each individual as unique and as having special characteristics that should guide an approach to staying healthy.'

Taking this into account, it seems only consequential for the pharmaceutical industry to take on the idea of individualised medication in order to move towards achieving its goal of preventing patients from side effects by giving specific therapeutics and, therefore, (after initially increasing the costs of all the -omics-based companion diagnostics) saving money for the health-care system in the long run:

> Individualized Medicine will surely change the costs within the health care system. The expenses for medical check-ups regarding predictive biomarkers, for instance, will increase. Consequently, the therapeutic wrongdoing will decrease at the same time. Therefore, Individualized Medicine does not automatically imply a more expensive but rather a more effective medicine. (Rieth, 2013)

Opposing these hopes are claims concerning the possibility that IM will encourage a transformation of the solidarity within our health-care system:

> It is argued that the ethical questions and challenges raised by the project of personalizing medicine are not sufficiently addressed without considering the possible effects of personalizing medicine on our system of health care ... Among the possible unintended consequences of the project to increase personal responsibility for health is reduced emphasis on the social determinants of health for which we are jointly responsible. The conclusion is that the benefits or damage that might result from personalizing medicine will depend no less upon political and policy decisions than on pharmacogenomic developments. (Árnason, 2012)

Nevertheless, according to other academics, this political and social discussion could itself lead to the trend of increasing public access to knowledge about one's own body:

> [T]he more we know about predispositions through genetic testing, the more our health and our diseases will seem to be results, products of our own actions, indeed as products of our own will ... In return, the person who is ill, will be confronted with the underlying question of why they became ill and, if not genetically advised, whether they could not have prevented the outbreak of the disease by taking a predictive genetic test. In this way, becoming ill will be moved into the personal responsibility of the patient. (Maio, 2012 [translated by the authors]; cf. Kollek and Lembke, 2008; in response, Langanke et al., 2011)

But do we actually have any reasons to believe that IM research will give us such a large scale of new information that we have to consider a transformation or even a shift in the 'paradigm' of the basic ways we think about health, solidarity and construction of our health system? No one will deny that there are successes in IM, but they still mainly focus on test-drug combinations of pharmacokinetics, especially in the field of oncology (Chapman et al., 2011; Young et al., 2012; André et al., 2013; Fan, 2013; Solus and Kraft, 2013), and these successes lack the prognostic power required to call for any behavioural changes. The German Association of Research-Based Pharmaceutical Companies (2014) presents an IM-labelled list of pharmaceuticals with obligatory/recommended test-drug combinations, which has been extended from 20 to 31 pharmaceuticals in the last five years. Of this total, 24 pharmaceuticals are oncological treatments and seven (an increase of four since 2009) are non-oncological treatments. The non-cancer treatments mainly include tests for side effects (Carbamazepine, Oxcarbazepine and Catalizumab), where an application should be avoided in case of a positive test – a result that is expected for 2–5 per cent of the patients tested. All of the IM-based drugs are connected to a predictive biomarker, which can be used to identify subpopulations of patients who are most likely to respond to a given therapy – and not a prognostic biomarker that provides information on the likely course of a disease in an untreated individual.

Hypothetical Ethics

This very short analysis of the ethical discourse about IM shows that the most extensively studied areas are still relatively far away from a practical implementation. A prime example of this is the discussion of IM as an engine of a 'dictatorship of prevention'. In this discussion, IM is placed in (1) the context of the ethical acceptability of mandatory screening tests or (2) the rejection of the principle of solidarity, while replacing it with the principle of personal health responsibility. However, such discussions are situated within the range of purely 'hypothetical ethics', since the extensive medical knowledge and applications they are based on exist merely in the anticipation of potential successes, rather than the outcome of the real research context of IM, which – particularly in the area of complex diseases – does not go far beyond the level of rather trivial recommendations for a fundamentally healthy lifestyle. On the other hand, if one focuses on reality in the field of IM research, it becomes evident that there are promising approaches mainly in two areas, both of which are not very promising for 'hypothetical ethics': the fields of biomarker-based prediction of disease trajectories and drug response, and non-pharmacological interventions.

The GANI_MED Approach

The progress in research in Germany's largest joint project for IM, the GANI_MED – Greifswald Approach to Individualized Medicine[3] – points exactly

---

3   The University Medicine Greifswald, Germany, has launched the GANI_MED-Project to address major challenges of IM by providing the implementation of the scientific and clinical infrastructure that allows the future implementation of findings relevant to IM into clinical practice (Grabe et al., 2014). Clinical patient cohorts (N > 4,500) with an emphasis on metabolic and cardiovascular diseases were established following a standardised protocol for the assessment of personal medical history, laboratory biomarkers and the collection of various biosamples for biobanking purposes. An extensive data management structure has been implemented to centralise all relevant clinical data for research purposes. In addition, ethical research projects on informed consent procedures, the reporting of incidental findings and economic evaluations were all launched at the same time (Langanke et al., 2011) as multiple omics-

in that direction: the promising studies within GANI_MED refer to limited and clearly defined questions. The (1) testosterone-based prediction about the onset and progression of metabolic syndrome and (2) the use of biomarkers for the prediction of treatment response for immunoadsorption in dilated cardiomyopathy are to be presented here as respective examples.

Individualised Testosterone Therapy in Men: Opportunities and Pitfalls

Testosterone (T) is the major circulating androgen in men with an age-related decline of about 2 per cent per year, starting at the age of 40 years (Haring et al., 2010). Observational research findings based on prospective epidemiological studies accumulated evidence suggesting low serum T concentrations as an independent predictor of various cardiovascular risk factors including hypertension (Torkler et al., 2011), dyslipidemia (Haring et al., 2011), metabolic syndrome (Brand et al., 2011) and diabetes mellitus (Ding et al., 2006). Furthermore, low T concentrations were independently associated with an increased mortality risk (Araujo et al., 2011). However, different from an aetiological, causal factor in the onset and progression of cardiometabolic disease, epidemiological data rather suggests T concentrations as a biomarker of good health and overall well-being in men (Haring et al., 2013).

In addition to the age-related T decline, the parallel onset of clinical symptoms, such as increased abdominal fat, decreased muscle mass and strength, decreased sexual interest and function, depressed mood and fatigue, known as the 'andropause hypothesis', combines these non-specific symptoms among aging men with low T concentrations to constitute the diagnosis of the late-onset hypogonadism (LOH) which is characterised by serum T concentrations < 10.4 nmol/L in combination with at least one clinical sign or symptom. Prevalence estimates for the LOH range is dependent on the definition and study sample from 5.6 per cent (Araujo et al., 2007) to 38.7 per cent (Mulligan et al., 2006) in patient-based samples. However, the concept of andropause is far from clear in endocrinology, and current clinical guidelines (Wang et al., 2009; Bhasin et al., 2010) provide only vague diagnostic criteria and weak evidence for the existence of LOH.

Thus, the speculative indication for testosterone replacement therapy (TRT) lacks not only a pathological basis, but also the evidence of the safety and effectiveness of its treatment. Recent reviews and meta-analyses of clinical TRT trials concluded that its safety and potential cardiometabolic effects are still unknown (Isidori et al., 2005; Haddad et al., 2007; Fernandez-Balsells et al., 2010). Furthermore, a recent meta-analysis (Corona et al., 2011) summarised

---

based biomarker assessments were made, which complement the search for biomarkers in widespread diseases.

that, given the small number of clinical trials conducted, the current evidence about the health consequences of low T concentrations, the diagnosis of LOH and, finally, the cardiometabolic effects and the long-term risk/benefit ratio of TRT is of low scientific quality or largely unknown (Handelsman, 2011). This is even more intriguing given the doubling in T product sales seen in the last two decades (Gan et al., 2012; Handelsman, 2012). Taken together, the important public health questions whether to treat aging men with low T, for what symptoms and at what T level, remain presently unanswered. Consequently, there is a strong need for a large, well-designed, long-term TRT trial to elucidate the cardiometabolic efficacy and safety of TRT in aging men (Cook and Romashkan, 2011).

With this in mind, emerging -omics technologies, including genomics, transcriptomics, proteomics and metabolomics, may advance the development of innovative molecular signatures to strengthen the diagnosis and treatment of LOH. A recent proof-of-principle study highlighted this potential using integrative personal omics profiling to analyse physiological states and their molecular changes during different health states, as well as to predict individual disease risks (Chen et al., 2012). Similarly, T assessment may play a role as a personalised risk marker and has a large potential for the integration of clinical and omics data specific to the diagnosis, treatment and monitoring of LOH to finally guide individualised treatment concepts (Haring, 2012).

These individualised treatment concepts are especially relevant to TRT, since the genetic background, comorbidities, medications and an adverse health-related lifestyle contribute significantly to a considerable interindividual variability of T concentrations at any age, resulting in persistent uncertainties with regard to the definition of normal T concentrations at different ages. In response to this lack of consensus about the definition of normal T concentrations in aging males, transparently defined treatment goals for men under TRT are missing to date. In conclusion, the assessment and integration of multi-omics molecular signatures from men under TRT has the great potential to translate recent advances in high-throughput omics technologies from 'bench to bedside' to advance individualised treatment concepts in hypogonadal men.

Biomarker-based Prediction of Therapy Response – Treatment Response after IA/IgG Treatment in Patients with Dilated Cardiomyopathy

Dilated cardiomyopathy (DCM) is a major cause of heart failure and is one of the leading reasons for heart transplantation (Maron et al., 2006). It is a disease of the cardiac muscle (myocardium), characterised by enlargement of the heart chambers (ventricles) and impaired myocardial function (Maron et al., 2006). The prevalence of this disorder in industrialised Western countries is approximately 36 patients for every 100,000 people, with an incidence of 5–8 new cases per year for every 100,000 people. Recent data suggest even higher actual prevalence rates of DCM (Miller and Missov, 2001). Besides genetic predisposition, viral infection and inflammation of the myocardium play a causal role in the disease process (Maron et al., 2006; Heymans et al., 2009). Moreover, it has been shown that autoimmune disorders and autoimmune processes are implicated in the development of DCM (Cihakova and Rose, 2008; Heymans et al., 2009). Thus, various cardiac-specific antibodies have been reported in DCM patients (Cihakova and Rose, 2008; Jahns et al., 2008). Their presence has also been described as an independent predictor of disease development and prognosis (Caforio et al., 2007). The potential pathogenic role of these cardiac antibodies has been proven in animal models by active immunisation or by transfer of antibodies against the corresponding epitopes, leading to DCM-specific alterations, such as dilatation of the left ventricle and a marked impairment of cardiac function (Jahns et al., 2004).

Circulating autoantibodies, however, can be removed by extracting immunoglobulins from the patient's plasma by immunoadsorption (IA), a method that can be simply described as an extracorporal blood purification procedure (Felix et al., 2008). Smaller randomised and non-randomised studies have indicated that IA with subsequent IgG substitution (IA/IgG) may result in a significant improvement of cardiac function and relief of symptoms in patients suffering from DCM (Felix et al., 2000; Staudt et al., 2001, 2004, 2006, 2010). However, response rates to this therapeutic intervention are characterised by a wide interindividual variability; approximately two-thirds of patients treated benefit from this therapy with respect to a significant improvement of cardiac function, while one-third does not (Staudt et al., 2010; Ameling et al., 2013). Thus, prediction of therapy response remains a great challenge, particularly in the face of the high treatment costs and the invasive character of this therapeutic option.

We recently developed a biomarker-based test for the prediction of therapy response to IA/IgG therapy in a pilot study for the first time, using data from 40 patients with DCM and severely reduced cardiac function (Ameling et al., 2013). From the baseline examinations, clinical data and data on the presence of antibodies with negative inotropic activity (NIA) (Staudt et al., 2004) were available for the analyses. Moreover, biopsies of the myocardial tissue (endomyocardial biopsies) were available from all patients before IA/IgG treatment. The genetic expression patterns of these endomyocardial biopsies have been profiled by established methods using chip arrays (Ameling et al., 2013). Data of responders (defined by a significant improvement of cardiac function after treatment; n = 24) and non-responders (n = 16) were compared for the prediction analyses.

Results of this pilot study showed that both the combination of clinical variables and the information on the NIA of antibodies did not allow reliable discrimination between responders and non-responders at the baseline, although there were some significant differences observed between the two groups (for example, shorter disease duration, diameter of the left chamber and stronger NIA of antibodies in responders). By contrast, the integration of information on the NIA of antibodies and expression levels of four genes that had been identified as being strongly related to therapy response allowed a very robust discrimination of responders from non-responders at the baseline (sensitivity of 100 per cent [95 per cent CI, 85.8–100 per cent]; specificity up to 100 per cent [95 per cent CI, 79.4–100 per cent]). Thus, this study could demonstrate for the first time that the combined assessment of the NIA of antibodies and gene expression patterns of DCM patients at the baseline enables the prediction of response to IA/IgG therapy and may, thus, facilitate appropriate selection of patients who will benefit from this therapeutic intervention. The data of this pilot study, moreover, provide new insights into disease pathophysiology and allow prediction of potential myocardial recovery of patients with DCM.

However, a major limitation of the approach that has been used in this pilot study is that it is based on analyses from endomyocardial biopsies, which may only be obtained by an invasive procedure. Thus, application of this prediction test is currently not feasible for clinical practice. Therefore, we are currently developing novel biomarker-based approaches for the prediction of therapy response to IA/IgG that are based on gene expression profiles derived from whole blood samples which can be much more easily obtained than biopsies. This approach will hopefully enable a broad application and will, thereby, facilitate identification of patients who will benefit from this promising treatment option, on the one hand, and avoid unnecessary treatments in those who will not, on the other hand.

In summary, analyses such as the presently illustrated pilot study constitute important components for the development of biomarker-based therapeutic approaches in IM.

Bridging the Gap?

Both examples clearly lead to and reiterate the ethical problems of marginal utility, but they certainly give no reason for an alarmist self-promotion of bioethics. One can concede that the alarm calls of bioethics have been provoked by an excessive promise of healing and output made by IM propagators and stakeholders in medicine and human biology. However, the current status of medical research raises a very differentiated and, in parts, decidedly clear-cut record. The biomarker-based IM is – according to the thesis of the authors – certainly not the new paradigm of medicine, but a research approach which may contribute to the progress in very limited areas of medical care.[4] We would like to sum this up in six final theses for further discussion:

Thesis I: IM shows respectable successes especially in the field of biomarker-based stratification of oncological entities and in the field of pharmacogenetic prediction.

Thesis II: regardless of this success, IM exhibits a much slower progress than anticipated in the heydays of the IM hype. The overall number of approved test and test-drug combinations which are examples of the successful implementation of IM into health care has primarily increased in the field of oncology over the last five years.

Thesis III: great clinical success has so far failed to materialise especially in the field of *prediction* of diseases or courses of diseases ('prognostic markers').

Thesis IV: the biomarker-based prediction of complex, lifestyle-dependent conditions, such as cardiovascular disease, especially appear to be surprisingly resistant to IM approaches. Up to the present day, the euphoria and the scepticism regarding a new medical culture of prevention are based more on conjectures than on facts.

Thesis V: theses I–IV do not imply that the paradigm of IM has failed. More precisely, the theses suggest a sober assessment of the potential application of a biomarker-based stratified medicine. Particularly, more specific and 'smaller' successes in the field of response prediction for treatment with and without drugs seem to be possible in the near future.

Thesis VI: IM is a far from successful implementation in many fields (in other words, fields of 'complex diseases' outside the field of oncology). Nevertheless, there is a continued need for accompanying bioethical research to realistically evaluate and benchmark actual and future results of IM research against its postulated hopes and promises.

---

4   For a discussion on the paradigm shift from another perspective, see Chapter 3, this volume.

References

Ameling, S., Herda, L.R., Hammer, E., Steil, L., Teumer, A., Trimpert, C., Dörr, M., Kroemer, H.K., Klingel, K., Kandolf, R., Völker, U. and Felix, S.B., 2013. Myocardial gene expression profiles and cardiodepressant autoantibodies predict response of patients with dilated cardiomyopathy to immunoadsorption therapy. *European Heart Journal*, 34(9), pp.666–75.

André, F., Ciccolini, J., Spano, J.P., Penault-Llorca, F., Mounier, N., Freyer, G., Blay, J.Y. and Milano, G., 2013. Personalized medicine in oncology: where have we come from and where are we going? *Pharmacogenomics*, 14(8), pp.931–9.

Araujo, A.B., Dixon, J.M., Suarez, E.A., Murad, M.H., Guey, L.T. and Wittert, G.A., 2011. Clinical review: endogenous testosterone and mortality in men: a systematic review and meta-analysis. *Journal of Clinical Endocrinology and Metabolism*, 96(10), pp.3007–19.

Araujo, A.B., Esche, G.R., Kupelian, V., O'Donnell, A.B., Travison, T.G., Williams, R.E., Clark, R.E. and McLinlay, J.B., 2007. Prevalence of symptomatic androgen deficiency in men. *Journal of Clinical Endocrinology and Metabolism*, 92(11), pp.4241–7.

Árnason, V., 2012. The personal is political: ethics of personalized medicine. *Ethical Perspectives*, 19(1), pp.103–22.

Ärzte Zeitung, 2013. Neue Chancen für die personalisierte Medizin. Politik kontra Kassen. *Ärzte Zeitung*. Available through: http://www.aerztezeitung. de/politik_gesellschaft/arzneimittelpolitik/article/837970/politik-kontra-kassen-neue-chance-personalisierte-medizin.html [Accessed 30 June 2014].

Bartens, W., 2011. Die Mogelpackung. *Sueddeutsche*. Available through: http://www.sueddeutsche.de/wissen/personalisierte-medizin-die-mogelpackung-1.1121890 [Accessed 30 June 2014].

Bhasin, S., Cunningham, G.R., Hayes, F.J., Marsumoto, A.M., Snyder, P.J., Swerdloff, R.S., Montori, V.M. and Task Force, Endocrine Society, 2010. Testosterone therapy in men with androgen deficiency syndromes: an endocrine society clinical practice guideline. *Journal of Clinical Endocrinology and Metabolism*, 95(6), pp.2536–59.

Brand, J.S., van der Tweel, I., Grobbee, D.E., Emmelot-Vonk, M.H. and van der Schouw, Y.T., 2011. Testosterone, sex hormone-binding globulin and the metabolic syndrome: a systematic review and meta-analysis of observational studies. *International Journal of Epidemiology*, 40(1), pp.189–207.

Caforio, A.L., Mahon, N.G., Baig, M.K., Tona, F., Murphy, R.T., Elliott, P.M. and McKenna, W.J., 2007. Prospective familial assessment in dilated cardiomyopathy: cardiac autoantibodies predict disease development in asymptomatic relatives. *Circulation*, 115(1), pp.76–83.

Chapman, P.B., Hauschild, A., Robert, C., Haanen, J.B., Ascierto, P., Larkin, J., Dummer, R., Garbe, C., Testori, A., Maio, M., Hogg, D., Lorigan, P., Lebbe,

C., Jouary, T., Schadendorf, D., Ribas, A., O'Day, S.J., Sosman, J.A., Kirkwood, J.M., Eggermont, A.M.M., Dreno, B., Nolop, K., Li, J., Nelson, B., Hou, J., Lee, R.J., Flaherty, K.T. and McArthur, G.A. for the BRIM-3 Study Group, 2011. Improved survival with vemurafenib in melanoma with BRAF V600E mutation. *New England Journal of Medicine*, 364(26), pp.2507–16.

Chen, R., Mias, G.L., Li-Pook-Than, J., Jiang, L., Lam, H.Y., Chen, R., Miriami, E., Karczewski, K.J., Hariharan, M., Dewey, F.E., Cheng, Y., Clark, M.J., Im, H., Habegger, L., Balasubramanian, S., O'Huallachain, M., Dudley, J.T., Hillenmeyer, S., Haraksingh, R., Sharon, D., Euskirchen, G., Lacroute, P., Bettinger, K., Boyle, A.P., Kasowski, M. Grubert, F., Seki, S., Garcia, M., Whirl-Carrillo, M., Gallardo, M., Blasco, M.A., Greenberg, P.L., Snyder, P., Klein, T.E., Altman, R.B., Butte, A.J., Ashley, E.A., Gerstein, M., Nadeau, K.C., Tang, H. and Snyder, M., 2012. Personal omics profiling reveals dynamic molecular and medical phenotypes. *Cell*, 148(6), pp.1293–307.

Cihakova, D. and Rose, N.R., 2008. Pathogenesis of myocarditis and dilated cardiomyopathy. *Advances in Immunology*, 99, pp.95–114.

Collins, F.S., 2010. *The language of life. DNA and the revolution in personalized medicine.* New York: Harper.

Cook, N.L. and Romashkan, S., 2011. Why do we need a trial on the effects of testosterone therapy in older men? *Clinical Pharmacology and Therapeutics*, 89(1), pp.29–31.

Corona, G., Monami, M., Rastrelli, G., Aversa, A., Tishova, Y., Saad, F., Lenzi, A., Forti, A., Mannucci, E. and Maggi, M., 2011. Testosterone and metabolic syndrome: a meta-analysis study. *Journal of Sexual Medicine*, 8(1), pp.272–83.

Ding, E.E., Song, Y., Malik, V.S. and Liu, S., 2006. Sex differences of endogenous sex hormones and risk of type 2 diabetes: a systematic review and meta-analysis. *Journal of the American Medical Association*, 295(11), pp.1288–99.

Fan, A.S., 2013. Companion diagnostic testing for targeted cancer therapies: an overview. *Genetic Testing and Molecular Biomarkers*, 17(7), pp.515–23.

Felix, S.B., Dörr, M., Herda, L.R., Beug, D. and Staudt, A., 2008. Immunoadsorption for treatment of dilated cardiomyopathy. *Internist (Berl)*, 49(1), pp.51–6.

Felix, S.B., Staudt, A., Dorffel, W.V., Stangl, V., Merkel, K., Pohl, M., Docke, W.D., Morgera, S., Neumayer, H.H., Wernecke, K.D., Wallukat, G., Stangl, K. and Baumann, G., 2000. Hemodynamic effects of immunoadsorption and subsequent immunoglobulin substitution in dilated cardiomyopathy: three-month results from a randomized study. *Journal of the American College of Cardiology*, 35(6), pp.1590–8.

Fernandez-Balsells, M.M., Murad, M.H., Lane, M., Lampropulos, J.F., Albuquerque, F., Mullan, R.J., Agrwal, N., Elamin, M.B., Gallegos-Orozco, J.F., Wang, A.T., Erwin, P.J., Bhasin, S. and Montori, V.M., 2010. Clinical review 1: adverse effects of testosterone therapy in adult men: a systematic review and meta-analysis. *Journal of Clinical Endocrinology and Metabolism*, 95(6), pp.2560–75.

Gadebusch Bondio, M. and Michl, S., 2010. Individueller, persönlicher, präziser. Die neue Medizin und ihre Versprechen. *Deutsches Ärzteblatt*, 107(21), pp.1062–4.

Gan, E.H., Pattman, S., Pearce, S. and Quinton, R., 2012. Many men are receiving unnecessary testosterone prescriptions. *British Medical Journal*, 345, p.e5469.

German Association of Research-Based Pharmaceutical Companies, 2014. Available through: http://www.vfa.de/de/arzneimittel-forschung/datenbanken-zu-arzneimitteln/individualisierte-medizin.html [Accessed 30 June 2014].

Grabe, H.J., Assel, H., Bahls, T., Dörr, M., Endlich, K., Endlich, N., Erdmann, P., Ewert, R., Felix, S.B., Fiene, B., Fischer, T., Flessa, S., Friedrich, N., Gadebusch Bondio, M., Salazar Gesell, M., Hammer, E., Haring, R., Havemann, C., Hecker, M., Hoffmann, W., Holtfreter, B., Kacprowski, T., Klein, K., Kocher, T., Kock, H., Krafczyk, J., Kuhn, J., Langanke, M., Lendeckel, U., Lerch, M.M., Lieb, W., Lorbeer, R., Mayerle, J., Meissner, K., Meyer zu Schwabedissen, H., Nauck, M., Ott, K., Rathmann, W., Rettig, R., Richardt, C., Saljé, K., Schminke, U., Schulz, A., Schwab, M., Siegmund, W., Stracke, S., Suhre, K., Ueffing, M., Ungerer, S., Völker, U., Völzke, H., Wallaschofski, H., Werner, V., Zygmunt, M.T. and Kroemer, H.K., 2014. Cohort profile: Greifswald Approach to Individualized Medicine (GANI_MED). *Journal of Translational Medicine*, 12(144), pp.1–15.

Grill, M. and Hackenbroch, V., 2011. Das große Versprechen. *Spiegel*, 32, pp.124–8. Available through: http://www.spiegel.de/spiegel/print/d-79805411.html [Accessed 30 June 2014].

Haddad, R.M., Kennedy, C.C., Caples, S.M., Tracz, M.J., Boloña, E.R., Sideras, K., Uraga, M.V., Erwin, P.J. and Montori, V.M., 2007. Testosterone and cardiovascular risk in men: a systematic review and meta-analysis of randomized placebo-controlled trials. *Mayo Clinic Proceedings*, 82(1), pp.29–39.

Handelsman, D.J., 2011. An old emperor finds new clothing: rejuvenation in our time. *Asian Journal of Andrology*, 13(1), pp.125–9.

Handelsman, D.J., 2012. Pharmacoepidemiology of testosterone prescribing in Australia, 1992–2010. *Medical Journal of Australia*, 196(10), pp.642–5.

Haring, R., 2012. Perspectives for metabolomics in testosterone replacement therapy. *Journal of Endocrinology*, 215(1), pp.3–16.

Haring, R., Baumeister, S.E., Völzke, H., Dörr, M., Felix, S.B., Kroemer, H.K., Nauck, M. and Wallaschofski, H., 2011. Prospective association of low total testosterone concentrations with an adverse lipid profile and increased incident dyslipidemia. *European Journal of Cardiovascular Prevention and Rehabilitation*, 18(1), pp.86–96.

Haring, R., Ittermann, T., Völzke, H., Krebs, A., Zygmunt, M., Felix, S.B., Grabe, H.J., Nauck, M. and Wallaschofski, H., 2010. Prevalence, incidence and risk factors of testosterone deficiency in a population-based cohort of men: results from the study of health in Pomerania. *Aging Male*, 13(4), pp.247–57.

Haring, R., Teumer, A., Völker, U., Dörr, M., Nauck, M., Biffar, R., Völzke, H., Baumeister, S.E. and Wallaschofski, H., 2013. Mendelian randomization suggests non-causal associations of testosterone with cardiometabolic risk factors and mortality. *Andrology*, 1(1), pp.17–23.

Heymans, S., Hirsch, E., Anker, S.D., Aukrust, P., Balligand, J.-L., Cohen-Tervaert, J.W., Drexler, H., Filippatos, G., Felix, S.B., Gullestad, L., Hilfiker-Kleiner, D., Janssens, S., Latini, R., Neubauer, G., Paulus, W.J., Pieske, B., Ponikowski, P., Schroen, B., Schultheiss, H.-P., Tschöpe, C., Van Bilsen, M., Zannad, F., McMurray, J. and Shah, A.M., 2009. Inflammation as a therapeutic target in heart failure? A scientific statement from the Translational Research Committee of the Heart Failure Association of the European Society of Cardiology. *European Journal of Heart Failure*, 11(2), pp.119–29.

Hudson, T.J., 2009. Personalized medicine: a transformative approach is needed. *Canadian Medical Association Journal*, 180(9), pp.911–13. Available through: http://www.cmaj.ca/cgi/content/full/180/9/911 [Accessed 30 June 2014].

Isidori, A.M., Giannetta, E., Greco, E.A., Gianfrilli, D., Bonifacio, V., Isidori, A., Lenzi, A. and Fabbri, A., 2005. Effects of testosterone on body composition, bone metabolism and serum lipid profile in middle-aged men: a meta-analysis. *Clinical Endocrinology*, 63(3), pp.280–93.

Jahns, R., Boivin, V., Hein, L., Triebel, S., Angermann, C.E., Ertl, G. and Lohse, M.J., 2004. Direct evidence for a beta 1-adrenergic receptor-directed autoimmune attack as a cause of idiopathic dilated cardiomyopathy. *Journal of Clinical Investigation*, 113(10), pp.1419–29.

Jahns, R., Boivin, V., Schwarzbach, V., Ertl, G. and Lohse, M.J., 2008. Pathological autoantibodies in cardiomyopathy. *Autoimmunity*, 41(6), pp.454–61.

Kollek, R. and Lemke, T. eds., 2008. *Der medizinische Blick in die Zukunft. Gesellschaftliche Implikationen prädiktiver Gentests*. Frankfurt: Campus Verlag.

Langanke, M., Brothers, K.B., Erdmann, P., Weinert, K., Krafczyk-Korth, J., Dörr, M., Hoffmann, W., Kroemer, H.K. and Assel, H., 2011. Comparing different scientific approaches to personalized medicine: research ethics and privacy protection. *Personalized Medicine*, 8(4), pp.437–44.

Langanke, M., Fischer, T. and Brothers, K. 2013. Public health – it is running through my veins: personalized medicine and individual responsibility for health. In: P. Dabrock, M. Braun and J. Ried, eds. *Individualized medicine between hype and hope: exploring ethical and societal challenges for healthcare?* Berlin, Münster, Wien, Zürich and London: LIT Verlag. pp.149–72.

Langanke, M., Lieb, W., Erdmann, P., Dörr, M., Fisher, T., Kromer, H., Flessa, S. and Assel, H., 2012. Was ist Individualisierte Medizin? Zur terminologischen Justierung eines schillernden Begriffs. *Zeitschrift für medizinische Ethik*, 58, pp.295–314.

Maio, G., 2012. Chancen und Grenzen der personalisierten Medizin – eine ethische Betrachtung. *GGW – Das Wissenschaftsforum in Gesundheit und Gesellschaft*, 12(1), pp.15–16.

Mancinelli, L., Cronin, M. and Sadée, W., 2000. Pharmacogenetics: the promise of personalized medicine. *AAPS PharmSci*, 2(1), p.E4. Available through: http://users.eecs.northwestern.edu/~yingliu/datamining_papers/ personalized.pdf [Accessed 30 June 2014].

Maron, B.J., Towbin, J.A., Thiene, G., Antzelevitch, C., Corrado, D., Arnett, D., Moss, A.J., Seidman, C.E., Young, J.B., American Heart Association, Council on Clinical Cardiology, Heart Failure and Transplantation Committee, Quality of Care and Outcomes Research and Functional Genomics and Translational Biology Interdisciplinary Working Groups, Council on Epidemiology and Prevention, 2006. Contemporary definitions and classification of the cardiomyopathies: an American Heart Association Scientific Statement from the Council on Clinical Cardiology, Heart Failure and Transplantation Committee; Quality of Care and Outcomes Research and Functional Genomics and Translational Biology Interdisciplinary Working Groups; and Council on Epidemiology and Prevention. *Circulation*, 113(14), pp.1807–16.

Miller, L.W. and Missov, E.D., 2001. Epidemiology of heart failure. *Cardiology Clinics*, 19(4), pp.547–55.

Mulligan, T., Frick, M.F., Zuraw, Q.C., Stemhagen, A. and McWhirter, C., 2006. Prevalence of hypogonadism in males aged at least 45 years: the HIM study. *International Journal of Clinical Practice*, 60(7), pp.762–9.

Nature Biotechnology, ed., 2012. What happened to personalized medicine? *Nature Biotechnology*, 30 (1). Available through: http://www.nature.com/nbt/journal/ v30/n1/full/nbt.2096.html [Accessed 8 June 2012].

Rieth, A. (Director Medical Development Therapeutic Amgen GmbH), 2013. Interview with Dr. Achim Rieth, Amgen. *VC-Magazin*. Available through: http://www.vc-magazin.de/technologien/life-sciences/item/2141- interview-mit-dr-achim-rieth-amgen [Accessed 30 June 2014].

Schleidgen, S. and Marckmann, G., 2013. Alter Wein in neuen Schläuchen? Ethische Implikationen der Individualisierten Medizin. *Ethik in der Medizin*, 25(3), pp.223–31.

Snyderman, R. and Langheier, J., 2006. Prospective health care: the second transformation of medicine. *Genome Biology*, 7(2), p.104. Available through: http://genomebiology.com/2006/7/2/104 [Accessed 30 June 2014].

Solus, J.F. and Kraft, S., 2013. Ras, Raf, and MAP kinase in melanoma. *Advances in Anatomic Pathology*, 20(4), pp.217–26.

Staudt, A., Herda, L.R., Trimpert, C., Lubenow, L., Lansberger, M., Dörr, M., Hummel, A., Eckerle, L.G., Beug, D., Müller, C., Hoffmann, W., Weitmann, K., Klingel, K., Kandolf, R., Kroemer, H.K., Greinacher, A. and Felix, S.B., 2010. Fcgamma-receptor IIa polymorphism and the role of immunoadsorption in cardiac dysfunction in patients with dilated cardiomyopathy. *Clinical Pharmacology and Therapeutics*, 87(4), pp.452–8.

Staudt, A., Hummel, A., Ruppert, J., Dörr, M., Trimpert, C., Birkenmeier, K., Krieg, T., Staudt, Y. and Felix, S.B., 2006. Immunoadsorption in dilated cardiomyopathy: 6-month results from a randomized study. *American Heart Journal*, 152(4), pp.712.e1–712.e6.

Staudt, A., Schaper, F., Stangl, V., Plagemann, A., Böhm, M., Merkel, K., Wallukat, G., Wernecke, K.D., Stangl, K., Baumann, G. and Felix, S.B., 2001. Immunohistological changes in dilated cardiomyopathy induced by immunoadsorption therapy and subsequent immunoglobulin substitution. *Circulation*, 103(22), pp.2681–6.

Staudt, A., Staudt, Y., Dörr, M., Böhm, M., Knebel, F., Hummel, A., Wunderle, L., Tiburcy, M., Wernecke, K.D., Baumann, G. and Felix, S.B., 2004. Potential role of humoral immunity in cardiac dysfunction of patients suffering from dilated cardiomyopathy. *Journal of the American College of Cardiology*, 44(4), pp.829–36.

Torkler, S., Wallaschofski, H., Baumeister, S.E., Völzke, H., Dörr, M., Felix, S., Rettig, R., Nauck, M. and Haring, R., 2011. Inverse association between total testosterone concentrations, incident hypertension and blood pressure. *Aging Male*, 14(3), pp.176–82.

Wang, C., Nieschlag, E., Swerdloff, R., Behre, H.M., Hellstrom, W.J., Gooren, L.J., Kaufman, J.M., Legros, J.J., Lunenfeld, B., Morales, A., Morley, J.E., Schulman, C., Thompson, I.M., Weidner, Wu, F.C., ISA, ISSAM, EAU, EAA and ASA, 2009. Investigation, treatment, and monitoring of late-onset hypogonadism in males: ISA, ISSAM, EAU, EAA, and ASA recommendations. *Journal of Andrology*, 30(1), pp.1–9.

Young, K., Minchom, A. and Larkin, J., 2012. BRIM-1, -2 and -3 trials: improved survival with vemurafenib in metastatic melanoma patients with BRAF(V600E) mutation. *Future Oncology*, 8(5), pp.499–507.

Chapter 3
Personalised Medicine: Getting Past the Controversies

George P. Browman[1]

Sources of Controversy in Personalised Medicine: A Personal View

New ideas and paradigms can be threatening as they replace old ways of thinking and prompt change in our actions that engenders controversy among proponents and sceptics. Personalised medicine, like evidence-based medicine (EBM) before it, has generated its share of controversy. EBM challenged a traditional expert, opinion-based paradigm rooted in a theoretical understanding about mechanisms of disease as an implied justification for clinical interventions, to be replaced by direct observations from clinical experiments as an explicit basis for clinical decision making. While there remain criticisms of EBM, in general, the concept has become influential for decision making at the clinical, regulatory and policy levels.

The erosion of scepticism and eventual broad acceptance of EBM came about as controversy was replaced by conversation, with key clarifications of assumptions, especially around the roles of inputs other than evidence (values, patient preferences, and real world circumstances) as complementary elements contributing to decision making (Sackett et al., 1996; Haynes et al., 2002). Additionally, a variety of tools were developed to help providers and policy makers cope with the new paradigm (Browman, 2012).

Another concept, comparative effectiveness research (CER) also met initially with controversy. CER is a research strategy for informing healthcare decision making based on analysis of data obtained from large populations. The population-level data is intended to be used to make inferences about cause and effect relationships (between exposures to treatments or environmental sources and outcomes); and inferences about appropriate healthcare for individuals. Ironically, its introduction through the American Reinvestment and Recovery Act (2009) was opposed by an influential consortium of stakeholders on the grounds that it threatened the evolution of personalised medicine for the

---

1 Thanks to Dr Jan Schildmann and Professor Jochen Vollmann for the opportunity to prepare this work.

individuals by emphasising population-level data (Garber and Tunis, 2009). Even evidence-based medicine, with its emphasis on clinical trials, was viewed by some as inconsistent with a personalised medicine approach for the individual.

As conversations replaced controversy, these apparent schisms have been reconciled with the understanding that evidence-based medicine, personalised medicine and CER are complementary and a mutually interdependent triad of approaches to clinical evaluation methods (Hahn and Schilsky, 2012; Nardini et al., 2012). Even calls for transformative clinical trial evaluation methods in light of the personalised medicine movement include features of EBM (Sleijfer et al., 2013).

Controversy that accompanies new ideas can be more positively framed as a necessary process of public discussion that leads to improvements in new ideas, moulds opinions, and nurtures adoption towards progress. At some point, the adoption of a new idea becomes inevitable and the debate turns towards constructive critical analysis and problem solving. The idea of personalised medicine may be at that point where controversy is being replaced by readiness for constructive action informed by the evolving conversation.

Criticism of personalised medicine seems to have fallen into three separate categories of complaint. The first category relates to the appropriation of the term itself, which some feel misrepresents the focus of personalised medicine as a 'patient centred' movement with all that is implied when in fact it is mainly a technological advance focused on laboratory-based findings to inform decisions about interventions. That the term 'personalised medicine' appropriates the popular concept of patient-centredness seems valid enough. In response, new more applicable monikers are being advanced, the most recent being 'precision medicine' (Mirnezami et al., 2012). We should now be past arguing the advance of personalised medicine on these semantic grounds as the terms are steadily clarified (for a detailed discussion on the definition of personalised medicine see Chapter 1, this volume).

The second category of complaint is that early enthusiasts of personalised medicine have been promising more than can be delivered (Browman et al., 2014). Considering the current evidence, this may be true, but the controversy is more related to the different time horizons of visionaries explaining the possibilities versus sceptics focusing on the limitations. This aspect of the controversy will be settled as time passes.

The third category of criticism, closely related to the second, concerns the feasibility of implementation of genomic medicine on a large population-level scale. In this chapter, we highlight conceptual advances that are enabling the promise of personalised medicine from a population perspective. We then highlight some remaining issues that still need to be addressed for the promise of personalised medicine to be fulfilled (for a discussion from another point of view on these topics see Chapter 2, this volume).

An oncology perspective is used to highlight many of the issues discussed as applications of personalised medicine are ubiquitous in the cancer literature.

Conceptual Advances from Controversy towards Adoption

There have been several conceptual developments and proposals to further enable research and practice in personalised medicine. None of these alone can provide the impact needed to advance the field; however, several of these can fit together as an enabling package for advancing personalised medicine. The synergy of several of these advances towards enabling personalised medicine has been acknowledged elsewhere (Ginsburg and Kuderer, 2012).

The emerging enabling concepts for facilitating genomic medicine at the population level are: 'comparative effectiveness research' and statistical modelling; 'big data' analytics; biobanking; communications infrastructure; 'the learning organisation' and 'rapid learning' healthcare. These enablers together with renewed conceptual explorations to clarify and redefine boundaries between healthcare and health research and between medical ethics and research ethics provide a framework for planning the future of personalised medicine.

This discussion does not cover technological advances in communications/information technology and genomic testing that often dominate the topic of personalised (genomic) healthcare. It is also important to acknowledge the future of personalised medicine and CER incremental advances in biostatistical methods associated with Bayesian analyses and adaptive trial designs (Tajik et al., 2013) as enabling, but these are beyond the scope of this discussion.

The developments listed above are combined below into two packages of interdependent conceptual advances. Each package represents a link among related concepts that together are enabling personalised medicine research, practice and evaluation that can translate the personalised medicine controversy into consensus.

Conceptual Package 1: 'Comparative Effectiveness Research', 'Big Data' Analytics, Biobanking and Institutional Communications Infrastructure

The common thread that ties together these enabling concepts is the evaluation challenge for personalised medicine. Envisioned initially as a movement for 'individuals', it became apparent that the application of genomic information to individuals' health required rapid acceleration in the acquisition of genomic information to tease out its clinical meaning. This process of acceleration in acquiring meaning began with several calls from a variety of sources for broad sharing of genomic data emanating initially from the human genome project to advance the science of genomics (Human Genome Organization, 2003; The Wellcome Trust, 2003; Arzberger et al., 2004; OECD, 2007).

Genomic information by itself provided limited information about its 'clinical' meaning, which requires the correlation of genomic data with individuals' personal and health-related characteristics and outcomes that can only be reliably analysed using larger population-level data; hence, the emergence of the movement towards 'big data' analytics research as a complement to the evidence-based movement (Raghupathi and Raghupathi, 2014).

The CER paradigm provides the link between genomic data per se, and the 'real world' outcome data being envisioned from CER (Sox, 2010). There is now a clear understanding of the necessity to link genomic information with clinical data from large population studies ('big data') in order to accelerate extraction of the meaning of genetic findings that will contribute to the evaluation of the interventions implied by the personalised medicine movement.

The biobanking movement represents an extension of the CER concept by providing safe storage of tissue linked to clinical and genomic information for future analysis, and to allow targeted research on emerging questions that are yet to be asked with our limited knowledge (Watson et al., 2009). Attention to strict operating procedures (SOPs), governance models, and quality control tools serve to ensure appropriate development of such resources while protecting donors' rights and privacy (Godard et al., 2003; Hawkins and O'Doherty, 2010; The Biobank Resource Centre, 2014).

Institutional initiatives and emerging collaborations across healthcare institutions, especially in the area of cancer genomics, demonstrate the need for and feasibility of large-scale information infrastructures to capture, store, share and analyse such information on a regional, national and potentially international scale (Meric-Bernstam et al., 2013; Sledge et al., 2013; Worldwide Innovative Networking in Personalized Cancer Medicine, 2014). (For additional thoughts on this topic see Chapter 12, this volume.)

Conceptual Package 2: The 'Learning Organisation'; 'Rapid Learning' Healthcare; the Medical/Research Ethics Boundary; the Clinical Practice/Research Boundary

The 'learning organisation' concept (Senge, 1990) is consistent with the quality improvement paradigm through which organisations commit to (preferably prospective) monitoring of the organisation's performance using several strategically selected and agreed-to indicators, one of which could be patient outcomes, but also involving other measures. As applied to personalised medicine, the concept is similar to the still controversial policy innovation of 'coverage with evidence development' designed to allow for early access to incompletely but continuously evaluated interventions under appropriate circumstances (Lexchin, 2011).

The quality improvement paradigm and 'coverage with evidence development' share the main feature of informing close to real-time decisions and actions based on appropriately collected and closely examined accumulating data. The underlying assumption is that policies and practices should not be static, but rather responsive to information deemed to be important and consequential. Responsiveness to accumulating data linked to well-articulated questions about performance (of a technology, a treatment, a programme or an individual) that allows for improvement is the essence of effective learning, but it must be accompanied by feedback loops for implementation and re-evaluation as modifications to processes are introduced.

The 'Rapid Learning Health Care (RLHC) Model' (Abernethy et al., 2010; Brody and Miller, 2013) is an extension of the 'learning organisation' philosophy and calls for real-time availability of data from CER to support practice and policy decisions. While the concepts of 'quality improvement' and a 'learning organisation' represent a culture of measurement, self-evaluation, reflection and action at the individual and collective organisational levels, the RLHC model is a call for more immediate data availability and subsequent action. According to its proponents, this more immediate responsiveness is made feasible through the availability of real-time data extracted automatically (depending on the programming) from comprehensive CER data infrastructures and networks. The strategy envisions continuous aggregation and analysis of clinically relevant data from point of care. Whether robust enough, compared with the limitations of administrative databases of the past, to inform clinical decision making is yet to be validated (Levine and Julian, 2008); but, at a minimum, such databases would serve as a useful platform for the translational research requirements of personalised medicine.

The use of real-time accumulating data from large, aggregated databases to make judgments about appropriate care for individuals represents the application of the research method to everyday clinical practice. As enabling concepts and technologies evolve to influence practice, the boundary between research and care blurs, and, at the same time, so does the boundary between clinical and research ethical frameworks. The implementation of a culture of continuous learning within a learning organisation naturally implies the use of the research method as a foundation of good practice. This raises the issue of whether current distinctions between research and practice are relevant today, particularly from an ethical perspective. Such distinctions have an important influence on how clinical care and clinical research are funded and may be obsolete barriers to the implementation of personalised medicine, where care and translational research dovetail. Calls for re-evaluation of these distinctions and the associated ethical frameworks for clinical care and human research represent important contributions to the conversation for the feasible implementation of personalised medicine (Faden et al., 2013; Kass et al., 2013).

Ironically, concerns about the schism between research and practice in medicine and its implications for medical education led to the influential Flexner Report of 1910 (Flexner, 1910) that recommended improved standards for medical education through the affiliation of medical schools with academic universities. The recommendations still serve as the dominant model for medical education worldwide (Flexner, 1910). The Report promoted the scientific basis of medicine and advocated that medical education should not only be university-based, but also be strongly underpinned by a scientific foundation of medical practice.

For various reasons, some related to the evolution of how healthcare and education are independently financed, including insurance arrangements, and some related to examples of ethically unacceptable research practices leading to evolving independent research ethics frameworks, the boundaries between research and care and between research ethics and medical ethics have hardened. The case could be made that the distinctness of these boundaries may be justifiable, especially as researchers, practitioners and the corporate sector have grown closer together creating more opportunities for inter-sectoral conflicts of interest that must be meticulously managed. On the other hand, the emergence of the conceptual advances related to personalised medicine does seem to call for a deeper exploration of the research-practice and associated ethics schism. At least, these issues are now being addressed with innovative proposals for new perspectives in the current conversation (Brody and Miller, 2013; Faden et al., 2013; Kass et al., 2013).

Residual Areas to be Addressed

Having reviewed the packages of interdependent concepts that promise to advance the application of personalised medicine past controversy to consensus, it is appropriate to review, in brief, some of the remaining challenges.

Ethical challenges associated with the advance of personalised medicine have been covered elsewhere (Browman et al., 2014), and so this discussion will focus on other issues. (For discussions on ethical issues see chapters 10, 11 and 18, this volume.)

To this point, the discussion has consistently referred to personalised medicine from a population (as opposed to an individual) perspective. This is because for personalised medicine to achieve the impact promised by its proponents, it must be available to all who can potentially benefit. This means addressing barriers related to access, and the competitive forces that could undermine cooperative or collaborative solutions to healthcare access and the application of new technologies. These may be the main barriers to the success of personalised medicine as other barriers are overcome by conceptual and technological advances.

Access Issues

Access issues relate to preferential access based on the ability to pay, which for the United States will hopefully be overcome with health insurance reform. Geographic barriers to access should not be very different from those for other sophisticated technologies; genomic technologies are portable, and, as they become more efficient and affordable, they will rely less on technical expertise allowing widespread adoption.

The Competitive, Entrepreneurial Healthcare Environment

Barriers related to unnecessary competitive forces within certain healthcare arrangements (restricted to only a few countries) may be more difficult to overcome as competitive models reside deeply within the psyche of the dominant market-based ideology of certain market-driven economies. However, even here, there may be reason for optimism because of the projected costs of infrastructure for personalised medicine that will require large investments and shared risk arrangements forcing cooperation among for-profit, not-for-profit, and public financing sectors. Formal collaborations of this type will require good governance around contractual arrangements and transparency to address the risks associated with conflicts of interest.

Privacy Protection and Trust

Another barrier to be overcome for the success of personalised medicine is how the informed public will view the checks and balances for the acquisition, storage and sharing of genomic and other linked personal information within alleged anonymised or deidentified large datasets (Browman et al., 2014). While revelations about government surveillance of citizens has heightened awareness of the importance of protecting one's own information, and warned citizens that privacy may be an illusion, there may be more realistic expectations of what can and cannot be protected. In addition, many already share their own private information through Facebook and other social networking sites, suggesting again the illusion of privacy. For these reasons, privacy per se may be more an issue of trust than of disclosure. While citizens reserve the choice of disclosing private personal information on their own in the interconnected electronic world, the burden still falls on those with the responsibility to protect such information in order to maintain trust, without which certain entities, such as biobanks, could not be successful (Browman et al., 2014). (For additional discussions on biobanking see chapters 7 and 8, this volume.)

Knowledge and Readiness for Personalised Medicine within the Medical Profession

A recently published survey of practising adult physicians within tertiary care US NCI (National Cancer Institute) -designated comprehensive cancer centres reported wide variation in how expert physicians were planning to use genomic results from predictive multiplex genomic testing in their practice (Gray et al., 2014). This included variations in attitudes about disclosure of such information to patients and families (Gray et al., 2014). Within these highly sophisticated clinical-research environments, 22 per cent of oncologists expressed low confidence in their ability to interpret and apply genomic information.

Other than paediatrics, cancer is perhaps the most active medical discipline for the current application of genomics for both preventative and therapeutic decision making. Comprehensive cancer centres are the most sophisticated environments for translational research and care. Given the uncertainties associated with the application of genomics in such environments, we can expect a much lower level of genomic expertise in other environments where predictive genetic testing, some prompted by patient demand, will occur.

The gap between genomic science and the education of practitioners, including experts, may be the most challenging barrier for the clinical application of genomics in healthcare (see also Chapter 11, this volume). In contrast to the intensive investments into research for improving the technologies associated with genomics, and the active conversations designed to overcome controversies associated with genomics, attention to education and preparation of the final delivery pathway of genomic practice is still in its infancy. This could represent the weak link that undermines the totality of effort in moving personalised medicine forward in a timely fashion.

Conclusion

The purpose of this chapter is to help change the conversation about personalised medicine from controversy to consensus. The chapter highlights active areas where controversial issues are being addressed through conceptual and technological advances as well as compromises, thus, improving chances for the appropriate wider spread adoption of personalised medicine. Continuing controversy seems a wasted effort except when it contributes to constructive solutions for the implementation of personalised medicine. The chapter points out how other new ideas/paradigms have faced similar criticism at their introduction, and the processes that eventually led to their acceptance. A brief review is presented of some of the important conceptual advances that together are contributing to a constructive conversation that can lead to the appropriate adoption of personalised medicine. Finally, the chapter highlights some remaining difficult challenges, many of them social, that must be addressed if personalised medicine is to evolve as predicted by its visionaries.

References

Abernethy, A.P., Etheredge, L.M., Ganz, P.A., Wallace, P., German, R.R., Neti, C., Bach, P.B. and Murphy, S.B., 2010. Rapid learning system for cancer care. *Journal of Clinical Oncology*, 28, pp.4268–74.

American Reinvestment and Recovery Act, 2009. Available at: http://www.recovery.gov/arra/About/Pages/The_Act.aspx#act [Accessed 18 June 2014].

Arzberger, P., Schroeder, P., Beaulieu, A., Bowker, G., Casey, K., Laaksonen, L., Moorman, D., Uhlir, P. and Wouters, P., 2004. An international framework to promote access to data. *Science*, 303, pp.1777–8.

The Biobank Resource Centre. Available at: http://www.biobanking.org/brc/webs/sops [Accessed 18 June 2014].

Brody, H. and Miller, F.G., 2013. The research-clinical practice distinction, learning health systems, and relationships. *Hastings Center Report*, September–October, pp.41–7.

Browman, G.P., 2012. Special series on comparative effectiveness research: challenges to real-world solutions to quality improvement in personalized medicine. *Journal of Clinical Oncology*, 30, pp.4188–91.

Browman, G.P., Vollmann, J., Virani, A. and Schildmann, J., 2014. Improving the quality of 'personalized medicine' research and practice – through an ethical lens. *Personalized Medicine*, 11(4), pp.413–23.

Faden, R.R., Kass, N.E., Goodman, S.N., Pronovost, P., Tunis, S. and Beauchamp, T.L., 2013. An ethics framework for a learning health care system: a departure from traditional research ethics and clinical ethics. *Hastings Center Report*, Jan–Feb, Spec. No., pp.S16–S27.

Flexner, A., 1910. *Medical education in the United States and Canada: a report to the Carnegie Foundation for the advancement of teaching*. Boston: The Merrymount Press.

Garber, A.M. and Tunis, S.R., 2009. Does comparative-effectiveness research threaten personalized medicine? *New England Journal of Medicine*, 360, pp.1925–7.

Ginsburg, G.S. and Kuderer, N.M., 2012. Comparative effectiveness research, genomics – enabled personalized medicine and rapid learning health care: a common bond. *Journal of Clinical Oncology*, 30, pp.4233–42.

Godard, B., Schmidtke, J., Cassiman, J.-J. and Ayme, S., 2003. Data storage and DNA banking for biomedical research: informed consent, confidentiality, quality issues, ownership, return of benefits. A professional perspective. *European Journal of Human Genetics*, 11(Suppl 2), pp.S88–S122.

Gray, S.W., Hicks-Courant, K., Cronin, A., Rollins, B.J. and Weeks, J.C., 2014. Physicians' attitudes about multiplex tumor genomic testing. *Journal of Clinical Oncology*, 32, pp.1317–23.

Hahn, O.M. and Schilsky, R., 2012. Randomized controlled trials and comparative effectiveness research. *Journal of Clinical Oncology*, 30, pp.4194–201.

Hawkins, A.K. and O'Doherty, K., 2010. Biobank governance: a lesson in trust. *New Genetics and Society*, 29, pp.311–27.

Haynes, R.B., Devereaux, P.J. and Guyatt, G.H., 2002. Clinical expertise in the era of evidence-based medicine and patient choice. *Evidence-Based Medicine*, 7, pp.36–8.

Human Genome Organization (Hugo), 2003. Statement on human genome databases. *Journal International de Bioéthique*, 14, pp.207–10.

Kass, N.E., Faden, R.R., Goodman, S.N., Pronovost, P., Tunis, S. and Beauchamp, T.L., 2013. The research-treatment distinction: a problematic approach for determining which activities should have ethical oversight. *Hastings Center Report*, Jan–Feb, Spec. No., pp.S4–S15.

Levine, M.N. and Julian, J.A., 2008. Registries that show efficacy: good, but not good enough. *Journal of Clinical Oncology*, 26, pp.5316–19.

Lexchin, J., 2011. Coverage with evidence development for pharmaceuticals: a policy in evolution? *International Journal of Health Services*, 41, pp.337–54.

Meric-Bernstam, F., Farhangfar, C., Mendels, J. and Mills, G.B., 2013. Building a personalized medicine infrastructure at a major cancer center. *Journal of Clinical Oncology*, 31, pp.1849–57.

Mirnezami, R., Nicholson, J. and Darzi, A., 2012. Preparing for precision medicine. *New England Journal of Medicine*, 366, pp.489–91.

Nardini, C., Annoni, M. and Schiavone, G., 2012. Mechanistic understanding in clinical practice: complementing evidence-based medicine with personalized medicine. *Journal of Evaluation in Clinical Practice*, 18, pp.1000–5.

OECD (Organisation for Economic Co-Operation and Development), 2007. *Principles and guidelines for access to research data from public funding*. Paris: OECD.

Raghupathi, W. and Raghupathi, V., 2014. Big data analytics in healthcare: promise and potential. *Health Information Science and Systems*, 2, p.3.

Sackett, D.L., Rosenburg, W.M., Gray, J.A., Haynes, R.B. and Richardson, W.S., 1996. Evidence based medicine: what it is and what it isn't. *British Medical Journal*, 312, pp.71–2.

Senge, P., 1990. *The fifth discipline: the art and practice of the learning organization*. 2nd edn. New York: Currency Doubleday.

Sledge, G.W., Hudis, C.A., Swain, S.M., Yu, P.M., Mann, J.T., Hauser, R.S. and Lichter, A.S., 2013. ASCO's approach to a learning health care system in oncology. *Journal of Oncology Practice*, 9, 145–8.

Sleijfer, S., Bogaerts, J. and Siu, L.L., 2013. Designing transformative clinical trials in the cancer genome era. *Journal of Clinical Oncology*, 31, pp.1834–41.

Sox, H.C., 2010. Defining comparative effectiveness research: the importance of getting it right. *Medical Care*, 48(6 Suppl.), pp.S7–8.

Tajik, P., Zwinderman, A.H., Mol, B.W. and Bossuyt, P.M., 2013. Trial designs for personalizing cancer care: a systematic review and classification. *Clinical Cancer Research*, 19, pp.4578–88.

Watson, P.H., Wilson-McManus, J.E., Barnes, R.O., Giesz, S.C., Png, A., Hegele, R.G., Brinkman, J.N., Mackenzie, I.R., Huntsman, D.G., Junker, A., Gilks, B., Skarsgard, E., Burgess, M., Aparicio, S. and McManus, B.M., 2009. Evolutionary concepts in biobanking – the BC BioLibrary. *Journal of Translational Medicine*, 7, p.95.

The Wellcome Trust, 2003. *Sharing data from large-scale biological research projects: a system of tripartite responsibility.* Available at: http://www.wellcome.ac.uk/About-us/Policy/Policy-and-position-statements/WTD002751.htm [Accessed 18 June 2014].

Worldwide Innovative Networking in Personalized Cancer Medicine: Overview and WIN report. Available at: http://www.winconsortium.org/page.jsp?id=200 [Accessed 18 June 2014].

Chapter 4

Patient as Person in Personalised Medicine: Autonomy, Responsibility and the Body

Thomas Wabel

Current debates on personalised medicine bring many of the underlying assumptions that shape our understanding of people as patients to the fore. Among these, respect of autonomy, including full information for the patient and the patient's opportunity and ability to make a responsible choice, range high. However, recent interview studies (Polzer, 2005; Wöhlke et al., 2013; see also Chapter 11, this volume) indicate that the sheer amount of information to be conveyed, the complexity of the treatment and high expectations on the patients' side make it hard to arrive at an informed consent in the full sense. Having the choice to make use of therapeutic and preventive means, it seems, can also be a burden for the patient.

In this chapter, I am arguing that a concept of autonomy as freedom from external constraint and as decision-making capacity (Beauchamp and Childress, 2008) is too narrow to describe and understand the patient's decision concerning their own body. I shall start with a brief glance at protection of the patient's autonomy in German legislation, before turning to some exemplary cases of the patients' perception of genetic information in 'personalised' cancer therapy. This is followed by discussing various concepts of autonomy. I suggest that one should understand autonomy essentially as embodied autonomy. Finally, preliminary considerations address the practical consequences resulting from such a concept.

This contribution argues from the perspective of (Protestant) theology and philosophy of religion. Its argument does not depend on the reader sharing the assumptions of Christian belief. It does claim, however, that within the Christian tradition, aspects of human self-understanding are developed that may become relevant for the understanding of the patient and the understanding of ourselves as patients.

The Patient's Autonomy in Personalised Medicine

At first sight, the achievements in genetic diagnostics, risk management and customised therapy that are connected with the term 'personalised medicine' clearly support the patient's autonomy. Early and individualised information on health risks increases the possibility of taking preventive measures. Yet, critics warn that this might lead to a shift of responsibility from a shared risk community to the individual patient (Lemke, 2004; Kollek and Lemke, 2008). This has, in turn, legitimately been criticised as projecting hypothetical scenarios onto a very different present state of development (Dabrock, 2011, pp.247–8; see also Fischer et al. on 'hypothetical ethics' in Chapter 2, this volume). However, there are more fundamental aspects of responsibility which shape the patients' self-perception with respect to an illness and which are relevant for their self-understanding as autonomous. These aspects have to do with the way genetic information is perceived.

German Legislation and Jurisdiction

While the debate on genomic medicine has moved away from claiming genetic exceptionalism in scientific discourse, exceptionalism still plays an important role in public awareness. Past debates and present concerns are reflected in the *German Genetic Diagnostics Act* (*Gendiagnostikgesetz*), passed in 2010. Its regulations concerning collection, dissemination and storage of genetic information, as well as the guidelines on genetic counselling, are so strict that it has been criticised for being impractical (Leopoldina et al., 2010).

Such regulations mirror the public perception of genomic medicine in Germany. To some extent, the wariness can be traced back to historical origins. 'Euthanasia' during the Third Reich has contributed to an oversensitivity concerning the use of genetic information for measures of individual and public health.[1] More importantly, the strict regulations of the *Genetic Diagnostics Act* aim at informational autonomy of the patient. This can lead to conflicts between the principle of autonomy and other bioethical principles.[2] Moreover, the principle of autonomy itself can produce certain inconsistencies. As German jurisdiction

---

1 A striking example of this is that the term *Public Health* normally remains untranslated in Germany, for its literal translation ('*Volksgesundheit*') is Nazi terminology and includes the extinction of genetic material that was regarded as non-Aryan from the 'racial corpus'.

2 In the German context, protection of privacy sometimes overrides the interest even of close relatives (Oberlandesgericht München: *Medizinrecht* 28/2010, p.645 – all subsequent references to legislation follow Rudnik-Schöneborn et al., 2013, pp.4–5). Only in cases of endangerment of oneself or of others may information be disclosed

has pointed out, autonomy of the patient also comprises decisions that, at first sight, do not seem rational. Not only is the 'right not to know' protected by constitutional law,[3] but patients also have the right to refuse treatment, even if this treatment is indicated.[4] In this sense, autonomy comprises 'freedom for disease' (Rudnik-Schöneborn et al., 2013, p.4).

The Patient's Voice

There is a certain 'dialectics of autonomy' to be noted here. On the one hand, all additional information is helpful for making a rational choice in a situation of incomplete information, thereby increasing autonomy. On the other hand, interview studies have shown that, for some patients, the possibility to choose is a burden rather than a benefit. In this, there is a considerable difference between physicians and patients in the perception of the chances of a 'personalised' treatment (Wöhlke et al., 2013, p.216). As one doctor recalls in the context of treating locally advanced rectal cancer: 'Most patients just want us to take the decision for them ... Rarely have I encountered patients who ... see something positive in the possibility to choose. Basically, it was rather too much of a burden for them' (Wöhlke et al., 2013, p.219 – physician 'A5').

Sometimes the sheer amount of information at hand is an ambiguous achievement for the patient. Some patients appreciate being better informed and being able to decide about preventive measures or the possibilities for treatment. As a participant in genetic testing for familial melanoma states: 'I think that we need to take an active role in our own health by getting as much information as we can' (Polzer, 2005, p.84 – 'Nicole', no previous melanoma). By the same token, the increase in complex information does not necessarily entail an increase in autonomy for the patient: 'To my mind, it's not that patients lose autonomy because of an increase in prognostic knowledge – but [this knowledge] is to the doctor's, not to the patient's benefit' (Wöhlke et al., 2013, p.219 – physician 'A11').

In the context of risk management and prevention, too, genetic knowledge is perceived to be ambivalent. In some cases, former melanoma patients are reluctant to acquire genetic risk information for their family members:

[W]hat do you do with that information once you have it? Yes, I ... could come home and say to the family, 'Okay, I have this in my DNA and chances are you do too and you have to watch for it'. The thing is, I've already done that in a

---

against the patient's will (Bundesgerichtshof: *Neue Juristische Wochenschrift*, 1983, p.350; Europäischer Gerichtshof: *Neue Juristische Wochenschrift*, 1994, p.3005).

3   Oberlandesgericht Celle: *Neue Juristische Wochenschrift*, 2004, p.449.
4   Bundesverfassungsgericht: *Neue Juristische Wochenschrift*, 2011, p.2113.

sense … [T]hey've watched me go through my own melanoma journey and we've discussed the fact that this can happen to anybody … On the one hand you want to keep the fear out of it … but at the same time you want to make them aware. (Polzer, 2005, p.86 – 'Melissa', previous melanoma)

The inconsistencies revealed in this statement are typical for the attitude some patients develop towards the character of genetic information. According to 'Melissa', the knowledge acquired from such a test is no different from the knowledge she and her family already have. At the same time, she refrains from such a test. The 'certainty' the test offers might fill her and her family with fear, which shows that, for her, knowing about a genetic risk *is* different from the risk they already know about.[5]

When focussing on patients as people in medicine, such inconsistencies have to be taken into account. On the one hand, patients want to make use of the possibilities that personalised medicine offers and are willing to undergo genetic analysis. On the other hand, a certain reluctance concerning genetic knowledge can be observed. The patient statements from which I have quoted can be seen as exemplary cases demonstrating an understanding of individuals regarding their physical condition that cannot easily be 'corrected' by better patient information. In this, they reveal inconsistencies regarding the understanding of 'autonomy'. On the one hand, patients explicitly want to exert their autonomy; on the other, they simply trust 'that the doctors will do the right thing'.[6]

Concepts of Autonomy

Autonomy as Informed Consent

According to the influential *Principles of Biomedical Ethics* (Beauchamp and Childress, 2008), the principle of respect of autonomy presupposes 'freedom from external constraint' and 'the presence of critical mental capacities such as understanding, intending, and voluntary decision-making capacity' (Beauchamp, 2003, p.24). Autonomy, in this sense, means freedom of choice concerning imminent decisions. Its opposite is paternalism on the side of the medical

---

5   It is instructive that 'Melissa' does not say, 'I might have passed it on to you', but rather, 'anyone can have it'.

6   Wöhlke et al., 2013, p.221 – patient 'P17'; translation mine. Following Ducournau and Strand (2009), the authors call this 'virtual trust', motivated neither by understanding nor by deep trust in the physician's competence, but by the hope for cure (Wöhlke et al., 2013, p.221).

expert. In this understanding, autonomy is realised by informed consent to a specific treatment in a specific context (Beauchamp and Childress, 2008, p.100).

This definition is workable and, indeed, indispensable for medical treatment, but it is necessarily narrow and, hence, limited. In some cases, a fully informed consent is difficult to achieve, for this would presuppose a complete understanding of the illness, of all the medical options, biological causes, etc. (Wöhlke et al., 2013, p.219). In the words of a physician concerning the treatment of rectal cancer: 'This is an elementary principle of therapy for me, to achieve … consent … But in an everyday situation, I encounter limits to that – because all this [genetics, methods] just can't be conveyed' (Wöhlke et al., 2013, p.219 – physician 'A8'; translation mine). While informed consent focuses on a specific decision concerning the choice of therapy, when dealing with the result of predictive diagnosis, there is often no direct connection between the patient's knowledge and their autonomy (Hildt, 2008, p.283f.).

To illustrate these shortcomings, I shall examine some of the underlying assumptions and ensuing limitations of a narrow concept of autonomy. My aim in this is to arrive at a broader understanding of autonomy that is still applicable for the medical context. To do both, it is necessary to draw attention to recent philosophical debates on the topic of autonomy.

Autonomy as Authenticity

The narrow concept of autonomy developed in Beauchamp's and Childress' *Principles* stands in the tradition of John Stuart Mill, insofar as it understands autonomy as freedom of paternalism and sovereignty over one's own body and mind (Mill, 1859; Rolf, 2008, p.203). The implications of this concept are easy to discover in present day society: to exert control over the body means to take responsibility for physical fitness and to manage possible health risks. Accordingly, to deal with a situation of crisis (say, a cancer diagnosis) autonomously, the patient can resort to well-established coping strategies from everyday life:

1. perceiving and *identifying* the problem realistically;
2. assessing the situation by *rational analysis*;
3. weighing the pros and cons of different *alternatives for action*; and
4. *managing* the situation by *controlled* and deliberate action.

Böttcher and Paul (2013) criticise the implications of a narrow concept of autonomy in a recent article on measures of fertility preservation for young cancer patients. In this concept, the process of reaching informed consent in patient–doctor consultations involves, above all, cognitive aspects as a basis for rational decision. The relation between body and psyche is neglected, even though it has often been shown that consciousness of one's body changes in the course of cancer diagnosis and treatment. In neglecting this aspect, a narrow conception of autonomy rests on a 'disembodied concept of humans' (Böttcher and Paul, 2013, p.50f.).

Here, the legacy of dualistic accounts of the human will becomes visible. Descartes' distinction of mental substances and material substances, and Kant's notion of freedom as the 'unconditional condition of any wilful act' (Kant, 1787, p.B 583) are cornerstones of our conception of autonomy, in that they claim the independence of human freedom from physical restraints. However, regarded in isolation, they have often led to dualistic positions which place mind over matter or freedom of rational choice over the limitations of physical conditions. Decisions of fundamental importance in life rest on more than just a rational basis.

> [R]egarding fertility protection, the bodily dimension can be of such relevance that in practice the ideal of autonomy founded on rationality is overcharged … Wanting a child is not exclusively a physical demand or an event in the biological course of one's life, but a realisation of aims in life that might also be irrational. (Böttcher and Paul, 2013, p.51)

Böttcher and Paul suggest a concept of *authenticity* to account for such choices. They identify aspects of authenticity following various philosophical approaches: the ability to relate to one's origin and biography, the social dimension of life, and the ability to distance oneself from immediate influences and from the perception of one's body (Böttcher and Paul, 2013, p.55). How does a concept of *embodied autonomy* tie into this?

Embodied Autonomy

The concept I am suggesting rests on anthropological considerations: how do we as human beings want to understand ourselves? When we seek medical advice, questions of understanding ourselves and our lives become particularly relevant. When our physical health is at stake, the body, the very basis of our existence in the world, is in danger. In a situation of severe illness, the elementary coping strategies mentioned above (identification – analysis – alternatives – management and control) are not sufficient. In these strategies – indispensable as they are – the body, the physical *condition* for existence, becomes the *object* of analysis and action. Hence, such strategies rest on a dualistic account of autonomy.

The concept of 'embodiment' has been introduced in recent philosophical discussion to avoid such dualism. Basically, the embodiment thesis holds that 'the body as it operates outside the subject's conscious awareness' influences and shapes the subject's experience, perception, cognition, decisions and actions (Gallagher, 2005, p.32). Hereby, *physical* aspects are reintroduced into processes that used to be regarded as purely *mental* phenomena, such as decision-making. The idea is not to reduce all mental phenomena to physical processes. Rather, what human beings do and say results from a constant interplay of body and mind. The mind is essentially *embodied* – and so are such central aspects of human self-understanding as freedom and autonomy. '[Free will] can only be understood as *embodied freedom*, resulting from the interdependency of personal intentionality and subpersonal mechanisms' (Jung, 2009, p.303, with reference to Gallagher, 2005, p.242; translation mine).

Autonomy, therefore, is realised in two directions: acting autonomously means being able to distance oneself from the immediate experience of a given situation. However, it also means being led back to the physical, bodily side of existence. Similarly, there is a double aspect to the body: the body *enables* me to act and communicate – and, at the same time, it *constrains* all such action and communication (Gallagher, 2005, p.149). Our body is never completely transparent to ourselves and we cannot escape the way it makes us experience the world. The body is the *basis* for all autonomous decisions – and, at the same time, it constitutes the *boundary* of all such decisions. Embodied autonomy consists of an interplay of enablement and limitation, of transformation and acceptance of a given situation.

Consequently, the concept of embodied autonomy takes into account that autonomy is not just about staying in control. Rather, autonomy, in the full sense, includes relating to a dimension of human existence that, for human beings, is beyond reach. This dimension is experienced immediately when the body is at stake.

The relevance of this concept for the medical context can be illustrated by distinguishing three different perspectives of the human body (Gallagher, 2005, p.31f.):

1. while autonomy in the narrow sense of informed consent is an adequate means to relate to the *body as an object of medical care*, it needs to be complemented by the aspects of
2. the *body as the centre of one's self-experience* and of
3. the *body as the basis of existence* and, hence, of all autonomous action.

These aspects can be distinguished terminologically – at least in German, which has two equivalents for 'body': *Körper* and *Leib*. *Körper* and *Leib* stand for different perspectives of the human organism, each in its own right:

1. To regard my body as the object of medical treatment, means to distance myself

from the body (*Körper*) I *have*.

2. To experience myself as 'I' within the world, presupposes feeling myself to be the body (*Leib*) I *am*.[7]

The way I act, speak and perceive myself is shaped by the way my body (*Körper*) operates outside my conscious experience. Bodily processes structure (preconsciously) what I consciously do and say: the sequence of my words (and, hence, thoughts) is structured by the rhythm of my speech, which, in turn, is dependent on my breathing. What I say and how I say it is formed in a way that can never be fully controlled by myself.[8]

From the physician's perspective, aspect (1) is perfectly adequate for medical treatment, and the corresponding concept of autonomy in the sense of informed consent is a workable approach. However, the case is different from the patient's perspective. What happens to the body directly influences the patient's self-perception in the sense of aspect (2). Finally, in some cases, aspect (3), which normally runs in the background of our self-perception without being noticed, becomes prevalent. It is easy to see that in cases such as 'stress, pain, hunger, fatigue, lability, and so forth', bodily processes influence the way I see the world even below the threshold of conscious self-perception (Gallagher, 2005, p.149). For example, I might lose concentration even before I realise that it is time to eat something. '[T]hese processes … condition, constrain, and color perception … If [the attunement of the body to the environment] were upset, if a certain process connected with respiration, for example, failed, then one's perception of the world would be different in some way' (Gallagher, 2005, p.150). It should be obvious that this also holds for the interplay of body, self-perception and autonomy in the case of severe illness, even in the absence of physical pain.

At this point, common elements and differences between Böttcher's and Paul's concept of *authenticity* and the concept of *embodied autonomy* can be highlighted. Embodied autonomy corresponds with an ethics of authenticity, in that the perspective of the body as the object of medical treatment (*Körper*) is complemented by the perspective of the body as the unity of a person's

---

7 Philosophically speaking, this is a phenomenological perspective of the world as I experience it (Waldenfels, 2000, p.248f.).

8 Jung (2009, p.298). This example shows that intentionality is embodied in a twofold sense: the expression of my thoughts and feelings is embodied in that it rests on a bodily foundation (a); in being uttered, my thoughts and feelings are embodied in my written or spoken words (b). It is this double aspect of embodiment, in which the body as *Körper* becomes relevant for intentionality and emotions, that distinguishes this concept from a phenomenology of the body (*Phänomenologie der Leiblichkeit*) like that of Hermann Schmitz, as presented by Mathias Wirth in Chapter 5, this volume.

self-perception, including their biography and the social dimension of their life (*Leib*). The idea of embodiment (*Verkörperung*) adds an aspect to this. As our life is essentially and inescapably embodied, so are our thoughts, wishes, plans, and the choices we take – in short, everything in which human autonomy is expressed. In a situation of illness, the preconscious iterative processes between body and self-perception which shape our understanding of ourselves come to the fore.[9] This opens up new possibilities for helping the patients to develop a relation to themselves as embodied people and, consequently, to take their decisions in a fuller, integrative sense of autonomy.

Consequences

What are the implications of a concept of embodied autonomy in the context of clinical counselling?

1. Böttcher and Paul (2013, pp.55–8) suggest that patient information and clinical counselling should enable the patient to make an *authentic choice* that considers a wider scope of wishes, desires and motives of both the patient and their relatives. For this, all relevant information – rational, emotional or social aspects – should be presented. The patient should be offered a network of interdisciplinary support and be encouraged to activate existing networks. Thus, helping the patient to realise autonomy in a broader sense includes developing their ability to cope with the diagnosis of a severe illness.

2. The concept of *embodiment* can complement this approach by drawing attention to the fact that conditions of health under which the body operates 'are not only objective, physical facts; they are facticities to which my body reacts and with which it copes' (Gallagher, 2005, p.151), and, within this process of coping, shapes my perception of life. In the case of illness, even basic ways of expressing oneself may reveal the extent to which the body enables and constrains personal autonomy. This helps one to understand that differences between the physician's and the patient's view of the options for treatment may arise at a very early stage,

---

9 An impressive example of the ambivalences resulting from this is Cathy's final monologue in season 1, episode 1 of the American TV series *The Big C*, in which a melanoma patient, upon receiving her diagnosis, starts to act in a seemingly irrational way. 'I'm living the dream! I'm here all year! … It's kind of funny – "Death Comedy". (*laughing*) I'm warning you – this laughter might turn into a sob in a second. (*sobbing*) – Yeah – here it goes' (http://www.movieweb.com/tv/TEswQsvwUWWTxu/pilot, accessed 2 April 2014). Laughing and crying have their common origin in situations in which all intentional action runs against a barrier to explanation and, since all answers fail, the body answers in place of the person (Plessner, 1941, pp.364–6).

long before reaching informed consent. Of course, this demands a considerable amount of sensitivity and judgment on the side of the physician.

3. For patients and clinical counsellors alike, developing autonomy in the full sense includes an understanding of what enables and constrains human freedom. Realising embodied autonomy means to establish a positive relation to the body as the basis of physical existence, while, at the same time, being aware of what escapes all medical care and surveillance (Wabel, 2013, p.13). In this, religion can play an important role. Religious practice and articulation can help to integrate what is beyond human reach into a person's self-understanding (Luhmann, 2000, pp.54f., 83f.). The experience of illness is embodied in a twofold sense in religious articulation: the bodily conditions of existence are expressed in religious language and, in turn, the articulation of religious experience can have bodily consequences.[10]

Autonomy in this sense neither results in complete control over the body, nor in passive resignation. Rather, it means to cherish the body as the basis of existence and to accept its constraints, knowing about the frailty of human existence. Accepting such limitations does not become less important with the progress of medical research. Autonomy is realised incompletely if it only aims at minimising the area that is beyond control. It is precisely *within* our attempts to stay in control (as doctors and as patients) that the dimension of what is beyond human reach needs to be acknowledged in order to gain a fuller understanding of autonomy.

References

Beauchamp, T.L., 2003. The origins, goals, and core commitments of The Belmont Report and Principles of Biomedical Ethics. In: J.K. Walter and E.P. Klein, eds. *The story of bioethics from seminal works to contemporary explorations*. Washington, DC: Georgetown University Press. pp.17–46.

Beauchamp, T.L. and Childress, J.F., 2008. *Principles of biomedical ethics*. Oxford: Oxford University Press.

Bester, D. and Janowski, B., 2009. Anthropologie des Alten Testaments. Ein forschungsgeschichtlicher Überblick. In: B. Janowski and K. Lien, eds. *Der*

---

10   Both dimensions come into play in verses such as, 'When I kept silence, my bones waxed old through my roaring all the day long' (Psalm 32:3) or 'I have set the Lord always before me ... Therefore my heart is glad and my glory rejoices, my flesh also shall dwell in safety' (Psalm 16, p.8f.). Here, 'bones', 'heart' and 'flesh' are 'aspects of a psychosomatic unity complementing each other' (Bester and Janowski, 2009, p.11; translation mine).

Mensch im Alten Israel. Neue Forschungen zur alttestamentlichen Anthropologie. Freiburg: Herder. pp.3–40.

Böttcher, B. and Paul, N., 2013. Personale Autonomie: Diskussion eines zentralen ethischen Konzepts von fertilitätsprotektiven Maßnahmen bei Krebspatienten. *Ethik in der Medizin*, 25(1), pp.47–59.

Dabrock, P., 2011. Die konstruierte Realität der sog. individualisierten Medizin. Sozialethische und theologische Anmerkungen. In: V. Schumpelick and B. Vogel, eds. *Medizin nach Maß. Individualisierte Medizin – Wunsch und Wirklichkeit.* Freiburg, Basel and Wien: Herder. pp.239–67.

Ducournau, P. and Strand, R., 2009. Trust, distrust and co-production. The relationship between research biobanks and donors. In: J.H. Solbakk, S. Holm and B. Hofmann, eds. *The ethics of research biobanking.* Dordrecht and Heidelberg: Springer. pp.115–30.

Gallagher, S., 2005. *How the body shapes the mind.* Oxford: Clarendon Press.

Hildt, E., 2008. Prädiktive Medizin und Patientenautonomie im Wandel. In: D. Schäfer, A. Frewer, E. Schockenhoff and V. Wetzstein, eds. *Gesundheitskonzepte im Wandel. Geschichte, Ethik und Gesellschaft.* Stuttgart: Steiner. pp.277–91.

Jung, M., 2009. *Der bewusste Ausdruck. Anthropologie der Artikulation.* Berlin and New York: de Gruyter.

Kant, I., 1787. Kritik der reinen Vernunft. Zweiter Teil. In: W. Weischedel, ed. 1956. *Immanuel Kant. Werke in zehn Bänden. Vol. IV.* Darmstadt: Wissenschaftliche Buchgesellschaft.

Kollek, R. and Lemke, T., 2008. *Der medizinische Blick in die Zukunft. Gesellschaftliche Implikationen prädiktiver Gentests.* Frankfurt and New York: Campus.

Lemke, T., 2004. *Veranlagung und Verantwortung. Genetische Diagnostik zwischen Selbstbestimmung und Schicksal.* Bielefeld: transcript.

Leopoldina, acatech and BBAW (2010). '*Gendiagnostikgesetz hält der Praxis nicht stand*' – *Wissenschaftsakademien fordern Novellierung*, [online] 10 November. Available at: http://www.leopoldina.org/de/presse/pressemitteilungen/pressemitteilung/press/865/ [Accessed 2 April 2014].

Luhmann, N., 2000. *Die Religion der Gesellschaft.* A. Kieserling, ed. Frankfurt/M.: Suhrkamp.

Mill, J.S., 1859. On Liberty. In: A. Ryan, ed. 2006. *John Stuart Mill. On liberty and the subjection of women.* London: Penguin.

Plessner, H., 1941. Lachen und Weinen. Eine Untersuchung der Grenzen menschlichen Verhaltens. In: G. Dux, O. Marquard and E. Ströker, eds. 1982. *Helmuth Plessner. Ausdruck und menschliche Natur. Gesammelte Schriften VII.* Frankfurt/M.: Suhrkamp. pp.201–387.

Polzer, J., 2005. Choice as responsibility. Genetic testing as citizenship through familial obligation and the management of risk. In: R. Bunton and A. Petersen, eds. *Genetic governance: health, risk and ethics in the biotech era.* London and New York: Routledge. pp.79–92.

Rolf, S., 2008. Respekt vor Patientenautonomie und Achtung der Menschenwürde. Beobachtungen zu anthropologischen Implikationen in deutscher und englischsprachiger Bioethik-Debatte. *Zeitschrift für Evangelische Ethik*, 52, pp.200–11.

Rudnik-Schöneborn, S., Langanke, M., Erdmann, P. and Robienski, J., 2013. Ethische und rechtliche Aspekte im Umgang mit genetischen Zufallsbefunden – Herausforderungen und Lösungsansätze. *Ethik in der Medizin*, 25(3), pp.1–15.

Wabel, T., 2013. Leibliche Autonomie. Zum Umgang mit Ambivalenzen des Autonomiebegriffs in der 'individualisierten Medizin'. *Zeitschrift für medizinische Ethik*, 59, pp.3–17.

Waldenfels, B., 2000. *Das leibliche Selbst. Vorlesungen zur Phänomenologie des Leibes.* R. Giuliani, ed. Frankfurt/M.: Suhrkamp.

Wöhlke, S., Heßling, A. and Schicktanz, S., 2013. Wenn es persönlich wird in der 'personalisierten Medizin': Aufklärung und Kommunikation aus klinischer Forscher- und Patientenperspektive im empirisch-ethischen Vergleich. *Ethik in der Medizin*, 25(3), pp.215–22.

Chapter 5

The Authority of Corporeality and Emotions: The New Phenomenology and its Relevance to the German Debate on Personalised Medicine

Mathias Wirth

A misunderstanding within medical ethics currently exists over what exactly is meant by the term 'personal' in personalised medicine. Does medical ethics, that notoriously accuses personalised medicine of not being personal, step into the dualistic segregation of material and immaterial, making the same misjudgements on the opposite side that they blame a molecular-oriented medicine for? Without saying personalised medicine was all negative, medical theorists such as Bergdolt (2011) and Gadebusch-Bondio and Michl (2010) hold *mutatis mutandis* that the term 'personal' is not used properly when only being related to a somatic-oriented medicine. Such vague statements made by Bergdolt, Gadebusch-Bondio and others only focus on an assumed public understanding, but are unjust to physicians who try to cure people, who do not fall into two separate parts of body and soul, by personalised medicine.

The argument that somatic and molecular-oriented medicine lack personalisation is based on René Descartes' juxtaposition of *res cogitans* (spirit) and *res extensa* (body) (Siep, 2001). The critics who doubt that personalised medicine is actually personal intend to warn of exclusively paying attention to the somatic side of sickness. When these ethics negate the use of the term 'personal' for the medical project which works in the field of more individualised medicine with respect to an individual's specific or even unique constitution, then they are saying that personal is just the *res cogitans*: the immaterial, the psychic part of the human. The proposition that somatic-dedicated medicine, that aims to improve treatment by paying close attention to the specific conditions of a patient's somatic constitution, cannot be called personal is a dualistic misjudgement. Suffering from sickness in pain and anger is highly personal, as its healing is of great importance for person, their autonomy, emotions and feeling.

Instead of wrongly blaming personalised medicine for its name, medical ethics could use this person-centred moment in the history of medicine in order to widen its focus on both the material and the immaterial, without reserving the 'personal' attribute for either side. The body belongs to the person as well as their feelings and thoughts. What definitely is a desire that medical anthropology and ethics emphasise is the interest in paying attention to the whole person and to the whole patient. Although there is no doubt whatsoever that sickness has a psychosomatic dimension to it, a widespread belief still exists that emotions or other immaterial situations are hopelessly private and have no direct effect on how to cure and treat patients as people. According to Herman Schmitz's (2003) philosophy, however, feelings gain authority because they are not just private but territorial atmospheres that take up room and can be even called half-things (*Halbdinge*). A glance, the voice and pressure are quite as real as normal things, but are different in their continuity. Atmospheres are classed as feelings in Schmitz's thinking (Schmitz, 2003): 'In my opinion, emotions are atmospheres poured out spatially that move the felt (not the material) body' (Schmitz et al., 2011, p.247; see also Böhme, 1993; Schmitz, 1994; Langewitz, 2007; Gugutzer, 2013). An example of such an atmosphere would be solemn silence or the pressure of sorrow (Schmitz et al., 2011). Suffering is not private but atmospheric, and neglecting it means not considering the reality of the sick person. Now the phenomenological philosophy of Schmitz helps us to see how corporeality (*Leiblichkeit*) is of great importance to personhood. Compared to the bodily sphere of the person, corporeality is the room where the person experiences pain, angst, shame or lust intensively and primarily, and in constant relation to the material body: 'Schmitz distinguishes *Leib* (personal body or flesh, corporeality) from the concept of *Körper* (physical body) … a *Leib* is the stratum of involuntary and immediate feeling (*Verspürung*)' (Blume, 2010, p.307). What Schmitz can teach in the entire debate on personalised medicine is how real immaterial occurrence of corporeality is, such as the experience of pain, angst, shame and lust, and that the dualistic concept of separated body and soul is a prejudice that lacks the dimension of corporeality (Blume, 2010). (For another concept of autonomy, see Chapter 4, this volume.)

As a first step, this chapter will show an ethical criticism of the claims that an all-encompassing focus on a person within personalised medicine cannot exist within a common dualistic perspective on what a person is. It follows a short introduction regarding the direction in which personalised medicine is moving: towards a person's specific somatic configuration. In the next step, the view of Schmitz's 'new phenomenology' will be presented. His position relates to the criticism of a too narrow perception of a concept of personhood. The last step will consist of showing the necessary medical ethical ramifications and how they can be realigned to a new conclusion in co-operation with Schmitz's question: what precisely is the personal with regard to illness and medicine?

What Signifies Personal?

From the beginning of mankind and culture, humans have paid attention to others' injuries and sickness and tried to heal them (Seidler, 1993). In order to give an idea of how deep the willingness to cure is implanted into man's constitution, you can go back to the years before 207 BC when the Roman author Hyginus wrote his Cura-tale about the beginning of man out of the hands of 'Cura', which means both care and concern. The German equivalent is the word *Sorge*, which encompasses both meanings. Hyginus fables that one day the goddess Cura wanted to cross a river and noticed plenty of loamy mud at the riverside. She carefully took some mud and formed a human out of it – not a precious origin with no promise of a divine life without suffering or sorrow. Then Jupiter came onto the scene and gave life to the muddy human and recommended that this creature be given a name. Cura wanted to name this being after herself, since she had made it, but Jupiter disagreed and wanted the creature to be named after him. All of a sudden, the god Earth rose to speak, declaring that it should be called Earth since it was made of earth. The three decided to call Saturn as a judge. He decided fairly: since Jupiter gave life to man, after death the soul returns to him. Since from Earth man was taken, man will return to it. However, since Cura formed man, man belongs to her throughout the entire life. This creature shall be called *homo*, because he looks like *humus* (earth) (Hyginus, 2007). What Hyginus is saying is that since humanity is made from the picture of Cura, caring is a sign of humanity (Haas, 2000). Hyginus's Cura-tale is a very early testimony to the alliance between personality and care that is prominently expressed in medical treatment, without saying that medicine is equal to care. What can be reviewed from here is that medicine, as basic care according to the early Roman writer Hyginus, belongs to the wider hermeneutic field of personhood.

Focusing on current perspectives on the conundrum person (Sturma, 2001a; Quante, 2007), instructions can also be found that reinforce the thesis that medicine is personal when trying to cure patients. This is not saying that an isolated focal point of the somatic sphere of sickness will lead to a recovery in a wider sense, but there is no doubt that the very beginning of healing the somatic wound is personal in two senses: in the sense that a physician acts as a person when treating sickness and in the sense that a person who is a patient gets back autonomy, or at least some of it, in the best case scenario; and when, finally, it might just be pain-realising drug therapy. This patient-personal dimension can best be understood when overcoming the dualistic scheme in anthropology. One way to do so is proposed by Schmitz.

One current perspective on the philosophy of person comes from Theo Kobusch (1993). Following his main findings, the term 'person' in the way it is understood today comes from the thirteenth century, not from ancient times, where *persona* meant the exact opposite of what we mean today. It was just the term for a theatrical mask (*prosopon/persona*) and not for a true character (Kobusch, 1993; Kreuzer, 2001; Mohr, 2001). The dignity of the person comes from freedom, because freedom is something absolute within the person (Kobusch, 1993; Sturma, 2001b), which means the capability to distance oneself from everything, including one's own thoughts and feelings (Kobusch, 1993). Within this distance, freedom is truly absolute, and, in a Kantian way of interpretation, this is what distinguishes humanity from all other forms of being. Nowadays, Kobusch states, 'person' is a universal concept of dignity that protects the individual, and this protection embraces the entire person which includes its material side that belongs, unsurprisingly, to the person (Kobusch, 1993). Exactly this dignity-concept of the person, according to Kobusch, was neither implied in the ancient use of person, nor within Plato, nor Aristotle, nor can this understanding be found in ancient Christian texts (Kobusch, 1993).

Another current perspective of the concept of 'person' that helps to clarify the meaning of 'personal' in the realm of medicine comes from Robert Spaemann (1996). Personhood to him is a *nomen dignitatis* and signifies a certain kind of behaviour towards people. This is not due to any quality one might have. Person does not refer to any specific feature, but rather to every human being (Spaemann, 1996). Generally speaking, people require attention. Spaemann reminds us of the narration of Cain and Abel in the book of Genesis (Gen. 4). When God lost Abel, he asked his brother Cain and he responded, 'Am I the keeper of my brother?' God's question shows he requires people to know where the other is; not knowing it means murder, Spaemann claims (1996). The appropriate answer to the personhood of the other (Spaemann, 1996; Quante, 2007), also without any religious framework, means that in a primary, yet unsatisfying sense, paying attention to a person's wellbeing begins with taking care of the material side of the person that would otherwise not exist.

There is also a perspective on personhood that casts light on the question of the meaning of medical intervention as being personal that comes from Hans Joas (2011). Joas's concept of sacredness of the person is the result of a long-lasting historical process that ended in the Universal Declaration of Human Rights and the conviction of the universality of humans' dignity (Kant, 1785). This came to pass within the history of an increasing understanding of the sacredness of the person (King, 1907; Joas, 2011). Joas emphasises that this is not only exclusively a religious affair, but is to be understood in a wider sense because the sacredness of the person derives from the person itself and not from any divine instruction (Joas, 2011). Joas verifies this phenomenologically when demonstrating the 'subjective evidence' and the 'affective intensity' people feel when facing a person, especially when the other is in danger or sorrow. According to Joas, these are the common responses to holiness, and thus, the person appears as a secularised God (Joas, 2011). Joas cites the famous French sociologist Émile Durkheim (1898), who also showed that the person is mostly seen as sacred. Durkheim elaborates: whenever we witness an offence against a person or their dignity, we gain feelings of averseness that are the same as when religious feelings get hurt (Durkheim, 1898; see also Habermas, 1981; Joas, 2004). Durkheim also names the practical consequence that follows from the sacredness of the person and helps to relate Durkheim's and Joas's theory of the holiness of the person to medical ethics. Durkheim lists the following reactions *face-à-face* with the person that is (implicitly) considered to be holy: 'sympathy for everything that is human', 'compassion for all pain and tragedy of the person', 'an intense desire of removing pain and tragedy' and 'thirst for justice' (Durkheim, 2010, p.60; Joas, 2011). What follows from this is once again the central meaning of medicine as a concrete answer to the dignity of the person and their pain, angst and suffering.

There are lots of reasons to not put health first, since it is incredibly fragile and, therefore, should not be the most important, as people do not lose what is most important to them in times of sickness. It would, however, be far from the desires of the person not to rank health as very important. Health is a *desideratum* of people; and this makes medicine personal, even in its fundamental sense of somatic medicine (Sturma, 2001b).

The Moving towards the Person in (Personalised) Medicine

Medicine has always had an individual character (Henke, 2011). One principle of medicine, Bergdolt (2011) holds, was the belief that the situation of the individual and their co-operation and mental capacity were needed for successful therapy. Bergdolt discusses dietetics, which means much more than a diet, also encompassing the person's habits, sleeping patterns, movements and work that were all addressed in the ancient book *Concerning the way of living (Perìdiaítes)* for instance. Medicine that accounts for all of these personal habits is already a personalised kind of medicine. Bergdolt can show the same pattern throughout the history of medicine: Galen's call for empathy and science in medicine, the observance of individual physical constitution of patients within the ancient medical school of Knidos, which was the first attempt at classifying diseases, and the advice of Giovanni Battista del Monte in 1575 that the physician is responsible for every single patient and their sickness (Bergdolt, 2011).

Nowadays, there are five areas in which personalised medicine tries to be especially keen on the individual constitution, aiming for better prevention and therapy and, therefore, referring to the patient's autonomy through: first, the use of biomarkers for stratification, testing whether a possible drug correlates with the genetic constitution of a patient or not and will only cause side effects ('customised drug design', 'targeted drug delivery'); second, general information about the genomic situation of a patient concerning their health, which can, for instance, be important for nutrition (nutri-genomics); third, assessing individual risks for certain diseases; fourth, individualised therapy and not a therapy of trial and error; and finally, individualised prosthesis – a fairly old idea that is, however, advancing with technology (Nordmann, 2006; Henke, 2011).

The Moving towards the Person in Hermann Schmitz's New Phenomenology

Schmitz's 'new phenomenology' finds its starting point in the observation that usually philosophical thought and life-experience do not communicate well. The tendency to consider personal experience as part of an inner world that is not worth discussing since it can offer nothing to our spheres of knowledge, is responsible for the *xenophobia* between philosophical thinking and personal living. Schmitz, therefore, stands against the dominant European intellectual culture (*Intellektualkultur*) that threw subjectivity out of the window to make more room for objectivity and rationalism. New phenomenology wants to bring these introjections of subjectivity back, stating the importance and factuality of subjectivity alongside objectivity (Schmitz, 2003). Due to his interest in the philosophical dimension of real-life challenges, Schmitz has also intervened in current ethical and medical-ethic debates (Düwell, 2007). Where science tries to come close to nature through experiments, phenomenology comes close to the nature of the person by careful and precise language that leaves behind the abstraction that could never quite capture people's feelings, or their behaviour (Schmitz, 2003).

Schmitz defines: corporeality absolutely requires the room; in the likes of pain or angst, everything is reduced to this and, for this moment, nothing else exists. Bodily impulse only has somewhat of a dependence on the room when, for instance, touching your skin leads to some pressure at a specific spot. Conditions of the soul do not require a room, which means that they are everywhere, such as in melancholia (*Schwermut*) where everything is befogged since there is no escape. Elsewhere Schmitz defines: corporeal is what is indivisible, expanded and local; and bodily is what is divisible, expanded and local. That which is without local determination belongs to the soul (*seelisch*). According to Schmitz, the following belong to the alphabet of corporeality: narrowness, wideness, direction, tension, swelling, intensity, rhythm, etc. (Schmitz, 1965).

Schmitz defines the corporeal as invisible and untouchable realities that afflict us as doubtlessly and intensely as pain, hunger, happiness, freshness, etc., that occur in the vicinity of our body but cannot be reduced to something somatic and, therefore, are called expanded and local (*absolute Örtlichkeit*) (Schmitz, 1965). This corporeality can only be felt by the first person's I, whereas the body can also be examined by a third party or by the self (Schmitz, 1992). Being corporal means you can be scared, as Schmitz puts it (1992). What follows from this view of human reality for ethics and medical ethics is that there is a true reality that makes us know that we are tangibly existing as a self, despite the fact that shame, for instance, an emotion that burns us and makes us aware of ourselves, is invisible and untouchable. Such everyday experiences teach us about the fallibility of the widespread reductionist opinion that claims that the real is what can be touched or measured. One's own feelings and emotions teach the opposite, and cannot be neglected as they last for space. Though corporeality is untouchable, this does not mean it is without needs. In fact, Schmitz emphasises the volume of corporeality asking for room, since the corps other than the body does not have skin that closes up (Schmitz, 1992).

Schmitz's idea of narrow and wide corporeality is equally important in order to understand his phenomenology and make it fruitful for unfolding personalised medicine. Both are the poles that mark the movement of corporeal experience: in angst and pain, one feels a narrow corporeality (*Enge*), and in lust, one feels a wide corporeality (*Schwellung*). Schmitz stresses the importance of narrowness because it keeps humans from living in the homogenous way plants do. The isolation and interruption of narrowness, that does not necessarily need to be caused by pain, leads to subjectivity and personality (Schmitz, 1992). In this area, Schmitz understands sickness as the experience of a foreign force to the person that narrows corporeality, and hence, casts light on the wide room in which the person acts (Schmitz, 1965). Though the reduction of wideness to narrowness (constriction) occurs regularly, for instance, in orgasm, in pain and sickness, an imbalance exists between wideness and narrowness, when it comes to pain and sorrow of severe illness, which depresses and reduces everything to the flesh. In the moments of panic that come with sickness and pain, complete loss of room-orientation occurs. Medicine, with its therapies, plays a vital part in re-establishing the balance between wideness and narrowness and is, therefore, important to the personal being of humans. Angst and pain narrow existence. Whoever fights against the 'fire' of pain and angst is an agent of the person (Schmitz, 1965). Medicine does this and, therefore, might be called an agent of the person.

Ethical Authority of both Material and Immaterial

According to Schmitz, feelings are not hopelessly private and so inward that they are of no actual importance (Löw, 2008; Slaby, 2014). Feelings are not nothing, but afflicting atmospheres that make us aware that we are ourselves (Schmitz, 1992): 'the mine-ness of one's being affectively involved remains and coincides with the contraction, which presents only this: itself in absolute identity without any further characterisation. In such cases, I speak of primitive present, in which the five elements here, now, being, this and I are fused' (Schmitz et al., 2011, p.249). It occurs within the intense experience of angst, pain and shame that makes humans lose their capacity of distance towards themselves and the situations they are in. Under such circumstances, the subject, as Schmitz puts it, falls down into what he above calls 'primitive present' (*primitive Gegenwart*), which is not meant negatively, but instead stresses the impossibility of escaping angst, pain and shame for the well-known ever-lasting moment (Schmitz et al., 2011, pp.75–6).

The effort medicine takes to cure patients appears to be personalised, since a successful therapy leads to the distance a person needs for being a person that is not bound to pain and angst (Schmitz, 2003; Schmitz et al., 2011). The ongoing debate about how personal personalised medicine is tends to overlook the natural connection of material and immaterial, such as the importance of physiology for a person's everyday cognitive ability.

However, it is not enough to work on the termination of suffering to be in accordance with a suffering person, although that is required and highly necessary as well as strictly personal, as explained before. Schmitz stressed the authority of sorrow, which is a well-known feeling of general grief within clinical practice. Sorrow is an atmosphere, and all atmospheres are mighty. They call for obedience, Schmitz stresses, and address both the sorrowful person and their surroundings. This tangible authority of feelings, however, leads to conflicts, since it is a popular fallacy that feelings are just private with no impression on others (Schmitz, 1992). Although they cannot be measured or made visible, their corporeality cannot be denied. Orientation on people implies the realisation of the authority of feelings that are felt within atmosphere they cause. In a clinical context, this means you should not class feelings such as angst, shame and sorrow as unimportant inner feelings, but as atmospheres that affect the whole scenery (Schmitz, 1992). It is an offence against the seriousness of suffering not to pay attention to a person and their feelings. To put it firmly, clinical practice as notorious personalised medicine can only treat patients within the belief of the seriousness of the circumstances. It is not required or even helpful to treat patients suffering from overwhelmingly deep regret, but it is a question of taking into account the whole atmosphere of the suffering of a person who needs silence, attention, help and, most of all, a cure.

There is no need for lots of money or special facilities to affirm corporeality of patients, but a certain habit. This habit might be summarised as respect, and this can be seen as the core issue of personalised medicine that is twofold and implies respect for both the somatic, molecular side of a person's sickness, and respect for the intense and atmospheric situation a patient goes through in corporeality (Schmitz, 2005).

Summary

Illness gains authority through the result of the element of suffering. On the basis of this authority, medicine follows the obligation to heal the source of a given illness. A number of developments being observed in the field of medicine allow for a medicine that is more and more personalised. The focus on the individual physiology and pathology has, so far, only concentrated on the somatic side, which is not reductionism but necessary. In order to do justice to the authority of suffering and its concrete shape, a more comprehensive appreciation of the place of suffering within a given illness is required. Medical ethics could help by taking advantage of the ever-growing importance of a personalised medicine that gives the complete physical dimensions of a given illness. With regard to the illness, it is not the tumour that suffers, but the actual person who is, by definition, corporeal (*leiblich*). The widely accepted dualistic view classifies the somatoform as score suffering. As opposed to this, there is the mental side, that concerns the individual and no one else. However, there is a third dimension: the corporeality; a dimension that is the particular focus of the philosopher Schmitz in his new phenomenology. Unlike the body, corporeality cannot be measured empirically, yet it is the actual place where emotions, such as shame, lust, fear and pain, are located; a place where a person is 'real'. To the patient, a respectful appreciation of their corporeality counts much more than the details of their diagnosis, the prognoses or their therapy regime. The authority of illness includes the relevance of 'emotions' and 'atmospheres' that have been strongly emphasised by Schmitz. The term 'personalised medicine' does not apply in a clinic that ignores the corporal needs for tranquillity, security, attention, best care and, above all, respect.

References

Bergdolt, K., 2011. Individualisierte Medizin. Historische und aktuelle Perspektive. In: V. Schumpelick and B. Vogel, eds, *Medizin nach Maß. Individualisierte Medizin – Wunsch und Wirklichkeit*. Freiburg i. Br.: Herder. pp.15–28.

Blume, A., 2010. Hermann Schmitz. In: H.R. Sepp and L. Embree, eds. *Handbook of phenomenological aesthetics*. London: Springer. pp.307–10.

Böhme, G., 1993. Fundamental concept of a new aesthetics. *Thesis Eleven*, 36, pp.113–26.

Durkheim, E., 1898. Der Individualismus und die Intellektuellen. In: H. Bertram, ed. 1986. *Gesellschaftlicher Zwang und moralische Autonomie*. Frankfurt a. M.: Suhrkamp. pp.54–70.

Durkheim, E., 2010. *Die elementaren Formen des religiösen Lebens*. Frankfurt a. M.: Verl. Der Weltreligionen [reprint].

Düwell, M., 2007. Zum moralischen Status des menschlichen Körpers – Eine Diskussion mit der 'Phänomenologie der Leiblichkeit'. In: J. Taupitz, ed. *Kommerzialisierung des menschlichen Körpers*. Heidelberg: Springer. pp.161–71.

Gadebusch-Bondio, M. and Michl, S., 2010. Individualisierte Medizin. Die neue Medizin und ihre Versprechen. *Deutsches Ärzteblatt*, 107, pp.934–6.

Gugutzer, R., 2013. Hermann Schmitz: Der Gefühlsraum. In: K. Senge and R. Schützeichel, eds. *Hauptwerke der Emotionssoziologie*. Wiesbaden: Springer. pp.304–10.

Haas, L., 2000. *Für kranke Menschen sorgen. Die Bedeutung der 'Cura' für ethisches Handeln im Gesundheitswesen*. Münster: Lit.

Habermas, J., 1981. *Theorie des kommunikativen Handelns, Volume 2: Zur Kritik der funktionalistischen Vernunft*. Frankfurt a. M.: Suhrkamp.

Henke, R., 2011. Individualisierte Medizin heute. In: V. Schumpelick and B. Vogel, eds. *Medizin nach Maß. Individualisierte Medizin – Wunsch und Wirklichkeit*. Freiburg i. Br.: Herder. pp.29–49.

Hyginus, 2007. *Fabulae*. Munich: dtv.

Joas, H., 2004. *Braucht der Mensch Religion? Über Erfahrungen der Selbsttranszendenz*. Freiburg i. Br.: Herder.

Joas, H., 2011. *Die Sakralität der Person. Eine neue Genealogie der Menschenrechte*. Berlin: Suhrkamp.

Kant, I., 1785. Grundlegung zur Metaphysik der Sitten. In: W. Weischedel, ed. 1982. *Werke, Volume VII*. Frankfurt a. M.: WBG. pp.11–102.

King, H.C., 1907. *Theology and the social consciousness: a study of the relations of the consciousness to theology*. 2nd edn. New York: Macmillan.

Kobusch, T., 1993. *Die Entdeckung der Person. Metaphysik der Freiheit und modernes Menschenbild*. Freiburg i. Br.: Herder.

Kreuzer, J., 2001. Der Begriff der Person in der Philosophie des Mittelalters. In: D. Sturma, ed. *Person. Philosophiegeschichte – Theoretische Philosophie – Praktische Philosophie*. Paderborn: Mentis. pp.59–78.

Langewitz, W., 2007. Beyond content analysis and non-verbal behavior – what about atmospheres? A phenomenological approach. *Patient Education and Counseling*, 53, pp.319–23.

Löw, M., 2008. The constitution of space: the structurisation of spaces through the simultaneity of effect and perception. *European Journal of Science and Theology*, 11, pp.25–49.

Mohr, G., 2001. Einleitung: Der Personbegriff in der Geschichte der Philosophie. In: D. Sturma, ed. *Person. Philosophiegeschichte – Theoretische Philosophie – Praktische Philosophie*. Paderborn: Mentis. pp.25–36.

Nordmann, A., 2006. Personalisierte Medizin? – Zum Versprechen der Nanomedizintechnik. *Hessisches Ärzteblatt*, 5, pp.331–3.

Quante, M., 2007. *Person*. Berlin: De Gruyter.

Schmitz, H., 1965. *System der Philosophie, Volume II/1: Der Leib*. Bonn: Bouvier.

Schmitz, H., 1992. *Leib und Gefühl. Materialien zu einer philosophischen Therapeutik.* 2nd edn. Paderborn: Junfermann.

Schmitz, H., 1994. Gefühle als Atmosphären und das affektive Betroffensein von ihnen. In: H. Fink-Eitel and G. Lohmann, eds. *Zur Philosophie der Gefühle.* 2nd edn. Frankfurt a. M.: Suhrkamp. pp.33–56.

Schmitz, H., 2003. *Was ist neue Phänomenologie?* Rostock: Koch.

Schmitz, H., 2005. *Die Person.* Bonn: Bouvier.

Schmitz, H., Müller, R.O. and Slaby, J., 2011. Emotions outside the box – the new phenomenology of feeling and corporeality. *Phenomenology and Cognitive Sciences,* 10, pp.241–59.

Seidler, E., 1993. *Geschichte der Medizin und der Krankenpflege.* 6th edn. Stuttgart: Kohlhammer.

Siep, L., 2001. Der Begriff der Person als Grundlage der biomedizinischen Ethik. Zwei Traditionslinien. In: D. Sturma, ed. *Person. Philosophiegeschichte – Theoretische Philosophie – Praktische Philosophie.* Paderborn: Mentis. pp.445–58.

Slaby, J., 2014. Emotions and the extended mind. In: C. von Scheve and M. Salmela, eds. *Collective emotions.* Oxford: Oxford University Press.

Spaemann, R., 1996. *Personen. Versuche über den Unterschied zwischen 'etwas' und 'jemand'.* Stuttgart: Klett-Cotta.

Sturma, D., 2001a. Person und Philosophie der Person. In: D. Sturma, ed. *Person. Philosophiegeschichte – Theoretische Philosophie – Praktische Philosophie.* Paderborn: Mentis. pp.11–22.

Sturma, D., 2001b. Person und Menschenrechte. In: D. Sturma, ed. *Person. Philosophiegeschichte – Theoretische Philosophie – Praktische Philosophie.* Paderborn: Mentis. pp.337–62.

Chapter 6

Towards Integration of 'Personalised' and 'Person-Centred' Medicine: The Concept of 'Integrative and Personalised Health Care'

Peter Heusser

The term 'personalised' or 'individualised medicine' is increasingly applied to designate the use of individual genetic and molecular markers for diagnostic, therapeutic and preventive purposes in medicine. Tremendous amounts of financial resources and research capacities are invested to improve risk prevention, diagnostic accuracy and treatment outcomes by developing more individually tailored biological problem solutions in medicine. However, this almost exclusively molecular and biological concept of 'personalisation' leads to a strong connotation – if not to a *de facto* identification – of 'person' with the molecular set-up of an individual's physical body. (For a more holistic discussion on the term 'person' see chapters 4 and 5, this volume.)

This is a pitfall which ought to be avoided. Evidence shows that patients do not identify themselves with their bodies and molecules alone, and that there is an increasing dissatisfaction among patients with the dominating one-sided physical and technical forms of medicine (Kaptchuk and Eisenberg, 1998; Handel, 2001). This is one of the reasons why many patients turn to complementary or alternative medicine (CAM), where they hope to find more holistic and more authentic patient-centred forms of care, including a better physician–patient relationship (Bishop et al., 2007).

For this reason, our research group wanted to find out what exactly patients who turn to CAM are missing in conventional medicine and what their own deeper understanding of person-centred or individualised care is. To this aim, we performed a systematic search for qualitative studies analysing patients' reasons for seeking CAM treatments, identified studies related to patients' reasons for seeking CAM using pre-defined quality of eligibility, and critically appraised the eligible studies. Finally, we conducted a meta-ethnographic study to translate key themes in patients' reasons for using CAM, and to identify, synthesise and interpret key concepts in patients' narratives associated with their concepts of individualised medicine. Out of 9,578 citations screened from 67 electronic databases, 30 publications could be included in the study. Key features of patients' concepts of individualised medicine that emerged were 'inner' or 'personal growth', 'holism', 'doctor–patient alliance', 'integrative care', 'self-activation' and 'wellbeing'. Thus, in contrast to the biologically and genetically oriented concept of 'individualised' or 'personalised' medicine of the medical and scientific community and the pharmaceutical industry, patients' conceptions of 'individualised medicine' are more humanistic in nature and reached beyond biology and molecules (Franzel et al., 2013). This finding concurs well with a representative study by the Swiss Academy of Medical Sciences published in 2002, in which the Swiss population was asked how medicine and health care ought to be constituted in the future. Sixty-nine per cent of the respondents wished for 'more humanism' in medicine, 58 per cent more complementary medicine, 27 per cent more family medicine, but only 21 per cent more 'high-tech' medicine. 'Holism' was one of the most important features desired in medicine (Leuenberger and Longchamp, 2002).

Based on this background, it is not surprising that the term 'personalised medicine' in the lay public does not match the biological meaning attributed to that term by the proponents of 'personalised medicine', but that it is automatically associated with a more holistic concept of 'person':

> For the public at large, the term 'personalised medicine' does not spark images of abstract science and technology. The image it creates is just the opposite: most people would conceive personalised medicine to be what's commonly called patient-centered or person-centered care – a more humane, empathetic approach to care focused on individuals and shaped by their needs and circumstances, rather than cell-level scientific manipulations. (Browman et al., 2011)

This shows that the words 'person' or 'individual' in the expression 'personalised or 'individualised' are instructive examples of what Hartzband and Groopman (2011) recently called the 'new language of medicine', namely the use of strong words that sound familiar and raise expectations and hope, but signify something else and lead to another direction. Indeed, according to the classical concepts of 'person' or 'individuality' in philosophical and medical anthropology, a human being or 'person' cannot be understood on the basis of molecular and biological variants alone, but as an individual in the wider context of its physical, biological, psychosocial and even spiritual dimensions (Kipke, 2001; Danzer, 2012).

In other words: the new, industrially promoted definition of 'personalisation' in medicine, with its confinement to the realms of biology and molecules, is unnatural and ahistorical, it contradicts the humanistic roots and goals of our culture and also the clearly articulated needs of patients. In this respect, 'personalised medicine' is one of the action fields of medicine – and a strongly growing one, too – that aggravates the process of 'dehumanisation in medicine' (Haque and Waytz, 2012) even more. Through ignoring the psychosocial, spiritual and contextual side of individuals and focusing on their molecular parts, 'personalised medicine' actually leads to a conceptual 'deindividuation' and 'mechanisation' of the concrete individual persons perceived, two of the main causes of dehumanisation in modern medicine, an increasingly discussed problem (Haque and Waytz, 2012; see Chapter 11, this volume). This indicates that the creation of a more humanistic health-care culture is at stake and that the focus of 'personalisation' on biology and molecules should be explicitly expanded to a more encompassing humanistic 'person-oriented' form of care.

It is such a form of patient- or person-centredness that was advocated in 2001 as a key quality of medical care in the Institute of Medicine's vision for a new health system in the twenty-first century. On the side of the physicians, this requires the development of personal qualities such as 'compassion, empathy, and responsiveness to the needs, values, and expressed preferences of the individual patient' (Institute of Medicine, Committee on Quality of Health Care in America, 2001).

This is not to say that the rationale and the goals of 'personalised medicine', as such, are not justified. They *are* justified, insofar as they can be based on realistic or already realised accomplishments. However, they should not be pursued in their biological isolation. Instead, they should be combined with the rationale and the goals of 'person-centred care' in the attempt to establish a more integrative form of individualisation in health care, including, of course, physical, but also psychosocial, environmental and existential issues. These factors constantly interplay with the biological processes. If they are left out of the picture, then 'personalisation' can even lead to 'depersonalisation', as was recently expressed by Horwitz et al. (2013):

> Personalised medicine is often described as genomic-based knowledge that 'promises the ability to approach each patient as the biological individual he or she is'. This is an appealing description, yet unless clinical, social, and environmental features that affect the outcomes of disease are also incorporated, the current approach may be carving a path to 'depersonalised' medicine, both in science and in its relevance to medical practice.

If, on the other hand, psychological and contextual factors in the sense of 'person-centredness' are included in the concept and practice of biological individualisation, this could possibly lead to more effective forms of health care than if the focus remained only on biology. In this respect, lessons can be learnt from the positive impact of individualised forms of psychosocial and existential patient management on the biological level of diabetes control. Several studies, for example, show that diabetes type-2 prevention can be realised successfully and economically if nutritional lifestyle changes among patients at risk can be achieved (Ausschuss für Bildung, Forschung und Technologiefolgenabschätzung (TAB) des Dt. Bundestags, 2009).

However, national campaigns with information and mentoring targeted at risk patients in Finland and Germany have also shown that the aim of motivating these patients can often not be reached, especially in men. For this reason, more 'personalised' forms of information with specific adaptations to gender, groups and risk levels are seen as a way out of this problem (Programme for the Prevention of Type 2 Diabetes in Finland, 2003–2010; Ausschuss für Bildung, Forschung und Technologiefolgenabschätzung (TAB) des Dt. Bundestags, 2009). Additionally, a person-specific exploration and an ensuing interventional modification of psychosocial and existential factors can effectively improve the motivation of individuals for and their adherence to lifestyle changes. It is known, for example, that psychosocial factors, such as emotional stress, can negatively influence glycemic control and self-management (Ogbera and Adeyemi-Doro, 2011). Conversely, a patient-centred communication and an individualised nutritional education can positively improve the competency of self-management, adherence and metabolic control (Lim et al., 2009; Croom et al., 2011). Furthermore, the spiritual practice of patients, social or group-based interventions, and an account of individual cultural factors in patient care can positively influence diabetes self-management and metabolic control (Deakin et al., 2005; Leeman et al., 2008; Casarez et al., 2010). Accordingly, the German government's Future report, 'Individualised medicine and health system' by the Ausschuss für Bildung, Forschung und Technologiefolgenabschätzung (TAB) des Dt. Bundestags (2009) explicitly emphasises the importance of including the psychological dimension, the questions of meaning, the biographical and existential dimensions, and the mobilisation of patients' resources in the context of individualised medicine.

Consequently, if 'personalised medicine' is to be pursued in accord with our cultural values and with the needs of patients treated as human people and not only as molecular individuals, the goals of 'personalised' and 'person-centred' medicine have to be united and harmonised in a more encompassing research and practice agenda of 'personalised medicine'. We have coined the term 'Integrative and Personalised Health Care' at Witten/Herdecke University to designate such an integrative form of individualised health care and research, and we have started to establish a common research focus of the different departments around this focal point (Heusser et al., 2012; Neugebauer and Heusser, 2014; Geraedts, 2014).

In this concept of 'Integrative and Personalised Health Care', the term *integrative* describes the meaningful integration of different medical disciplines and treatment options in a patient-centred health-care policy, based on a comprehensive perception of the patient, an intact practitioner–patient relationship, scientific evidence and inter-professional co-operation, much in the sense of the definition of the American Consortium of Academic Health Centers for Integrative Medicine: 'Integrative medicine is the practice of medicine that reaffirms the importance of the relationship between practitioner and patient, focuses on the whole person, is informed by evidence, and makes use of all appropriate therapeutic approaches, healthcare professionals and disciplines to achieve optimal health and healing' (Consortium of Academic Health Centers for Integrative Medicine, 2004).

The term *personalised medicine* (or *individualised medicine*) is used in a wider, more encompassing sense than usual. On the one hand, it corresponds to the well-known meaning designating the use of individual genetic and molecular markers for diagnostic, preventive and therapeutic purposes (Hempel, 2009). On the other hand, it is used in an explicitly extended humanistic sense, accounting for the individuals in the context of their biological, psychological, mental, social, economic, cultural and spiritual dimensions (Dörner et al., 1999).

The term *health care* encompasses systemic aspects of health care, including the necessary co-operation between different health professions, the different health-care areas where individualisation plays a role, such as the promotion and maintenance of health, prevention, diagnosis and treatment of disease, curative care, rehabilitation and palliative care, and also those systemic aspects where the aspects of individuality have to be integrated into the collective system, such as the functionality of health-care systems, economic and other societal resources, demographic change and education of health-care professionals (Geraedts, 2014). Presently, there are around 40 externally funded research projects related to 'integrative and personalised health care', ranging from basic and clinical research to health systems research and medical education, comprising medicine, dentistry and nursing, and including complementary medicine (Heusser et al., 2012; Neugebauer and Heusser, 2014).

References

Ausschuss für Bildung, Forschung und Technologiefolgenabschätzung (TAB) des Dt. Bundestags. 2009. *Zukunftsreport 'Individualisierte Medizin und Gesundheitssystem' [Future report 'Individualised medicine and health system']*. 17 February 2009, Drucksache 16/12000.

Bishop, F.L., Yardley, L. and Lewith, G.T., 2007. A systematic review of beliefs involved in the use of complementary and alternative medicine. *Journal of Health Psychology*, 12, p.251.

Browman, G., Hébert, P.C. and Coutts, J., 2011. Personalized medicine: a windfall for science, but what about patients? *Canadian Medical Association Journal*, 183(18), p.1277.

Casarez, R.L., Engebretson, J.C. and Ostwald, S.K., 2010. Spiritual practices in self-management of diabetes in African Americans. *Holistic Nursing Practice*, 2(4), pp.227–37.

Consortium of Academic Health Centers for Integrative Medicine 2004. Available at: www.imconsortium.org [Accessed 12 August 2013].

Croom, A., Wiebe, D.J., Berg, C.A., Lindsay, R., Donaldson, D., Foster, C., Murray, M. and Swinyard, M.T., 2011. Adolescent and parent perceptions of patient-centered communication while managing type 1 diabetes. *Journal of Pediatric Psychology*, 36(2), pp.206–15.

Danzer, G., 2012. *Personale Medizin [Personal medicine]*. Bern: Hans Huber.

Deakin, T., McShane, C.E., Cade, J.E. and Williams, R.D., 2005. Group based training for self-management strategies in people with type 2 diabetes mellitus. *The Cochrane Database of Systematic Reviews*, 18(2), p.CD003417.

Dörner, G., Hüllemann, K.D., Tembrock, G., Wessel, K.F. and Zänker, K.S., eds, 1999. *Menschenbilder in der Medizin, Medizin in den Menschenbildern [Concepts of the human being in medicine, medicine in concepts of the human being]*, Berliner Studien zur Wissenschaftsphilosophie & Humanontogenetik, Band 16. Bielefeld: Kleine Verlag.

Franzel, B., Schwiegershausen, M., Heusser, P. and Berger B., 2013. Individualized medicine from the perspectives of patients using complementary therapies: a meta-ethnography approach. *BMC Complementary and Alternative Medicine*, 13(1), p.124.

Geraedts, M., 2014. Integrative und personenzentrierte Gesundheitsversorgung aus der Perspektive des Gesundheitssystems [Integrative and Person-centred Health Care from a Health System Perspective]. *Gesundheitswesen*, 76, pp.705–6.

Handel, D.L., 2001. Complementary therapies for cancer patients. What works, what doesn't, and how to know the difference. *Texas Medicine*, 97, pp.68–72.

Haque, O.S. and Waytz, A., 2012. Dehumanization in medicine: causes, solutions, and function. *Perspectives on Psychological Science*, 7(2), pp.176–86.

Hartzband, P. and Groopman, J., 2011. The new language of medicine. *New England Journal of Medicine*, 365(15), pp.1372–3.

Hempel, U., 2009. Personalisierte Medizin I: Keine Heilkunst mehr, sondern rationale, molekulare Wissenschaft [Personalised medicine I: no longer an art of healing, but rational, molecular science]. *Deutsches Ärzteblatt*, 106(42), p.A–2068.

Heusser, P., Neugebauer, E., Berger, B. and Hahn E., 2012. Integrative und personalisierte Gesundheitsversorgung – Forderungen für ein zeitgemäßes Gesundheitssystem [Integrative and personalised health care – requirements for a timely health-care system]. *Gesundheitswesen*, 75(3), pp.151–4.

Horwitz, R.I., Cullen, M.R. and Christian, J.B., 2013. (De)personalized medicine. *Science*, 339, pp.1155–6.

Institute of Medicine, Committee on Quality of Health Care in America, 2001. *Crossing the quality chasm: a new health system for the 21st century.* Washington, DC: National Academy Press.

Kaptchuk, T.J. and Eisenberg, D.M., 1998. The persuasive appeal of alternative medicine. *Annals of Internal Medicine*, 129, pp.1061–5.

Kipke, R., 2001. *Mensch und Person [Man and person].* Berlin: Logos Verlag.

Leeman, J., Skelly, A.H., Burns, D., Carlson, J. and Soward, A., 2008. Tailoring a diabetes self-care intervention for use with older, rural African American women. *The Diabetes Educator*, 34(2), pp.310–17.

Leuenberger, P. and Longchamp, C., 2002. Was erwartet die Bevölkerung von der Medizin? Ergebnisse einer Umfrage des GfS-Forschungsinstitutes, Politik und Staat, Bern, im Auftrag der SAMW [What does the population expect from medicine? Results of a survey of the GfS-Research Institute, Politics and State, Bern, commissioned by the Swiss Academy of Medical Sciences]. In: W. Stauffacher and J. Bircher, eds. *Zukunft der Medizin Schweiz.* Basel: Schweizerischer Ärzteverlag. pp.181–235.

Lim, H.M., Park, J.E., Choi, X.J., Huh, K.B. and Kim, W.Y., 2009. Individualized diabetes nutrition education improves compliance with diet prescription. *Nutrition Research and Practice*, 3(4), pp.315–22.

Neugebauer, E. and Heusser, P., 2014. Personalisierte oder Personenzentrierte Medizin? Ihre Synthese in einer Integrativen und Personalisierten Medizin [Personalized or Person-centred Medicine? Their Synthesis in an Integrative and Personalized Health Care]. *Gesundheitswesen*, 76, pp.694–5.

Ogbera, A. and Adeyemi-Doro, A., 2011. Emotional distress is associated with poor self-care in type 2 diabetes mellitus. *Journal of Diabetes*, 3(4), pp.348–52.

Programme for the Prevention of Type 2 Diabetes in Finland 2003–2010. Available at: www.diabetes.fi/files/1108/Programme_for_the_Prevention_of_Type_2_Diabetes_in_Finland_2003–2010.pdf [Accessed 3 October 2013].

PART II
Personalised Medicine in Clinical and Practical Research

Chapter 7

Ethical Considerations for Developing a Best-Practice Guideline for Next Generation Sequencing in Oncology[1]

Eva C. Winkler, Klaus Tanner, Hanno Glimm and Christof von Kalle[2]

A key goal in current cancer research is decoding the molecular mechanisms of tumour genesis, including how the tumour genome is affected by therapy. There are two main developments contributing to the dynamic in this field of research. First, new molecular techniques, such as high-throughput sequencing, make whole-genome analysis possible within increasingly shorter timeframes. Whereas the sequencing of the first human genome took seven years, today it can be done in just a few days, and it is expected that such sequencing will soon play a role in everyday clinical practice.

Second, systematic efforts by internationally co-operating consortia are creating the infrastructure for sharing the data of a larger proportion of samples of certain tumour entities. This is necessary in order to search for driving mutations of different tumour entities in a systematic way and compare them with the constitutional genome of healthy cells. The International Cancer Genome Consortium (ICGC), for example, co-ordinates such genetic tumour mapping. It is a stated goal of the consortium to make all data available to all researchers as quickly as possible and with as few restrictions as possible to speed up the research progress (ICGC, 2012). At the National Center for Tumor Diseases (NCT) in Heidelberg results of the tumour genome analysis of all consenting patients' cancer tissue are collected in a biobank and research

1 This chapter was originally published in German in a slightly modified form, under the title 'Personalisierte Medizin und Informed Consent: Klinische und ethische Erwägungen im Rahmen der Entwicklung einer Best Practice Leitlinie für die biobankbasierte Ganzgenomforschung in der Onkologie' in: *Ethik in der Medizin* 2013, 25, 195–203. With kind permission of Springer Science+Business Media.

2 This work was one of the results of a Faculty Fellowship of the Marsilius-Kolleg Heidelberg.

database, and these results can be correlated with patients' clinical data. In order to identify the changes that might explain tumour growth, the whole genome of healthy cells from the same patient is sequenced and compared with the tumour genome. Clinical and molecular data are saved in de-identified (pseudonymised) form, allowing re-identification of patients and re-contacting in the event that a suitable treatment concept should emerge. This method of handling the data also permits the correlation of genetic variations with the clinical course of the disease.

Ethical and Legal Considerations of Biobank-Based Genome Research

High-resolution genomics is associated not only with great hopes for medical and pharmaceutical research, but also with concerns about discrimination on grounds of genetics or misuse of data. A Nondiscrimination Act was passed in the United States in 2008 to provide patients with protection from misuse of genetic data by the insurance industry and employers (Institute NHGR, 2008). Intensive international debate is ongoing as to how the ethical and legal frameworks and the infrastructure of the intersection between clinical practice and Genomic (-OMIC) research should be designed to achieve an acceptable balance between protection of the patient's interests and those of the research community (Treloar et al., 2007; Metcalfe et al., 2009; Streicher et al., 2011; Zika et al., 2011). There is a particular sensitivity in Germany in light of the background of abuse of power by physician scientists during the Nazi era. Patient autonomy lies at the centre of the ethical and legal discussion. This is normatively protected through the general right of personality as established in Art. 2, Sec. 2, Sentence 1 of the German Constitution (Grundgesetz, GG). This is also the basis on which the right to self-determination regarding personal data was developed in law. It is also a central component of the German Genetic Diagnostics Act (Gendiagnostikgesetz), which applies to diagnostics in the clinical context, but not, however, in the research context (Hoeyer et al., 2005).

According to the medical research principles of the World Medical Association, a consent to a research project is only legally valid and ethically justifiable if the participant is capable of giving informed consent and has been informed of the aims, methods, benefits and risks of the study, has understood this information and has then freely given consent (WMA Declaration of Helsinki, 1964). Research and clinical sequencing examining the whole genome is challenging the conventional concept of informed consent and raises ethical and practical questions: how should incidental findings arising from research studies be communicated? Is it permissible to depart from the principle of genetic counselling, in which comprehensive and specific information must be provided before the genetic testing takes place? How might it be possible to counsel patients in advance with regard to the many potentially disease-relevant findings? How can the patient's right not to know be respected? These normative questions are being addressed in Heidelberg by the EURAT Project 'Ethical and Legal Aspects of Whole Human Genome Sequencing' (EURAT, 2013). This project brings together scientists from normative and scientific disciplines of the University of Heidelberg, the NCT, the University Hospital, the German Cancer Research Center, the European Molecular Biology Laboratory, the Max Planck Institute for Comparative Public Law and International Law, and the Center for Health Economics Research at Leibniz University, Hannover. The aim of the project is to work on possible responses to the ethical and legal question. One result of this work has been a position statement with the quality of a best-practice guideline, which has been adopted by the senate of the University and the German Cancer Research Center.

This chapter sets out to give an overview of the ethical and clinical questions that are relevant for the process of informing participants and securing consent in biobank-based genomics research. Furthermore, it examines the question pertaining to the organisational ethics of how to guarantee responsible handling of genetic data in biobanks, taking into account the numerous professions and institutions involved. Both of these problem areas – the normative/practical and the organisational/ethical – are examined below, and possible approaches to solutions are offered.

Ethical and Practical Requirements of the Informed Consent Process

As a general principle, the classical concept of informed consent as described above is not directly applicable to biomaterial banks, since such repositories are designed to facilitate procedures and infrastructure for an unspecified number of future research projects and, therefore, study-specific information on the purpose, significance and scope of future projects cannot be provided at the point of acquiring consent in the narrow sense.

The relevant issues applicable to the use of whole-genome sequencing in cancer research are discussed below and are also reflected in a Code of Conduct in the second part of the chapter.

Data Protection and Protection of Privacy

The human genome is inherently self-identifying. Therefore, conventional data protection measures of de-identification (pseudonymisation) and anonymisation become invalid as soon as a patient's name is made available in connection with just one sequence of their genome and this can be compared against a second, anonymised, genetic database. A working group from Boston recently showed that it is technically possible to discover the identity of individual participants in public genome sequencing projects through comparison with data freely available on the Internet (Gymrek et al., 2013). While re-identification needs quite an effort and someone who does this purposely, the patient must be informed about this issue. Data protection is, therefore, of great significance concerning the whole processing chain. Information provided to patients should include: measures for anonymisation or pseudonymisation of data, conditions for potential sharing of samples and data, particularly internationally, and the data protection standards applicable to potential international co-operation partners, forms of publication of sequencing results, protocols for handling samples and data following withdrawal of consent, as well as potential commercial uses of the results of research. Currently, evidence of data abuse or discrimination arising from biobank data or by insurers is rather thin (Barlow-Stewart et al., 2008). Nevertheless, the potential for misuse may increase in line with the increasing scale of genomic data shared globally, depending on the ease of access to whole-genome datasets.

Handling and Communication of Incidental Findings to the Patient

Incidental findings are findings that were not sought in the original diagnostic or research question. They also arise increasingly in the context of modern imaging techniques (Berland, 2011). What is novel in whole-genome sequencing is that it is certain that findings beyond the primary intended scientific or diagnostic question will be made. Instead of incidental findings, it is, therefore, more appropriate to refer to additional findings. These are findings situated outside the original diagnostic or research context, for example, mutations in healthy cells of the patient (germline mutations). Additional findings may be of importance for future screening or treatment measures, so that a duty to communicate relevant findings to the patient may apply legally. Even where there are no treatment options, the findings may at least be of considerable relevance for life planning. To date, no standard exists setting out which findings should be communicated to the patient and by which criteria (Wolf et al., 2012). Whether to receive any such findings, and if so, which ones, should be discussed with the patient in the initial counselling about participating in clinical or research genome sequencing. Because of the wide range of findings with vastly varying penetrance and relevance for the patient and their relatives, advance information cannot be provided in detail, but only in the form of examples from specific disease categories. In the counselling process, the patient should have the opportunity to fundamentally consent to or decline the communication of additional findings. The EURAT project is pursuing a tiered approach. This distinguishes between the communication of findings of direct relevance for treatment or screening, and those which might affect the individual's life plans.

Patients' Understanding of the Counselling Process

There have been few studies to date examining the study participants' need for information. These show that patients and donors are frequently altruistically motivated to donate their tissue samples, have limited understanding of genetic research, and only around half of the participants wish to be informed about findings with therapeutic relevance. Ideally, the information should be comprehensible, and the facts and circumstances should be presented in a manner fitting the patient's need for information. Nevertheless, we know from the information process for clinical studies with much less complex content that many participants doubt that they have understood all relevant aspects of the study (Raich et al., 2001). Studies show very clearly that written information material is too complicated, too long and, overall, insufficiently oriented towards patients' needs (Grossman et al., 1994). Furthermore, difficulties in comprehension are frequently a consequence of limited reading ability and a level of health literacy that excludes comprehension of genetics and cell-level processes (Wallmann, 2012). The concrete information requirements of patients for a decision regarding tissue donation for whole-genome sequencing have not yet been researched. One EURAT subproject is, therefore, developing and validating a procedure to support this decision-making process (Brown et al., 2011). Looking at current practice, an analysis of the contents of consent documents for sequencing projects shows that, for example, the critical issue of feedback of clinically relevant findings is rarely addressed in the informed consent process. Overall there is great variation across patient information and consent documentation and, to date, there is no discernible trend towards a consistent standard (Allen and Foulkes, 2011; Hirschberg et al., 2013, see also Chapter 8, this volume). A survey of 126 biobanks in 23 countries found that the requirements for donor consent and data protection varied considerably (Zika et al., 2011). The EURAT project, therefore, has developed various models of patient information and consent materials which will cover various research fields in the form of framework protocols (e.g. cancer research, human genetic research), but will not specify concrete study projects within the framework protocol (see position statement).

A 'Code of Conduct' as an Organisational-Ethics Response to a Field of Action in which Ethical and Legal Standards are yet to be Determined

The first regulatory proposals for biobanks in Germany were published by the National Ethics Council in 2004, and a concept for legal regulation of human biobanks was added in 2010 (TMF Arbeitsgruppe Biomaterialbanken, 2014). Debate is ongoing, however, as to whether legal regulation is necessary or whether, in fact, donor protection cannot also be achieved safely and more efficiently through non-statutory self-regulation by the biobanks (DFG, 2011; TMF Arbeitsgruppe Biomaterialbanken, 2014). In the United States, there have also been proposals for regulation to introduce structures and criteria for the supervision and governance of biobanks (Issues PCftSoB, 2012; Wolf et al., 2012). Such regulation would also include establishing procedures to guarantee the analysis, validation and feedback of findings, as well as data protection measures. The National Human Genome Research Institute and research consortia, such as the ICGC, have adopted recommendations on the consent process and are applying these within their own work programmes (ICGC, 2012; Institute NHGR, 2014).

A research institution that wishes to shape the framework conditions for biobank-based whole-genome sequencing must be concerned not only with a well-founded response to the new ethical and legal considerations arising. Rather, institutions are also faced with the challenge of how they can promote responsible handling of ethically sensitive topics within their spheres of competence. For this reason, the NCT decided to formulate a guideline for dealing with ethically controversial questions in biobank-based genome research as a code of conduct for medical and non-medical staff.

Effective codices operate on two levels: the content level and the ideational. On the content level, they formulate the core desired behaviours in ethically relevant situations and clearly delimit undesired behaviours. On the ideational level, they formulate how those addressed by the code wish to view themselves as a profession. This not only defines an ideal conception of professional behaviour for the individual, but is also significant from an organisational ethics viewpoint. The code is a symbol that this organisation takes the topics that are dealt with in the code seriously. A consistent guideline for all those who work with genetic data within the NCT is intended to foster responsible behaviour along the whole chain of activity. From the patient information process to data analysis, this chain includes a wide range of institutions and professions: physicians, study nurses, medical-technical assistants, molecular biologists, geneticists and bioinformatics specialists. The goal, therefore, is also to bring together the varied professional groups, some of which have no developed or articulated codes of professional ethics, with a view to a common professional standard. In this very dynamic field of activity, the NCT code of conduct is not conceived as a static document, but is to be updated whenever new aspects of ethical and legal considerations emerge from practice and prove relevant to the responsible handling of genetic data.

Excerpt of the Code of Conduct for the handling of genetic information in the context of biobank-based whole-genome sequencing:

Code of Conduct of the Personalised Oncology Programme – National Center for Tumor Diseases, Germany

In order to set the stage of how we approach this field of activity, the NCT agrees on a consensus in the form of a code of conduct: The code of conduct will be updated constantly according to new insights from genomic research and bioinformatics, as well as from ethical and legal discussions and feedback from the clinical encounter. An accompanying research project yields at optimising a patient-centred information procedure and analyses ethically challenging situations. This code of conduct applies to all employees who contribute to the programme 'personalised oncology' and should determine our attitude towards our patients.

The NCT Personalized Oncology Programme aims at … .
[…]
In doing so, the NCT takes the following points seriously.

The informed consent process will be tailored to the needs of our patients.
The informed consent process should respect patient autonomy and empower patients to represent their interests. Within an accompanying research project, we will investigate the information needs of our patients with a focus on the return of potentially actionable information. The results should help to improve the informed consent process in daily clinical routine.

We will offer to re-contact patients for participation in clinical trials and for reporting oncologically relevant findings.
We ask patients whether they want to be re-contacted if we have a clinical trial to offer. In accordance with the preferences patients stated during the informed consent process, we will also contact them for validated cancer-related findings which might become relevant for prevention or therapy. In the long-term, all datasets should be systematically screened for tumour mutations that can be therapeutically targeted.

We do not search for non cancer-related mutations in patients' healthy cells (germline mutations).
Since the question of how to handle genetic germline information is ethically and legally contested, we will use germline analysis only as a means for subtraction and for checking for known tumour-related mutations according to the actual state of science. Thereby, we reduce the likelihood of incidental or additional findings in germline cells.

continued …

We consult with the Returnable Results Committee if a result leaves the diagnostic context of the study.

Genetic data that might become relevant for the patient or their family is sensitive information and the terms of returning potentially relevant information are under dispute. We have, therefore, set up a governance structure that represents clinicians, geneticists, researchers, bioinformaticians, ethicists and patient representatives. Depending on the kind and frequency of additional findings in the pilot phase, the 'Returnable Results Committee' will meet on a regular basis and might generate a positive roster of returnable results from the results compiled.

In a case where the return is deemed appropriate, we will consult with our genetic consultation service about how to best approach the patient with the information. This committee will start working with the approval of the institutional review board – until then, the practice of returning results as recommended by the IRB is to be followed.

The germline row data will be pseudonymised and stored disconnected from networks that are accessible via Internet.

All data will be pseudonymised in order to enable the re-contacting of patients. After substraction, the germline data will be archived on storage media that are separated from the Internet and will be physically secured. Until further notice, we are not building a cohesive germline databank. Research projects that use the biobank need to be approved by the institution's Review Committee. With this governance structure, we want to make sure that the patient's interest will be represented even though the 'informed consent' was given before details of concrete research projects emerged.

Conclusion

Biobank-based genomic research and data-sharing generates a specific set of ethical challenges. They mainly pertain to data protection due to the risk of re-identification and the return of results. These questions not only need to be addressed in the informed consent process, but also along the entire chain of data production, analysis and publication. One possibility for how an institution or a research consortium can be responsive to the ethical challenges is a code of conduct that defines appropriate handling of genomic information. This code constitutes an important element of a best-practice guideline complemented by envisioned standards of an ethically and legally sound informed consent process that is also oriented towards the needs of the individual patient.

References

Allen, C. and Foulkes, W.D., 2011. Qualitative thematic analysis of consent forms used in cancer genome sequencing. *BMC Medical Ethics*, 12, p.14.

Barlow-Stewart, K., Taylor, S., Treloar, S., Stranger, M. and Otlowski, M., 2008. Verification of consumers' experiences and perceptions of genetic discrimination and its impact on utilisation of genetic testing. *Psycho-oncology*, 17, pp.S161–2.

Berland, L.L., 2011. The American College of Radiology strategy for managing incidental findings on abdominal computed tomography. *Radiologic Clinics of North America*, 49(2), pp.237–43.

Brown, R.F., Shuk, E., Butow, P., Edgerson, S., Tattersall, M.H. and Ostroff, J.S., 2011. Identifying patient information needs about cancer clinical trials using a Question Prompt List. *Patient Education and Counseling*, 84(1), pp.69–77.

DFG, 2011. *Die Stellungnahme der DFG-Senatskommissionen.* [online] Available at: http://www.dfg.de/service/presse/pressemitteilungen/2011/presse mitteilung_nr_12/ [Accessed 15 April 2014].

EURAT, 2013. *Ethical and legal aspects of whole genome sequencing.* [online] Avaliable at: http://www.uni-heidelberg.de/totalsequenzierung/english.html [Accessed 15 April 2014].

Grossman, S.A., Piantadosi, S. and Covahey, C., 1994. Are informed consent forms that describe clinical oncology research protocols readable by most patients and their families? *Journal of Clinical Oncology*, 12(10), pp.2211–15.

Gymrek, M., McGuire, A.L., Golan, D., Halperin, E. and Erlich, Y., 2013. Identifying personal genomes by surname inference. *Science*, 339(6117), pp.321–4.

Hirschberg, I., Knuppel, H. and Strech, D., 2013. Practice variation across consent templates for biobank research. A survey of German biobanks. *Frontiers in Genetics*, 4, p.240.

Hoeyer, K., Olofsson, B.O., Mjorndal, T. and Lynoe, N., 2005. The ethics of research using biobanks: reason to question the importance attributed to informed consent. *Archives of Internal Medicine*, 165(1), pp.97–100.

ICGC, 2012. *Goals, structure, policies and guidelines.* [online] Available at: http://www.icgc.org/icgc/goals-structure-policies-guidelines [Accessed 15 April 2014].

Institute NHGR, 2008. *Genetic Information Nondiscrimination Act (GINA).* [online] Available at: http://www.genome.gov/24519851 [Accessed 15 April 2014].

Institute NHGR, 2014. *Policy, legal and ethical issues in genetic research.* [online] Available at: http://www.genome.gov/Issues/ [Accessed 15 April 2014].

Issues PCftSoB, 2012. *Privacy and progress in whole genome sequencing.* [online] Available at: http://bioethics.gov/cms/node/764 [Accessed 15 April 2014].

Metcalfe, A., Werrett, J., Burgess, L., Chapman, C. and Clifford, C., 2009. Cancer genetic predisposition: information needs of patients irrespective of risk level. *Familial Cancer*, 8(4), pp.403–12.

Raich, P.C., Plomer, K.D. and Coyne, C.A., 2001. Literacy, comprehension, and informed consent in clinical research. *Cancer Investigation*, 19(4), pp.437–45.

Streicher, S.A., Sanderson, S.C., Jabs, E.W., Diefenbach, M., Smirnoff, M., Peter, I., Horowitz, C.R., Brenner, B. and Richardson, L.D., 2011. Reasons for participating and genetic information needs among racially and ethnically diverse biobank participants: a focus group study. *Journal of Community Genetics*, 2(3), pp.153–63.

TMF Arbeitsgruppe Biomaterialbanken (AG BMB), 2014. *Infrastruktur und Rahmenbedingungen für Biobanken [Infrastructure and framework for biobanks].* [online] Available at: http://tmf-ev.de/Arbeitsgruppen_Foren/AGBMB. aspx [Accessed 15 April 2014].

Treloar, S.A., Morley, K.I., Taylor, S.D. and Hall, W.D., 2007. Why do they do it? A pilot study towards understanding participant motivation and experience in a large genetic epidemiological study of endometriosis. *Community Genetics*, 10(2), pp.61–71.

Wallmann, B., 2012. Gesundheitskompetenz – Aufbauen auf einem starken Fundament [Health literacy – building on a strong foundation]. *Prävention und Gesundheitsförderung*, 7(1), p.3.

WMA Declaration of Helsinki – Ethical Principles for Medical Research Involving Human Subjects, 1964. [online] Available at: http://www.wma. net/en/30publications/10policies/b3/ [Accessed 15 April 2014].

Wolf, S., Crock, B., Van Ness, B., Lawrenz, F., Kahn, J., Beskow, L., Cho, M., Christman, M., Green, R., Hall, R., Illes, J., Keane, M., Knoppers, B., Koenig, B., Kohane, I., Leroy, B., Maschke, K., McGeveran, W., Ossorio, P., Parker, L., Petersen, G., Richardson, H., Scott, J., Terry, S., Wilfond, B. and Wolf, W., 2012. Managing incidental findings and research results in genomic research involving biobanks and archived data sets. *Genetics in Medicine*, 14(4), pp.361–84.

Zika, E., Paci, D., Braun, A., Rijkers-Defrasne, S., Deschenes, M., Fortier, I., Laage-Hellman, J., Scerri, C.A. and Ibarreta, D., 2011. A European survey on biobanks: trends and issues. *Public Health Genomics*, 14(2), pp.96–103.

Chapter 8

Practice Variation across Consent Templates for Biobank Research: A Survey of German Biobanks[1]

Irene Hirschberg, Hannes Kahrass and Daniel Strech

Introduction

Biobanks are collections of human biological samples and related health and personal information. A high quality biobank that organises samples for use by biomedical researchers is seen as an important resource for health research, including basic research, questions in personalised or stratified medicine (genetic and other biomarkers) and research in widespread diseases (Asslaber and Zatloukal, 2007; Zika et al., 2010).

The development of large-scale population-based as well as disease-specific biobanks also implies several new ethical, legal and social challenges. These comprise, for example, issues around the role of ethics committees, data protection, dealing with incidental findings, public involvement measures, and particularly regarding the need for new or at least modified models of informed consent of the donors (Budimir et al., 2011; Gottweis and Kaye, 2012). As acquired for diagnostic and therapeutic procedures in clinical as well as in research settings, informed, voluntary and valid consent is a precondition for the collection of samples and clinical data of donors in a biobank. It also tends to protect donors' rights and autonomy and to maintain public trust in biobank research. Crucial points include the scope and content of consent forms, for example, how do consent forms address potential future research projects that might involve the donated biomaterials (broad/general versus narrow/specific consent) (Cambon-Thomsen et al., 2007; Greely, 2007; Hansson, 2009; OECD, 2009; Budimir et al., 2011; German Ethics Council, 2010). Additionally, biobank research consent procedures and documentation involve different or

---

1   This chapter is a slightly revised version of the following article published in *Frontier Genetics*: Hirschberg, I., Knüppel, H., Strech, D. 2013: Practice variation across consent templates for biobank research. A survey of German biobanks. *Front. Genet.* 4:240. doi: 10.3389/fgene.2013.00240.

additional aspects compared with clinical research, for example, concerning data protection and data sharing with other researchers (Hoeyer et al., 2005; Beskow et al., 2010; McGuire and Beskow, 2010; Pawlikowski et al., 2011). Besides, the harmonisation of consent templates, at least of the most important criteria, is essential for future cooperation and networking at the national and international level.[2]

Though information and consent documents do certainly not substitute the discussion between clinician/researcher and patient/participant, they are an important component within the informed consent procedure and its documentation, as well as for legal aspects. Regarding quality and performance of consent forms in clinical or research contexts, several empirical studies demonstrated that consent forms are often not adequate in content, comprehensibility or practicability and do not meet participants' needs. Improvements are necessary within consent procedure and documents to support an adequately well-balanced and evidence-based decision-making process by participants (Jefford and Moore, 2008; Padhy et al., 2011; Brehaut et al., 2012; Mandava et al., 2012).

Several ethical guidelines define the required criteria for consent in clinical research (see, for example, Council for International Organizations of Medical Sciences (CIOMS), 2002; World Medical Association (WMA), 2013). Some guidelines also explicitly mention required criteria for consent in biobank research (see, for example, OECD, 2009). Nevertheless, there is no specific guideline for biobank research and consent procedures that can be employed as a tool for the assessment of consent forms' content in clinical or biobank research. Furthermore, we currently lack a broadly accepted 'best practice' model for consent forms in biobank research (Gottweis and Kaye, 2012).

Also in Germany, the number and importance of biobank facilities and projects with similar requirements is increasing, for example, in population-wide studies such as KORA and popgen, and the National Biobank Initiative ('Nationale Biomaterialbanken Initiative') funded by the German Federal Ministry of Education and Research (Bundesministerium für Bildung und Forschung, BMBF).

Existing studies that describe different biobanks and their governance strategies also indicate challenges in consent procedures (Hirtzlin et al., 2003; Zika et al., 2010; Gottweis and Kaye, 2012). Some research groups propose a unified consent model or possible content for a consent form in biobank research (Porteri and Borry, 2008; Salvaterra et al., 2008) or for whole-genome sequencing studies in the clinical context (Ayuso et al., 2013). Besides, there are studies comparing participant information and consent forms in genetic

---

2   For a discussion of similar topics from another perspective see Chapter 7, this volume.

research (Mascalzoni et al., 2010) or in clinical trials (Hüppe et al., 2014). But so far, no study has assessed and compared the content of consent forms for biobank research. The objective of this study was to perform a survey and content analysis of currently used consent forms in German biobanks.

Methods

To improve the comprehensiveness, reliability, validity and objectivity of our assessment of biobank specific consent forms, we first systematically developed an assessment matrix of potentially relevant issues that might be addressed in consent documents for biobank research. We then applied this assessment matrix to a sample of consent forms from German biobanks.

Development of the Assessment Matrix

To identify issues that might be addressed in consent documents for biobank research, we referred to frequently cited policies, guidelines and regulations dealing with general recommendations for consent procedures in biomedical research (mainly clinical studies) and/or biobank research. More specifically, we used nine prominent guidelines for biomedicine (Council of Europe, 1997), biomedical research with humans in general (European Parliament and the Council of the European Union, 2001; European Medicines Agency (EMEA), 2002; Council for International Organizations of Medical Sciences (CIOMS), 2002; Council of Europe, 2005; World Medical Association (WMA), 2013; US Department of Health and Human Services, 2009), and biobank or biomaterial research in particular (Council of Europe, 2006; OECD, 2009). For the national (German) context, we referred to a 'commented checklist' of issues in patient information and consent for clinical studies with an annex for biobank research (Harnischmacher et al., 2006). The set of selected guidelines is a purposive sample. Most of the chosen guidelines are for instance indicated as important legal and ethical frameworks in other sources such as the *Oxford Textbook of Clinical Research Ethics* (Capron, 2008; Emanuel et al., 2008). We have discussed the selection of guidelines and the resulting construct validity of the matrix of consent issues internally and with experts from the fields of law and biobank research.

In all 10 documents, one author (IH) searched for text passages that explicitly or implicitly mentioned issues of potential relevance to the content of consent forms in biomedical research in general and applicable to biobank research. Examples mentioned as necessary information for consent included 'general procedures and safeguards used to protect privacy and confidentiality', the 'policy with respect to benefit sharing' and 'information on the human biological material and data to be collected, their intended uses, storage, transfer and their disposal technique' (OECD, 2009). An example of a relevant but implicitly mentioned issue dealt with the removal of biological materials after death: 'Biological materials should not be removed from the body of a deceased person for research activities without appropriate consent or authorisation' (Council of Europe, 2006). Other issues were mentioned only in relation to the research protocol, such as 'incentives for subjects' (World Medical Association (WMA), 2013), or came under the discussion of policy, but indicated as relevant to participants: 'The HBGRD's[3] policy should also address the situation where participants become legally incapacitated or die. It is essential that the HBGRD provide information on their policy to the participant or the appropriate substitute decision-maker at the time of consenting' (OECD, 2009). The results and any ambiguity were discussed with the other authors (HK, DS). We excluded generally important aspects of biomedical research that were mentioned in one or more guidelines but were not considered relevant to the content of consent forms in biobank research, for example, 'trial treatment and random assignment' (European Medicines Agency (EMEA), 2002) and 'alternative procedures or courses of treatment' (US Department of Health and Human Services, 2009). We also excluded formal aspects such as 'title of the document' or 'date/signature' (Harnischmacher et al., 2006).

We compared the mentions of issues relevant to consent forms in biobank research in different guidelines, and developed categories for similar mentions of issues. During the development of these categories, we slightly adapted the issues arising from the clinical study context to the biobank context. For instance, we revised the wording 'duration of participation in trial/study' to 'duration of participation or storage'. In some cases we performed a synthesis of issues, for example, subsuming 'money or material goods' (Council for International Organizations of Medical Sciences (CIOMS), 2002), 'payment' and 'expenses' (European Medicines Agency (EMEA), 2002), 'additional costs' (US Department of Health and Human Services, 2009), 'incentives' (World Medical Association (WMA), 2013), and 'allowance' (Harnischmacher et al., 2006) under 'Payment/allowance and additional costs'. We finally obtained 41 issues grouped under four main headings (see results section and Table 8.1). Each of the 41 issues derives from at least two guidance documents.

Biobank Survey and Analysis of the Consent Documents

To get an overview of consent documents and templates currently used in biobank research in Germany, we considered all biobanks registered in the German

---

3   HBGRD stands for Human Biobanks and Genetic Research Database (authors' note).

Biobank Registry ('Deutsches Biobanken-Register', http://www.biobanken.de) in July 2012. We excluded six of the 108 registered biobanks because they were either doubly mentioned in the register or did not exist anymore (or their website could not be accessed). Nine of the remaining 102 biobanks had consent forms publicly available on their websites. We asked the heads of the other 93 biobanks via email to send us their consent documents. In this email we made clear that German biobanks will not be named individually in the dissemination of findings from our study. The response rate after repeated contact was 48 per cent (44/90 biobanks, three mailing addresses were incorrect). Not all biobanks were willing to provide their consent document; some biobanks used a shared consent form, and two biobanks provided two documents for different purposes. At last, we were able to include 30 consent documents of 33 biobanks in our analysis. If the biobanks provided additional participant information and a consent form, we included both documents in the analysis.

The representation of all 41 issues in each of the 30 consent documents was assessed according to standards in thematic text analysis (Dixon-Woods et al., 2005). All researchers were experienced in thematic text analysis and research ethics. The consent forms were read in full by two authors (IH, HK) independently to identify and extract text passages corresponding to each of the 41 consent issues for biobank research. For the purpose of this study the authors only rated whether the issues were mentioned or not. For example, the authors did not evaluate in depth whether these issues were sufficiently comprehensible. After the independent text extraction and rating the researchers compared their results. Discrepancies between the resulting spreadsheets were identified in 114 (9.3 per cent) of all 1,230 ratings (41 ratings for each of the 30 consent forms). These discrepancies were discussed and resolved with the third author (DS).

Results

Assessment Matrix

Our assessment matrix comprises 41 issues in four categories: (A) 'General information' covering for example, explanation of the type of research and its purpose; (B) 'Conditions of participation' including background on voluntary participation, consent conditions and scope; (C) 'Consequences of participation' comprising issues on for example, risks and benefits, and (D) 'Dealing with data and biomaterial' encompassing issues on, for example, data protection measures and cooperation with other parties. Table 8.1 presents the 41 issues of the assessment matrix for consent in biobank research, the number of guidelines from which each issue derived, and the extent to which the issues were mentioned in the German biobank sample.

Table 8.1 **Representation of 41 consent issues for biobank research in 30 German consent documents**

Consent issues for biobank research		Origin: mention in guidelines for the regulation of biomedical research (n = 10)		Application: mention in biobank-specific consent documents (n = 30)	
		N	%	N	%
(A) General information					
A.1	Research explanation and purpose	10	100	28	93
A.2	Future development and changes	5	50	9	30
A.3	Biobank design and structure	5	50	21	70
A.4	Funding and (conflict of) interests	6	60	6	20
A.5	Duration of participation or storage	7	70	15	50
A.6	Biomaterial: types and quantity of specimen	3	30	27	90
A.7	Data: type and quantity of data	3	30	19	63
A.8	Description of collection procedures and additional tests	8	80	26	87
A.9	Sample collection: further examination needed/follow up-points	2	20	23	77
A.10	Rights/ownership of samples and data and their transfer	2	20	17	57
A.11	Opinion or approval of Ethical Review Board/Committee	5	50	16	53
(B) Conditions of participation					
B.1	Dimension of consent: scope, safeguards and conditions	5	50	15	50
B.2	Free and voluntary participation	10	100	24	80
B.3	Right to withdraw or alter consent (without disadvantage)	10	100	29	97
B.4	Withdrawal: modalities and consequences regarding biomaterial and data	5	50	24	80
B.5	Decision on participation/withdrawal without affecting medical care or relationship to physician	5	50	15	50
B.6	Compensation and insurance cover	8	80	5	17
B.7	Options (partial consent)	3	30	16	53
(C) Consequences of participation					
C.1	Direct benefit for participant	10	100	15	50
C.2	Indirect benefit for subgroups or society	10	100	19	63
C.3	Risk	10	100	21	70
C.4	Payment/allowance or additional costs	6	60	10	33
C.5	Benefit-sharing	3	30	18	60
C.6	Feedback on findings or incidental findings	6	60	20	67

Consent issues for biobank research		Origin: mention in guidelines for the regulation of biomedical research (n = 10)		Application: mention in biobank-specific consent documents (n = 30)	
		N	%	N	%
C.7	Publication of data only unlinked	2	20	17	57
C.8	Re-contacting of participant: purpose and conditions	4	40	18	60
C.9	Contact person/point	5	50	18	60
(D) Dealing with data and biomaterial					
D.1	Confidentiality of records and data/extent and limits of confidentiality	9	90	24	80
D.2	Privacy rights and procedures/safeguards, data processing, and identifiability of data and samples	6	60	27	90
D.3	Use of health data and records and their purpose	4	40	20	67
D.4	Storage of data and biomaterial	5	50	20	67
D.5	Policy for genetic information/consent to genetic analyses	4	40	12	40
D.6	Contact (with) or disclosure to/of participants' physician	3	30	19	63
D.7	Policy on use/disclosure to third parties for non-research purpose	3	30	7	23
D.8	Sharing data and material with other researchers/policy and process	2	20	24	80
D.9	International cooperation/trans-border use	2	20	7	23
D.10	Commercialisation and collaboration with for-profit entities	5	50	17	57
D.11	Right of access to personal data	3	30	5	17
D.12	Disposal or destruction of data and material	3	30	21	70
D.13	Dealing with data and material after participants die or become incapacitated	2	20	0	0
D.14	Removal of material after death	2	20	1	3

German Consent Documents for Biobank Research

Our sample comprised 30 consent documents from 33 German biobanks registered in the German Biobank Registry in July 2012. The sample includes different types of biobank with varying characteristics as type (population-wide or disease-specific biobank, or clinical study with sample collections), number of participants, organisation and funding, and inclusion of healthy probands or patients (for example, inclusion of all admitted patients). However, all registered biobanks are considered to perform biobank research. The German Biobank Registry is operated by the TMF (Technology, Methods, and Infrastructure for Networked Medical Research) and is funded by the German Federal Ministry of Education and Research.

Most of the biobanks had developed their own consent documents; one biobank just used a consent form for genetic diagnostic similar to a template of the German Society of Human Genetics. The consent documents (participant information and consent form) varied in several characteristics, for example, in length of document (one to five pages), target group (patient, healthy participant, next of kin, children or parents), scope of consent, content, complexity and comprehensibility.

The coverage of the 41 issues by the 30 consent documents was very variable. One issue (B.3 'Right to withdraw or alter consent (without disadvantage)') was addressed in 97 per cent, another issue (D.13 'Dealing with data and material after participants die or become incapacitated') was not addressed by any consent form (see Table 8.1). Though for the interpretation of the results, it has to be considered that a few issues – as D.14 'Removal of samples after death' – are not applicable to all biobanks. Nevertheless, in these cases the issues were counted as 'not mentioned'.

A large majority of the German consent documents referred to issues as A.1 'Research explanation and purpose' (93 per cent) and A.6 'Biomaterial: types and quantity of specimen' (90 per cent), to elementary conditions such as B.2 'Free and voluntary participation' (80 per cent) or B.3 'Right to withdraw or alter consent (without disadvantage)' (97 per cent) and to basic aspects such as D.1 'Confidentiality of records and data/extent and limits of confidentiality' (80 per cent) and D.2 'Privacy rights and procedures/safeguards, data processing, and identifiability of data and samples' (90 per cent).

Information on some controversially discussed or partly not foreseeable issues was given less frequently, for example, for general information (section A) such as A.2 'Future development and changes' (30 per cent) or information on A.10 'Rights/ownership of samples and data and their transfer' (57 per cent). Also some points regarding the conditions of participation (section B) were considered by just half of the documents, for example, B.5 'Decision on participation/withdrawal without affecting medical care or relationship to physician' (50 per cent) or B.7 'Options/partial consent' (53 per cent). Of the issues regarding the consequences of participation (section C), the most mentioned was C.3 'Risk' (70 per cent) and the least-mentioned C.4 'Payment/ allowance or additional costs' (33 per cent). The mentioning of risks ranged from: no any mentioned risks at all over minimal risks for the sample/blood-taking procedure to a very detailed description of the risks using genetic data. (The latter refer to, for example, the knowledge as such and the related psychological burdens for the donor or family members, implication on re-identifiability of 'anonymised' data, and potential implications on health insurance and employment.)

Some issues of presumably high importance for biobank research (in section D: 'Dealing with data and biomaterial') were mentioned infrequently, for example, D.9 'International cooperation/trans-border use' (23 per cent), D.11 'Right of access to personal data' (17 per cent) or D.7 'Policy on use/disclosure to third parties for non-research purpose' (23 per cent).

The number of issues found also varied widely among the 30 consent documents (see Table 8.2), from a minimum of 9 (22 per cent) to a maximum of 36 (88 per cent). The median of issues addressed across all 30 consent forms was 25.5 issues (62 per cent).

Table 8.2   Distribution of consent issues for biobank research
            (n = 41, divided into five ranges), found in consent
            documents of a German biobank sample (n = 30)

Consent issues for biobank research	Mention in German biobank consent documents	
Range	N	%
33–41 (approx. 80–100%)	3	10
25–32 (approx. 60–80%)	14	47
17–24 (approx. 40–60%)	6	20
9–16 (approx. 20–40%)	7	23
0–8 (approx. 0–20%)	0	0

Discussion and Conclusion

This study illustrates that consent documents from 30 German biobanks differ widely in the range of issues that they address. Out of 41 potentially relevant issues (systematically identified in leading guidelines on consent in biomedical research) only three consent forms (10 per cent) address more than 80 per cent while another seven consent forms (23 per cent) address less than 40 per cent.

One should bear in mind that the consideration of more issues does not facilitate consent or increase its validity per se. Nevertheless, one should have reasonable motives to minimise the extent of content and leave out relevant issues.

With respect to the existing heterogeneity and different types of biobanks, it has to be considered that not all of the mentioned issues must be applicable or equally relevant to each biobank. Nevertheless, core criteria for consent in biobank research and consent forms could be harmonised on an at least abstract level. Such abstract templates could then be adapted to the individual national or local context. In the German sample it is remarkable that issues with a presumably high significance for biobank research in general (Cambon-Thomsen et al., 2007; Hansson, 2009; OECD, 2009; Budimir et al., 2011) were mentioned in less than 25 per cent of all consent forms, for example, D.9 'International cooperation/trans-border use', D.11 'Right of access to personal data' and D.7 'Policy on use/disclosure to third parties for non-research purpose'. The low coverage of such issues in consent forms may be partly because new developments in data protection law and research agendas are not foreseeable in detail. But it may be also because of a still limited awareness of legal, ethical and practical challenges in biobank research and the need for their transparent communication to potential participants (Gottweis and Kaye, 2012).

Concerning the complexity of information, empirical studies need to assess which potentially relevant content issues for consent forms in biobank research can be condensed or simplified without minimising the validity of the consent and the tissue donors' understanding of biobank research. For a first step in this direction see Beskow et al. (2010).

Our study has the following limitations: As a demand of further research it would be worthwhile to expand or modify the guideline-based assessment matrix for consent in biobank research in the following way: (1) to define a set of ethically reasoned core criteria or balance the assessment issues regarding their importance or relevance; (2) to outline explaining dimensions for these issues; and (3) to further analyse which aspects are not covered sufficiently by the matrix respectively by the included guidelines (for example, diagnostic/therapeutic misconception). (For further remarks see Hirschberg et al. (2014). Such conceptual and empirical research would provide the basis for a deeper evaluation of existing consent documents and for the development of new consent documents. Within our explorative study of German biobank consent documents we only considered whether a potentially relevant content issue was mentioned in a consent form at all. We evaluated neither the accuracy of the explanation of this issue nor its quality, comprehensibility or readability. Furthermore, we did not assess criteria for supportive decision-making (for example, IPDAS-criteria (IPDAS, 2005; Elwyn et al., 2006)). These assessment criteria are certainly important for the development and evaluation of valid consent procedures as shown for example by Beskow et al. (2010) and Brehaut et al. (2012). Another limitation arises from the fact that we could only include 32 per cent of consent forms from the full sample of 102 biobanks registered in the German Biobank Registry. However, our sample of 30 consent forms included all leading German biobanks with relatively high quality standards (including all six biobanks that are part of the National Biobank Initiative funded by the German Federal Ministry of Education and Research, BMBF). We suppose that the inclusion of further consent forms would not have changed the overall picture of the strong heterogeneity of consent forms for biobank research. Moreover, we would even expect a wider variation in content issues. Other investigations have reached similar results and support the finding that consent material in general, or in biomedical and biobank research in particular, needs improvement (Padhy et al., 2011; Pawlikowski et al., 2011; Brehaut et al., 2012; Mandava et al., 2012).

Taking into account the widely shared vision of national and international networking of biobanks and increased activities in data and sample sharing, our findings demonstrate the need of improvement and harmonisation of consent procedures in the field of biobank research. Furthermore, such improvements are important to fulfil the demand of responsible biobank governance and to maintain public trust in biobank research (Gottweis and Kaye, 2012). This does also include transparent communication on consent procedures. As described in the methods section only nine consent templates (8.8 per cent) of the 102 initially identified biobanks were available publically on the biobanks' websites. Furthermore, even after repeated contact and the guarantee to anonymise the results for our assessment of consent forms only 32 per cent of registered German biobanks were willing to provide their present consent form. Beside the need to improve and harmonise consent procedures, increased transparency of such basic information should become a major aim of German biobanks, to demonstrate appropriate standards of governance.

When it comes to future improvement and harmonisation of consent forms, public attitudes and expert opinion in relevant fields such as law, ethics, medicine, natural and social science, etc., should be sought to define core criteria for consent. It may also help to overcome the lack of awareness of potentially relevant consent issues and to address them in an appropriate way.

Conclusion

Our findings serve as a starting point to reflect upon the spectrum of relevant consent issues in biobank research. The present study supports the systematic and transparent development of a 'best practice' model of consent for biobank research. The findings show that at least the majority of consent documents in German biobanks should be improved and harmonised to better support an informed and balanced choice by potential donors and to facilitate research cooperation and networking. Further steps of such a best practice model would include the development of a best practice consent template (considering content, adherence to quality and language criteria) followed by a discussion and review of the template with other stakeholders (for example, researchers, research ethics committees, potential biobank participants, patients' representatives and ethicists). A first step towards harmonisation in the German context has been done with the development of a broad consent template by the German Working Group of Research Ethics Committees (Arbeitskreis Medizinischer Ethik-Kommissionen, 2013). Especially for a best practice model for consent forms, the understanding and validity of the text should be tested empirically (Sugarman et al., 2005; Flory et al., 2008). Finally, its use should be accompanied by continuous evaluation.

References

Arbeitskreis Medizinischer Ethik-Kommissionen in der Bundesrepublik Deutschland 2013. Mustertext zur Spende, Einlagerung und Nutzung von Biomaterialien sowie zur Erhebung, Verarbeitung und Nutzung von Daten in Biobanken (empfohlen vom Arbeitskreis Medizinischer Ethik-Kommissionen gemäß Beschluss vom 09.11.2013). Available at: http://www.ak-med-ethik-komm.de/formulare.html (accessed 1 April 2014).

Asslaber, M. and Zatloukal, K. 2007. Biobanks: transnational, European and global networks. *Brief Funct Genomic Proteomic*, 6, 193–201.

Ayuso, C., Millan, J.M., Mancheno, M. and Dal-Re, R. 2013. Informed consent for whole-genome sequencing studies in the clinical setting. Proposed recommendations on essential content and process. *Eur J Hum Genet*, 21, 1054–1059.

Beskow, L.M., Friedman, J.Y., Hardy, N.C., Lin, L. and Weinfurt, K.P. 2010. Developing a simplified consent form for biobanking. *PLoS ONE*, 5, e13302.

Brehaut, J.C., Carroll, K., Elwyn, G., Saginur, R., Kimmelman, J., Shojania, K., Syrowatka, A., Nguyen, T., Hoe, E. and Fergusson, D. 2012. Informed consent documents do not encourage good-quality decision making. *J Clin Epidemiol*, 65, 708–724.

Budimir, D., Polasek, O., Marusic, A., Kolcic, I., Zemunik, T., Boraska, V., Jeroncic, A., Boban, M., Campbell, H. and Rudan, I. 2011. Ethical aspects of human biobanks: a systematic review. *Croat Med J*, 52, 262–279.

Cambon-Thomsen, A., Rial-Sebbag, E. and Knoppers, B.M. 2007. Trends in ethical and legal frameworks for the use of human biobanks. *Eur Respir J*, 30, 373–382.

Capron, A.M. 2008. Legal and regulatory standards of informed consent in research. In: E.J. Emanuel, C. Grady, R.A. Crouch, R.K. Lie, F.G. Miller and D. Wendler, eds. *Oxford Textbook of Clinical Research Ethics*. Oxford: Oxford University Press, pp. 613–32.

Council for International Organizations of Medical Sciences (CIOMS) 2002. *International Ethical Guidelines for Biomedical Research Involving Human Subjects*. Geneva: CIOMS. Available at: http://www.cioms.ch/publications/guidelines/guidelines_nov_2002_blurb.htm (accessed 1 April 2014).

Council of Europe 1997. Convention for the Protection of Human Rights and Dignity of the Human Being with regard to the Application of Biology and Medicine: Convention on Human Rights and Biomedicine. Strasbourg. Council of Europe. Available at: http://conventions.coe.int/Treaty/EN/Treaties/Html/164.htm (accessed 1 April 2014).

Council of Europe 2005. Additional Protocol to the Convention on Human Rights and Biomedicine Concerning Biomedical Research. Strasbourg. Council of Europe. Available at: http://conventions.coe.int/treaty/en/Treaties/Html/195.htm (accessed 1 April 2014).

Council of Europe 2006. Recommendation Rec(2006)4 of the Committee of Ministers to member states on research on biological materials of human origin. Strasbourg. Council of Europe. Available at: https://wcd.coe.int/ViewDoc.jsp?id=977859&BackColorInternet=9999CC&BackColorIntranet=FFBB55&BackColorLogged=FFAC75 (accessed 1 April 2014).

Dixon-Woods, M., Agarwal, S., Jones, D., Young, B. and Sutton, A. 2005. Synthesising qualitative and quantitative evidence: a review of possible methods. *J Health Serv Res Policy*, 10, 45–53.

Elwyn, G., O'Connor, A., Stacey, D., Volk, R., Edwards, A., Coulter, A., Thomson, R., Barratt, A., Barry, M., Bernstein, S., Butow, P., Clarke, A., Entwistle, V., Feldman-Stewart, D., Holmes-Rovner, M., Llewellyn-Thomas, H., Moumjid, N., Mulley, A., Ruland, C., Sepucha, K., Sykes, A. and Whelan, T. 2006. Developing a quality criteria framework for patient decision aids: online international Delphi consensus process. *BMJ*, 333, 417.

Emanuel, E.J., Grady, C., Crouch, R.A., Lie, R.K., Miller, F.G. and Wendler, D., eds. 2008. *Oxford Textbook of Clinical Research Ethics*. Oxford: Oxford University Press.

European Medicines Agency (EMEA) 2002. CPMP/ICH/135/95 Guideline for good clinical practice, ICH Topic E 6 (R1). London: EMEA. Available at: http://www.emea.europa.eu/docs/en_GB/document_library/Scientific_guideline/2009/09/WC500002874.pdf (accessed 1 April 2014).

European Parliament and the Council of the European Union 2001. Directive 2001/20/EC on the approximation of the laws, regulations and administrative provisions of the Member States relating to the implementation of good clinical practice in the conduct of clinical trials on me-dicinal products for human use. Luxembourg. Available at: http://eur-lex.europa.eu/LexUriServ/LexUriServ.do?uri=OJ:L:2001:121:0034:0044:EN:PDF (accessed 1 April 2014).

Flory, Jh., Wendler, D. and Emanuel, E. 2008. Empirical issues in informed consent for research. In: E.J. Emanuel, C. Grady, R.A. Crouch, R.K. Lie, F.G. Miller and D. Wendler, eds. *Oxford Textbook of Clinical Research Ethics*. Oxford: Oxford University Press, pp. 645–660.

German Ethics Council 2010. Human biobanks for research. Opinion. Berlin: Deutscher Ethikrat. Available at: http://www.ethikrat.org/files/der_opinion_human-biobanks.pdf (accessed 1 April 2014).

Gottweis, H. and Kaye, J. 2012. *Biobanks for Europe: A Challenge for Governance.* Report of the Expert Group on Dealing with Ethical and Regulatory Challenges of International Biobank Research. Luxembourg: European Commission.

Greely, H.T. 2007. The uneasy ethical and legal underpinnings of large-scale genomic biobanks. *Annu Rev Genomics Hum Genet*, 8, 343–364.

Hansson, M.G. 2009. Ethics and biobanks. *Br J Cancer*, 100, 8–12.

Harnischmacher, U., Ihle, P., Berger, B., Goebel, J. and Scheller, J. 2006. *Checkliste und Leitfaden zur Patienteneinwilligung. Grundlagen und Anleitung für die Klinische Forschung.* Berlin: Medizinisch Wissenschaftliche Verlagsgesellschaft.

Hirschberg, I., Kahrass, H. and Strech, D. 2014: International requirements for consent in biobank research: qualitative review of research guidelines. *J Med Genet*, 51, 773–781.

Hirtzlin, I., Dubreuil, C., Preaubert, N., Duchier, J., Jansen, B., Simon, J., Lobato De Faria, P., Perez-Lezaun, A., Visser, B., Williams, G.D. and Cambon-Thomsen, A. 2003. An empirical survey on biobanking of human genetic material and data in six EU countries. *Eur J Hum Genet*, 11, 475–488.

Hoeyer, K., Olofsson, B.O., Mjorndal, T. and Lynoe, N. 2005. The ethics of research using biobanks: reason to question the importance attributed to informed consent. *Arch Intern Med*, 165, 97–100.

Hüppe, A., Dziubek, K. and Raspe, H. 2014. Zum Verbesserungspotenzial schriftlicher Aufklärungsmaterialien zu (bio)medizinischen Forschungs vorhaben – Empirische Analyse von Antragsunterlagen einer Forschungs ethikkommission. *Ethik in der Medizin*, 26(3), 211–224.

IPDAS 2005. Criteria for judging the quality of patient decision aids. Checklist. International Patient Decision Aids Standards (IPDAS) Collaboration. Available at: http://ipdas.ohri.ca/IPDAS_checklist.pdf (accessed 1 April 2014).

Jefford, M. and Moore, R. 2008. Improvement of informed consent and the quality of consent documents. *Lancet Oncol*, 9, 485–493.

Mandava, A., Pace, C., Campbell, B., Emanuel, E. and Grady, C. 2012. The quality of informed consent: mapping the landscape. A review of empirical data from developing and developed countries. *J Med Ethics*, 38, 356–365.

Mascalzoni, D., Janssens, A.C., Stewart, A., Pramstaller, P., Gyllensten, U., Rudan, I., Van Duijn, C.M., Wilson, J.F., Campbell, H. and Quillan, R.M. 2010. Comparison of participant information and informed consent forms of five European studies in genetic isolated populations. *Eur J Hum Genet*, 18, 296–302.

McGuire, A.L. and Beskow, L.M. 2010. Informed consent in genomics and genetic research. *Annu Rev Genomics Hum Genet*, 11, 361–381.

OECD 2009. *Guidelines on Human Biobanks and Genetic Research Databases*. Paris: Organisation for Economic Co-Operation and Development (OECD). Available at: http://www.oecd.org/sti/biotech/44054609.pdf (accessed 1 April 2014).

Padhy, B.M., Gupta, P. and Gupta, Y.K. 2011. Analysis of the compliance of informed consent documents with good clinical practice guideline. *Contemp Clin Trials*, 32, 662–666.

Pawlikowski, J., Sak, J. and Marczewski, K. 2011. Biobank research and ethics: the problem of informed consent in Polish biobanks. *Arch Med Sci*, 7, 896–901.

Porteri, C. and Borry, P. 2008. A proposal for a model of informed consent for the collection, storage and use of biological materials for research purposes. *Patient Educ Couns*, 71, 136–142.

Salvaterra, E., Lecchi, L., Giovanelli, S., Butti, B., Bardella, M.T., Bertazzi, P.A., Bosari, S., Coggi, G., Coviello, D.A., Lalatta, F., Moggio, M., Nosotti, M., Zanella, A. and Rebulla, P. 2008. Banking together. A unified model of informed consent for biobanking. *EMBO Rep*, 9, 307–313.

Sugarman, J., Lavori, P.W., Boeger, M., Cain, C., Edsond, R., Morrison, V. and Yeh, S.S. 2005. Evaluating the quality of informed consent. *Clinical Trials*, 2, 34–41.

US Department of Health and Human Services 2009. Code of Federal Regulations. Title 45 Part 46. Protection of Human Subjects. Washington, DC. Available at: http://www.hhs.gov/ohrp/humansubjects/guidance/45cfr46.html (accessed 1 April 2014).

World Medical Association (WMA) 2013. Declaration of Helsinki: Ethical Principles for Medical Research Involving Human Subjects. Fortaleza: WMA. Available at: http://www.wma.net/en/30publications/10policies/b3/ (accessed 7 February 2015).

Zika, E., Paci, D., Schulte in Den Bäumen, T., Braun, A., Rijkers-Defrasne, S., Deschênes, M., Fortier, I., Laage-Hellman, J., Scerri, C. and Dolores, I. 2010. *Biobanks in Europe: Prospects for Harmonisation and Networking*. EU-Report. Luxembourg: EU Joint Research Centre: Institute for Prospective Technological Studies.

Chapter 9

Individualised Medicine in the Diagnosis and Prognosis of Patients Younger than 65 Years with Normal Karyotype Acute Myeloid Leukemia: A Systematic Review and Meta-Analysis of the Impact of Fms-Related Tyrosine Kinase 3 Internal Tandem Duplication (FLT3-ITD)[1]

Matthias Port[*], Miriam Böttcher[*], Felicitas Thol, Nicole Trachte, Jürgen Wasem, Arnold Ganser, Laura Pouryamout[*] and Anja Neumann[*2]

Introduction

Individualised and personalised medicine has gained an important role in the current research into oncological and haematological diseases. The definition

[*]   These authors contributed equally to the work.

1   This chapter was originally published in German in a slightly modified form, under the title 'Individualisierte Medizin in der Diagnostik und prognostischen Einschätzung in der akuten myeloischen Leukämie mit normalem Karyotyp bei Erwachsenen unter 65 Jahren: eine systematische Literaturrecherche und Metaanalyse zu FLT3-ITD' in: *Ethik in der Medizin* 2013, 25, 183–193. With kind permission of Springer Science+Business Media.

2   This study was conducted in the research network Personalised Medicine in Oncology: An Interdisciplinary Study on Ethical, Medical, Economical and Legal Aspects (Grant project number: 01 GP 1001A-C), which is supported by the German Federal Ministry of Education and Research (Bundesministerium für Bildung und Forschung – BMBF). None of the authors have any conflict of interest to declare.

of 'individualised and personalised medicine' is still controversial. The term as used in this article is based on biological findings leading to stratification of subgroups (for a detailed discussion on the definition of personalised medicine see Chapter 1, this volume).

Biological characteristics, such as morphology or karyotype, have been used to classify and treat diseases like acute myeloid leukaemia (AML) for many years. With the progressive developments in gene analysis, the biological knowledge about acquired genetic abnormalities has increased dramatically at this time (Hanahan and Weinberg, 2011). Examples of the scientific and medical progress over the last few years are the treatment of chronic myeloid leukaemia (O'Brien et al., 2003), malignant melanoma (Chapman et al., 2011) or the adenocarcinoma of the lung (Bareschino et al., 2011); whereby it is becoming especially obvious in the latter that the currently remarkable improvements in prognosis are only achievable for subgroups. The implementation of these new insights into the daily clinical routine is a big challenge for health professionals and health-care systems.

This article focuses on the insights in AML and particularly on the subgroup of AML with normal karyotype (CN-AML).

AML is a clonal disease of haematopoietic progenitor cells that accumulate a variety of mutations and epigenetic events leading to increased proliferation, disruption of differentiation, lack of apoptosis, and suppression of normal haematopoietic progenitor cells (Dohner et al., 2010). Diagnosis and classification were based on cytological criteria and cytogenetic alterations until the recent developments in molecular genetics. In particular, the cytogenetic karyotype has enabled physicians to classify AML patients as 'low-', 'intermediate-' and 'high-risk AML'; the CN-AML is associated with an intermediate risk. AML patients are treated with chemotherapy. Therapy in adult patients younger than 60 years includes an induction chemotherapy followed by post-remission therapy. The strategies available for post-remission therapy are high-dose cytarabine-based chemotherapy or high-dose chemotherapy with/without total body irradiation followed by autologous or allogeneic stem cell transplantation (Dohner et al., 2010). The optimal therapy for individual patients is chosen based on the risk classification.

About 40 per cent of patients younger than 60 years have a normal karyotype (Grimwade et al., 2010). A multitude of genetic alterations, such as mutations of genes or quantitative changes in gene expression in the leukemic cells, have been described in recent years and their impact on prognosis has been evaluated (Marcucci et al., 2011). The findings have already been used to select the type of consolidation therapy for the patient. In this systematic review, we focus on the frequent mutations of fms-related tyrosine kinase 3 (FLT3), in detail, on internal tandem duplications (FLT3-ITD) (Vardiman et al., 2009) in CN-AML in patients aged between 15 and 65 years. FLT3-ITD plays a role in the proliferation, survival and differentiation of haematopoietic progenitor cells and, currently, is the most important biomarker to identify high-risk AML in patients with normal karyotype.

Materials and Methods

A systematic literature search was conducted using the databases Embase, Pubmed, Healthstar, BIOSIS, ISI Web of Knowledge, and Cochrane, including publications published between 1 January 2000 and 31 March 2012.

We used the string of keywords shown in Table 9.1, with the appropriate Medical Subject Heading (MeSH) terms and the original words.

Table 9.1   String of keywords used for literature search

Disease	Acute myeloid leukemia OR AML OR Cytogenetically Normal Acute Myeloid Leukemia OR CNAML OR AkutemyeloischeLeukämie OR normalkaryotypische AML
AND	
Genetic markers	NPM1 OR FLT3 OR CEBPA
AND	
Therapy	Treatment OR Outcome OR Clinical Outcome OR Prognosis OR Transplantation OR Therapie OR Behandlung OR Prognose

Using the reference lists of the articles included, the systematic literature search was extended by a manual search.

Publications were included if data about (1) treatment options, clinical outcome and prognosis with regard to (2) the molecular genetic marker FLT3-ITD (3) in patients with CN-AML (4) aged between 15 and 65 years were available. A deviation of 5 per cent of patients older than 60 years was accepted. The study population had to include (5) at least 100 patients. (6) Publications in the German and English language were included. Those publications not limited to a population of patients with CN-AML only were included if patients with CN-AML represented a subgroup for which discrete results were available. Studies involving animal experiments or *in vitro* studies were excluded.

Four reviewers (M.P., M.B., L.P. and A.N.) independently scanned the titles and abstracts to determine the eligibility of articles identified by the search described. The screening was followed by an analysis at a full-text level.

Data extraction was carried out focusing on the following domains:

1. study reference (bibliographical notes, setting and year);
2. study framework (target population, allocation of molecular markers); and
3. results (hazard ratios for overall survival (OS) and relapse-free survival (RFS) for FLT-ITD).

Relevant data were extracted into tables using standardised documentation sheets (Table 9.2). In addition to the qualitative data synthesis, a meta-analysis was performed with the aid of specific software (RevMan 5.1, available at http://ims.cochrane.org/revman/download).

Results

Systematic Literature Search

A total of 3,470 publications were identified within the systematic literature search. Duplicates (n=1,677) were removed, resulting in 1,793 publications passing the title and abstract screening. A total of 1,614 additional papers did not meet the inclusion criteria and were excluded. The remaining 179 full-text articles were analysed. A total of 18 publications (Fröhling et al., 2004; Boissel et al., 2005; Dohner et al., 2005; Heuser et al., 2006; Thiede et al., 2006; Gale et al., 2008a; Langer et al., 2008; Marcucci et al., 2008; Paschka et al., 2008; Schlenk et al., 2008; Virappane et al., 2008; Whitman et al., 2008; Langer et al., 2009; Dunna et al., 2010; Kim et al., 2010; Taskesen et al., 2010; Wagner et al., 2010; Chapman et al., 2011) (Figure 9.1) met the inclusion criteria and were included in the systematic review. Data of three publications related to CN-AML could be included in the quantitative analysis (Marcucci et al., 2008; Virappane et al., 2008; Taskesen et al., 2010).

Systematic Description of the Publications

Relevant information has been summarised out of the 18 publications that could be analysed in terms of CN-AML in Table 9.2.

The patient populations of the publications identified could be assigned to various study groups and countries. There were numerous publications from large clinical study groups with overlapping study populations (see Figure 9.2).

The question of the prognostic significance of FLT3-ITD was evaluated *post hoc* in all studies identified. No prospective trials were identified with regard to the key question of this paper. Seven publications were from the 'German-Austrian Study Group Acute Myeloid Leukaemia (AMLSG)' and related study

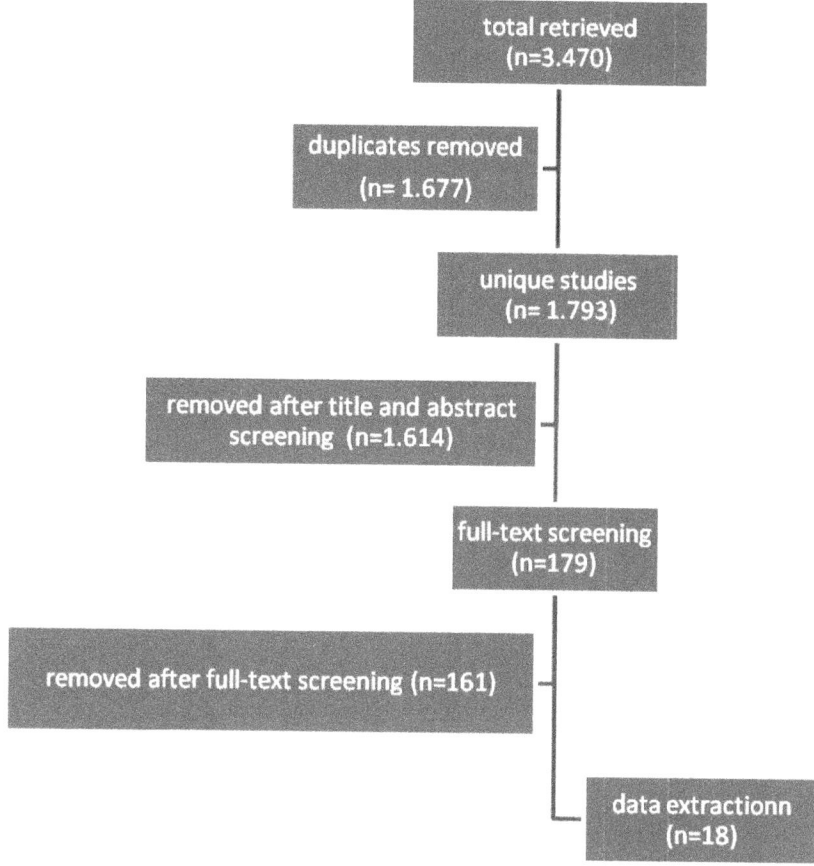

Figure 9.1 Flow chart of study selection from literature search 01/2000 – 03/2012

groups (Fröhling et al., 2004; Dohner et al., 2005; Heuser et al., 2006; Schlenk et al., 2008; Damm et al., 2010; Taskesen et al., 2010; Wagner et al., 2010). Three of the seven papers derive from their institutions' predecessors 'AMLSG-Ulm' and 'SHG-Hannover/Frankfurt', both from Germany (Heuser et al., 2006; Damm et al., 2010; Wagner et al., 2010), and one from the 'Haemato-Oncology Foundation for Adults in the Netherlands (HOVON)' and the 'Swiss Group for Clinical Cancer Research (SAKK)' (Taskesen et al., 2010). A total of five articles of the American study group 'The Cancer and Leukaemia Group B (CALGB)' (Langer et al., 2008; Marcucci et al., 2008; Paschka et al., 2008; Whitman et al., 2008; Langer et al., 2009) were included. Two publications were from the 'Medical Research Council (MRC)' in the UK (Gale et al., 2008b; Virappane et al., 2008), one each from the 'German Study Initiative Leukaemia (DSIL)'

Table 9.2 Descriptive statistics of studies meeting the inclusion criteria

First author	Year	Country	Study population	Patients CN-AML	FLT3 ITD (%)	HR OS FLT3 ITD	HR DFS FLT3 ITD	HR RFS FLT3 ITD
Fröhling, S.	2004	Germany	AMLSG HD93/98A	236	32.6	2.03		2.25
Kim, Y.K.	2010	Korea	Korean study population	121	38.0	OR 2.4 (1.3–4.3)		OR 3.13 (1.67–5.88)
Langer, C.	2008	United States	CALGB 9621, 19808	172	36.0	2.29		
Langer, C.	2009	United States	CALGB 9621, 19808	119	45.0	2.70 (1.41–5.17)	2.18 (1.03–4.61)	
Marcucci, G.	2008	United States	CALGB 9621, 19808	175	40.0	2.1 (1.2–3.7)	1.9 (1.1–3.4)	
Taskesen, E.	2010	Germany, Netherlands, Switzerland	AMLSG HD93, HD98A, 07-04; AMLSHG 02-95, 01-99; HOVON-SAKK -04, -04A, -29, -42	1182	31.4	1.78 (1.49–2.14)		1.75 (1.45–2.12)
Virappane, P.	2008	United Kingdom	UK MRC AML10 UK MRC AML12	470	37.0	5.56 (1.91–16.16)		7.73 (2.57–23.25)
Wagner, K.	2010	Germany	AMLSHG 0295, 0199	273	30.2	1.69 (1.2–2.4)		1.37 (0.93–2.01)

Author	Year	Country	Trial/Protocol	N	%
Boissel, N.	2005	France	ALFA 90, ALFA 9802	106	31.0
Damm, F.	2010	Germany	AMLSHG 0199, 0295	249	32.4
Döhner, K.	2005	Germany	AMLSG HD93/98A	300	32.3
Dunna, N.	2010	India	India, Nizam's Institute of Medical Sciences	128	20.4
Gale, R.	2008	United Kingdom	UK MRC AML10 UK MRC AML12	1124	26.0
Heuser, M.	2006	Germany	AML-SHG 01/99	142	29.0
Paschka, P.	2008	United States	CALGB 9621, 19808	196	38.0
Schlenk, R.	2008	Germany	AMLSG HD93, AML-2/95, HD98A, AML-1/99	872	31.0
Thiede, C.	2006	Germany	AML 96 (DSIL)	387	30.7
Whitman, S.P.	2008	United States	CALGB 9621, 19808	139	34.6

min	20.4
max	45.0
median	32.4
mean	33.1

1.69	**1.90**	**1.37**
5.56	**2.18**	**7.73**

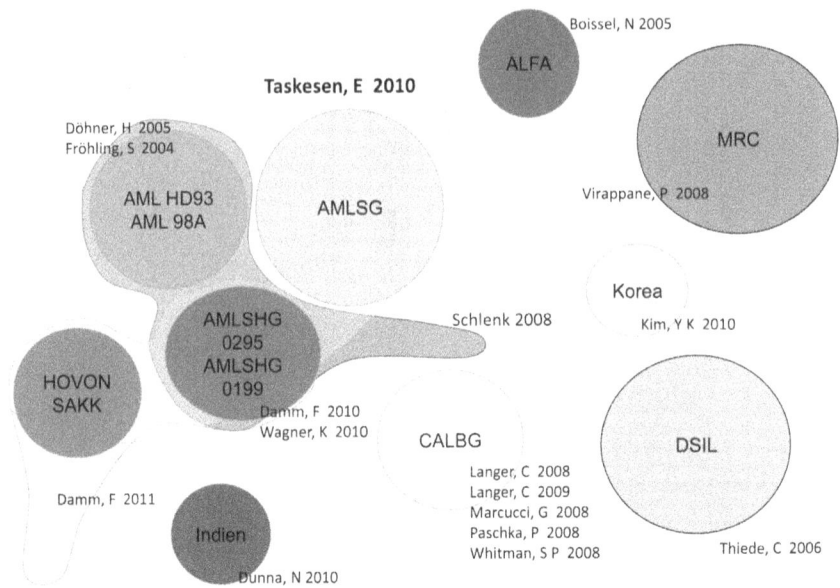

Figure 9.2   **Representation of the evaluated studies and display of overlapping populations**

(Thiede et al., 2006) and the French study group 'Acute Leukaemia French Association-90 (ALFA90)' (Boissel et al., 2005), a Korean (Kim et al., 2010) and an Indian working group (Dunna et al., 2010).

All papers included AML patients with a normal karyotype. The latter could comprise a subgroup of the total if discrete results for this subcategory were provided (see Table 9.2). The size of the study population with a normal karyotype ranged from 106 to 1,182 patients.

In all of the patients with normal karyotype, FLT3-ITD was found in 20 to 45 per cent (median, 32 per cent; mean, 33 per cent; Table 9.2). With regard to FLT3-ITD, the hazard ratio for OS was provided in seven papers and ranged between 1.69 and 5.56 (Fröhling et al., 2004; Gale et al., 2008b; Langer et al., 2008; Marcucci et al., 2008; Virappane et al., 2008; Langer et al., 2009; Dunna et al., 2010; Taskesen et al., 2010; Wagner et al., 2010). The impact of FLT3-ITD on disease-free-survival (DFS) was provided in two papers with hazard ratios of 1.9 (Marcucci et al., 2008) and 2.18 (Langer et al., 2009). Two papers reported FLT3-ITD impact on event-free survival (EFS), with hazard ratios of 1.56 (Taskesen et al., 2010) and 2.10 (Marcucci et al., 2008). Three papers also provided hazard ratios for relapse-free survival (RFS) (1.37: Wagner et al., 2010, 1.75: Taskesen et al., 2010 and 7.73: Virappane et al., 2008).

FLT3-ITD OS

Study or Subgroup	log[Hazard Ratio]	SE	FLT3-ITDmut Total	FLT3-ITDwt Total	Weight	Hazard Ratio IV, Random, 95% CI
Virappane 2008	1.7156	0.5452	176	288	13.6%	5.56 [1.91; 16.19]
Marcucci 2008	0.7419	0.2855	70	105	31.1%	2.10 [1.20; 3.67]
Taskesen 2010	0.5766	0.0907	372	810	55.2%	1.78 [1.49; 2.13]
Total (95% CI)			618	1203	100.0%	2.19 [1.40; 3.43]

Heterogeneity: Tau² = 0.09; Chi² = 4.45, df = 2 (P = 0.11); I² = 55%
Test for overall effect: Z = 3.42 (P = 0.0006)

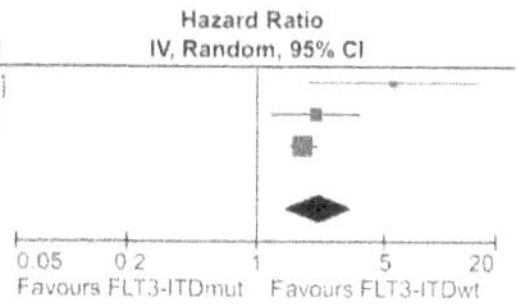

Favours FLT3-ITDmut   Favours FLT3-ITDwt

FLT3-ITD RFS/DFS

Study or Subgroup	log[Hazard Ratio]	SE	FLT3-ITDmut Total	FLT3-ITDwt Total	Weight	Hazard Ratio IV, Random, 95% CI
Virappane 2008	2.0451	0.5618	176	288	17.6%	7.73 [2.57; 23.25]
Marcucci 2008	0.6419	0.2789	70	105	34.5%	1.90 [1.10; 3.28]
Taskesen 2010	0.5598	0.0959	372	810	47.9%	1.75 [1.45; 2.11]
Total (95% CI)			618	1203	100.0%	2.34 [1.32; 4.14]

Heterogeneity: Tau² = 0.17; Chi² = 6.81, df = 2 (P = 0.03); I² = 71%
Test for overall effect: Z = 2.91 (P = 0.004)

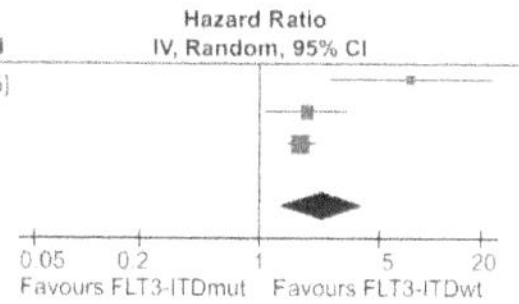

Favours FLT3-ITDmut   Favours FLT3-ITDwt

Figure 9.3   **Forrest plots of the hazard ratios (HRs) and 95 per cent confidence intervals for overall survival and relapse-free survival for FLT3-ITD**

Meta-Analysis

The overlap of the study populations with regard to the qualitative and quantitative analysis for CN-AML is illustrated in Figure 9.2. Eleven publications could not be used for the quantitative analysis due to a lack of data concerning hazard ratio (HR) (Boissel et al., 2005; Dohner et al., 2005; Heuser et al., 2006; Thiede et al., 2006; Gale et al., 2008b; Paschka et al., 2008; Schlenk et al., 2008; Whitman et al., 2008; Damm et al., 2010; Dunna et al., 2010) or odds ratios (OR) (Kim et al., 2010). Furthermore, only data of non-overlapping study populations were analysed. The clinical outcome was always worse for patients with FLT3-ITD. The overall HR was 2.19 (95 per cent CI 1.40 to 3.43, P < 0.0006) for OS and 2.34 (95 per cent CI 1.32 to 4.14, P < 0.004) for RFS compared to the wild type with a total of 1,203 patients analysed (Marcucci et al., 2008; Virappane et al., 2008; Taskesen et al., 2010) (Figure 9.3).

Discussion

The analysis for the presence of FLT3-ITD in leukemic cells at diagnosis provides important prognostic information for patients with acute myeloid leukaemia. FLT3-ITD is already in use for the treatment decision, for example, the recommendation for allogeneic stem cell transplantation as a post-remission therapy in first complete remission (Arber et al., 2008; Dohner and Dohner,

2008). Therefore, the mutation analysis of this gene belongs to the urgently recommended procedures to be carried out at the time of initial diagnosis. It is classified as mandatory within clinical trials (Dohner and Dohner, 2008). Nonetheless, the mutation analysis is not yet a generally accepted standard in the diagnosis of AML, leading to problems in the reimbursement of molecular diagnostics through health insurance.

The focus on 'younger' adults up to 60 years of age was chosen because an important option for consolidation therapy, that is, stem cell transplantation, is usually limited to this patient group during the time period examined. Due to competing risks and a relatively clear classification based on cytogenetic alterations, we only included CN-AML patients for whom the optimal decision with regard to chemotherapy-based consolidation therapy and allogeneic transplantation remains unclear.

Our meta-analysis demonstrated a clearly negative impact of FLT3-ITD on both OS and RFS. This is in accordance with most publications cited in the classification of the WHO (Arber et al., 2008) and with a previous meta-analysis published by Yanada et al. (2005), which encompassed a more heterogeneous patient population with regard to age and karyotype.

A significant limitation of this type of meta-analysis is the lack of prospective controlled studies. The usual study design with *post hoc* analysis for FLT3-ITD, the moderate to high heterogeneity of the meta-analysis depending on the selected outcome parameter which arose mainly from the publication of Virappane et al. (2008) and – due to lack of important data – the impossibility for detailed assessment of confounders are further limitations. Numerous questions remain unanswered regarding the importance of FLT3-ITD as a predictive marker. Among others, a prospective testing of FLT3-ITD is desirable and studies with this focus are in the recruitment and evaluation phase. In addition, not only has the presence or absence of the FLT3-ITD a prognostic impact, but also the allelic burden which can vary considerably. Thus, patients with a low allelic burden have a much better prognosis even though their leukemic cells carry the FLT3-ITD (Pratcorona et al., 2013). The favourable outcome of patients with AML harbouring a low-allelic burden FLT3-ITD mutation and concomitant NPM1 mutation is relevant for choosing the optimised post-remission therapy. The optimal integration of competing prognostic risk factors, which act as confounders, into the treatment decisions still have to be defined. Currently, more than 20 mutations and genes that influence the prognosis of AML are under discussion (Marcucci et al., 2011).

The integrative evaluation and analysis of mutations and classical prognostic markers (such as age, cytogenetics, leukaemia cell count and treatment response to induction chemotherapy) is a challenge for the upcoming years and underlines the need for collaboration of the large study groups (see chapters 7 and 8, this volume, for a discussion on these topics in regard to biobanks).

Molecular heterogeneity of tumours, uncertainty of diagnostics, molecular progression, cost of analysis, and the increasing complexity of diagnosis and treatment decisions might have a negative impact on the usage of personalised medicine.

This work supports the prognostic significance of the marker FLT3-ITD. A careful and rapid initial work-up is mandatory in each patient with CN-AML not only because of the very different effects of post-remission therapy (chemotherapy versus allogeneic stem cell transplantation) in terms of the chances of cure, but also the associated treatment-related long-term morbidity and mortality. Therefore, the molecular analysis has to be included in the supply and reimbursement structures.

References

Arber, D.A., Brunning, R.D., Le Beau, M.M., Falini, B., Vardiman, J.W., Porwit, A., Thiele, J. and Bloomfield, C.D., 2008. Acute myeloid leukaemia and related precursor neoplasms. In: S.H. Swerdlow, E. Campo, N.L. Harris, E.S. Jaffe, S.A. Pileri, H. Stein, J. Thiele and J.W. Vardiman, eds. *WHO classification of tumours of haematopoietic and lymphoid tissues*, 4th edn. Lyon: IARC Press, Lyon, pp.109–66.

Bareschino, M.A., Schettino, C., Rossi, A., Maione, P., Sacco, P.C., Zeppa, R. and Gridelli, C., 2011. Treatment of advanced non small cell lung cancer. *Journal of Thoracic Disease*, 3(2), pp.122–33.

Boissel, N., Renneville, A., Biggio, V., Philippe, N., Thomas, X., Cayuela, J.-M., Terre, C., Tigaud, I., Castaigne, S., Raffoux, E., De Botton, S., Fenaux, P., Dombret, H. and Preudhomme, C., 2005. Prevalence, clinical profile, and prognosis of NPM mutations in AML with normal karyotype. *Blood*, 106(10), pp.3618–20.

Chapman, P.B., Hauschild, A., Robert, C., Haanen, J.B., Ascierto, P., Larkin, J., Dummer, R., Garbe, C., Testori, A., Maio, M., Hogg, D., Lorigan, P., Lebbe, C., Jouary, T., Schadendorf, D., Ribas, A., O'Day, S.J., Sosman, J.A., Kirkwood, J.M., Eggermont, A.M.M., Dreno, B., Nolop, K., Li, J., Nelson, B., Hou, J., Lee, R.J., Flaherty, K.T. and McArthur, G., 2011. Improved survival with vemurafenib in melanoma with BRAF V600E mutation. *New England Journal of Medicine*, 364(26), pp.2507–16.

Damm, F., Heuser, M., Morgan, M., Yun, H., Grosshennig, A., Göhring, G., Schlegelberger, B., Döhner, K., Ottmann, O., Lübbert, M., Heit, W., Kanz, L., Schlimok, G.G., Raghavachar, A., Fiedler, W., Kirchner, H., Döhner, H., Heil, G., Ganser, A., Krauter, J.J., Goehring, G., Doehner, K., Luebbert, M. and Doehner, H., 2010. Single nucleotide polymorphism in the mutational hotspot of WT1 predicts a favorable outcome in patients with cytogenetically normal acute myeloid leukemia. *Journal of Clinical Oncology*, 28(4), pp.578–85.

Dohner, H., Estey, E.H., Amadori, S., Appelbaum, F.R., Büchner, T., Burnett, A.K., Dombret, H., Fenaux, P., Grimwade, D., Larson, R.A., Lo-Coco, F., Naoe, T., Niederwieser, D., Ossenkoppele, G.J., Sanz, M., Sierra, J., Tallman, M.S., Löwenberg, B. and Bloomfield, C.D., 2010. Diagnosis and management of acute myeloid leukemia in adults: recommendations from an international expert panel, on behalf of the European LeukemiaNet. *Blood*, 115(3), pp.453–74.

Dohner, K. and Dohner, H., 2008. Molecular characterization of acute myeloid leukemia. *Haematologica*, 93(7), pp.976–82.

Dohner, K., Schlenk, R.F., Habdank, M., Scholl, C., Rucker, F.G., Corbacioglu, A., Bullinger, L., Frohling, S. and Dohner, H., 2005. Mutant nucleophosmin (NPM1) predicts favorable prognosis in younger adults with acute myeloid leukemia and normal cytogenetics: interaction with other gene mutations. *Blood*, 106(12), pp.3740–6.

Dunna, N.R., Rajappa, S., Digumarti, R., Vure, S., Kagita, S., Damineni, S., Rao, V.R., Yadav, S.K., Ravuri, R.R. and Satti, V., 2010. Fms like tyrosine kinase (FLT3) and nucleophosmin 1 (NPM1) mutations in de novo normal karyotype acute myeloid leukemia (AML). *Asian Pacific Journal of Cancer Prevention*, 11(6), pp.1811–16.

Fröhling, S., Schlenk, R.F., Stolze, I., Bihlmayr, J., Benner, A., Kreitmeier, S., Tobis, K., Döhner, H. and Döhner, K., 2004. CEBPA mutations in younger adults with acute myeloid leukemia and normal cytogenetics: prognostic relevance and analysis of cooperating mutations. *Journal of Clinical Oncology*, 22(4), pp.624–33.

Gale, R., Hills, R., Green, C., Patel, Y., Gilkes, A., Lazenby, M., Wheatley, K., Linch, D.C. and Burnett, A., 2008a. The impact of FLT3-ITD and NPM1 mutational status on the outcome of ATRA therapy in patients with non-APL AML: Results of the UK MRC AML12 trial abstract No. 554. *Blood*, 112(11), p.207.

Gale, R.E., Green, C., Allen, C., Mead, A.J., Burnett, A.K., Hills, R.K., Linch, D.C., Medical Research Council Adult Leukaemia Working, P., Hils, R.K. and Wo, M.R.C.A.L., 2008b. The impact of FLT3 internal tandem duplication mutant level, number, size, and interaction with NPM1 mutations in a large cohort of young adult patients with acute myeloid leukemia. *Blood*, 111(5), pp.2776–84.

Grimwade, D., Hills, R.K., Moorman, A. V, Walker, H., Chatters, S., Goldstone, A.H., Wheatley, K., Harrison, C.J., Burnett, A.K. and Group N.C.R.I.A.L.W., 2010. Refinement of cytogenetic classification in acute myeloid leukemia: determination of prognostic significance of rare recurring chromosomal abnormalities among 5876 younger adult patients treated in the United Kingdom Medical Research Council trials. *Blood*, 116(3), pp.354–65.

Hanahan, D. and Weinberg, R.A., 2011. Hallmarks of cancer: the next generation. *Cell*, 144(5), pp.646–74.

Heuser, M., Beutel, G., Krauter, J., Döhner, K., von Neuhoff, N., Schlegelberger, B., Ganser, A. and Doehner, K., 2006. High meningioma 1 (MN1) expression as a predictor for poor outcome in acute myeloid leukemia with normal cytogenetics. *Blood*, 108(12), pp.3898–905.

Kim, Y.K., Kim, H.J.N., Lee, S.R., Ahn, J.S., Yang, D.H., Lee, J.J., Lee, I.K. and Shin, M.G., 2010. Prognostic significance of nucleophosmin mutations and FLT3 internal tandem duplication in adult patients with cytogenetically normal acute myeloid leukemia. *Korean Journal of Hematology*, 45(1), pp.36–45.

Langer, C., Marcucci, G., Holland, K.B., Radmacher, M.D., Maharry, K., Paschka, P., Whitman, S.P., Mrózek, K., Baldus, C.D., Vij, R., Powell, B.L., Carroll, A.J., Kolitz, J.E., Caligiuri, M.A., Larson, R.A. and Bloomfield, C.D., 2009. Prognostic importance of MN1 transcript levels, and biologic insights from MN1-associated gene and microRNA expression signatures in cytogenetically normal acute myeloid leukemia: a cancer and leukemia group B study. *Journal of Clinical Oncology*, 27(19), pp.3198–204.

Langer, C., Radmacher, M.D., Ruppert, A.S., Whitman, S.P., Paschka, P., Mrózek, K., Baldus, C.D., Vukosavljevic, T., Liu, C.G., Ross, M.E., Powell, B.L., de la Chapelle, A., Kolitz, J.E., Larson, R.A., Marcucci, G., Bloomfield, C.D., Cancer and Leukemia Group B (CALGB), 2008. High BAALC expression associates with other molecular prognostic markers, poor outcome, and a distinct gene-expression signature in cytogenetically normal patients younger than 60 years with acute myeloid leukemia: a Cancer and Leukemia Group B (CALGB) study. *Blood*, 111(11), pp.5371–9.

Marcucci, G., Haferlach, T. and Dohner, H., 2011. Molecular genetics of adult acute myeloid leukemia: prognostic and therapeutic implications. *Journal of Clinical Oncology*, 29(5), pp.475–86.

Marcucci, G., Maharry, K., Radmacher, M.D., Mrózek, K., Vukosavljevic, T., Paschka, P., Whitman, S.P., Langer, C., Baldus, C.D., Liu, C.-G., Ruppert, A.S., Powell, B.L., Carroll, A.J., Caligiuri, M.A., Kolitz, J.E., Larson, R.A. and Bloomfield, C.D., 2008. Prognostic significance of, and gene and microRNA expression signatures associated with, CEBPA mutations in cytogenetically normal acute myeloid leukemia with high-risk molecular features: a Cancer and Leukemia Group B study. *Journal of Clinical Oncology*, 26(31), pp.5078–87.

O'Brien, S.G., Guilhot, F., Larson, R.A., Gathmann, I., Baccarani, M., Cervantes, F., Cornelissen, J.J., Fischer, T., Hochhaus, A., Hughes, T., Lechner, K., Nielsen, J.L., Rousselot, P., Reiffers, J., Saglio, G., Shepherd, J., Simonsson, B., Gratwohl, A., Goldman, J.M., Kantarjian, H., Taylor, K., Verhoef, G., Bolton, A.E., Capdeville, R. and Druker, B.J., 2003. Imatinib compared with interferon and low-dose cytarabine for newly diagnosed chronic-phase chronic myeloid leukemia. *New England Journal of Medicine*, 348(11), pp.994–1004.

Paschka, P., Marcucci, G., Ruppert, A.S., Whitman, S.P., Mrózek, K., Maharry, K., Langer, C., Baldus, C.D., Zhao, W., Powell, B.L., Baer, M.R., Carroll, A.J., Caligiuri, M.A., Kolitz, J.E., Larson, R.A. and Bloomfield, C.D., 2008. Wilms' tumor 1 gene mutations independently predict poor outcome in adults with cytogenetically normal acute myeloid leukemia: a Cancer and Leukemia Group B study. *Journal of Clinical Oncology*, 26(28), pp.4595–602.

Pratcorona, M., Brunet, S., Nomdedéu, J., Ribera, J.M., Tormo, M., Duarte, R., Escoda, L., Guàrdia, R., Queipo de Llano, M.P., Salamero, O., Bargay, J., Pedro, C., Martí, J.M., Torrebadell, M., Díaz-Beyá, M., Camós, M., Colomer, D., Hoyos, M., Sierra, J. and Esteve, J., 2013. Favorable outcome of patients with acute myeloid leukemia harboring a low-allelic burden FLT3-ITD mutation and concomitant NPM1 mutation: relevance to post-remission therapy. *Blood*, 121(14), pp.2734–8.

Schlenk, R.F., Dohner, K., Krauter, J., Frohling, S., Corbacioglu, A., Bullinger, L., Habdank, M., Spath, D., Morgan, M., Benner, A., Schlegelberger, B., Heil, G., Ganser, A., Dohner, H. and German-Austrian Acute Myeloid Leukemia Study Group, 2008. Mutations and treatment outcome in cytogenetically normal acute myeloid leukemia. *New England Journal of Medicine*, 358(18), pp.1909–18.

Taskesen, E., Bullinger, L., Corbacioglu, A., Sanders, M., Erpelinck, C.A., Wouters, B.J., van der Poel-van de Luytgaarde, S., Damm, F., Krauter, J., Ganser, A., Schlenk, R.F., Löwenberg, B., Delwel, R., Dohner, H., Valk, P.J. and Dohner, K., 2010. Prognostic impact, concurrent genetic mutations and gene expression features of AML with CEBPA mutations in a cohort of 1182 cytogenetically normal AML patients: further evidence for CEBPA double mutant AML as a distinctive disease entity. *Blood*, 117(8), pp.2469–75.

Thiede, C., Koch, S., Creutzig, E., Steudel, C., Illmer, T., Schaich, M., Ehninger, G. and Leukami, D.S., 2006. Prevalence and prognostic impact of NPM1 mutations in 1485 adult patients with acute myeloid leukemia (AML). *Blood*, 107(10), pp.4011–20.

Vardiman, J.W., Thiele, J., Arber, D.A., Brunning, R.D., Borowitz, M.J., Porwit, A., Harris, N.L., Le Beau, M.M., Hellström-Lindberg, E., Tefferi, A. and Bloomfield, C.D., 2009. The 2008 revision of the World Health Organization (WHO) classification of myeloid neoplasms and acute leukemia: rationale and important changes. *Blood*, 114(5), pp.937–51.

Virappane, P., Gale, R., Hills, R., Kakkas, I., Summers, K., Stevens, J., Allen, C., Green, C., Quentmeier, H., Drexler, H., Burnett, A., Linch, D., Bonnet, D., Lister, T.A. and Fitzgibbon, J., 2008. Mutation of the Wilms' tumor 1 gene is a poor prognostic factor associated with chemotherapy resistance in normal karyotype acute myeloid leukemia: the United Kingdom Medical

Research Council Adult Leukaemia Working Party. *Journal of Clinical Oncology*, 26(33), pp.5429–35.

Wagner, K., Damm, F., Goehring, G., Goerlich, K., Heuser, M., Schaefer, I., Ottmann, O., Luebbert, M., Heit, W., Kanz, L., Schlimok, G.G., Raghavachar, A.A., Fiedler, W., Kirchner, H.H., Brugger, W., Zucknick, M., Schlegelberger, B., Heil, G., Ganser, A., Krauter, J.J., Göhring, G., Görlich, K., Schäfer, I. and Lübbert, M., 2010. Impact of IDH1 R132 mutations and an IDH1 single nucleotide polymorphism in cytogenetically normal acute myeloid leukemia: SNP rs11554137 is an adverse prognostic factor. *Journal of Clinical Oncology*, 28(14), pp.2356–64.

Whitman, S.P., Ruppert, A.S., Radmacher, M.D., Mrózek, K., Paschka, P., Langer, C., Baldus, C.D., Wen, J., Racke, F., Powell, B.L., Kolitz, J.E., Larson, R.A., Caligiuri, M.A., Marcucci, G. and Bloomfield, C.D., 2008. FLT3 D835/I836 mutations are associated with poor disease-free survival and a distinct gene-expression signature among younger adults with de novo cytogenetically normal acute myeloid leukemia lacking FLT3 internal tandem duplications. *Blood*, 111(3), pp.1552–9.

Yanada, M., Matsuo, K., Suzuki, T., Kiyoi, H. and Naoe, T., 2005. Prognostic significance of FLT3 internal tandem duplication and tyrosine kinase domain mutations for acute myeloid leukemia: a meta-analysis. *Leukemia*, 19(8), pp.1345–9.

Chapter 10

Taking it Personally: Patients' Perspectives on Personalised Medicine and its Ethical Relevance

Sabine Wöhlke, Julia Perry and Silke Schicktanz[1]

Introduction

The terms *personalised* or *individualised* medicine advertised and promoted by German (for example, http://www.gesundheitsforschung-bmbf.de/) and international (for example, http://www.p-medizine.eu/) research programmes, seem to be the biomedical buzzwords of the twenty-first century (Hayes, 2010; Langanke et al., 2012). The future differentiation of patients with regard to their response to treatment (for example, on the basis of their pharmacogenetic profile or their gene expression) is an essential aim. These terms are frequently described as misleading (Schleidgen et al., 2013; see also Chapter 1, this volume). Therefore, justifiably, it was proposed to use the term *stratified* medicine (Hüsing et al., 2008). However, this has thus far not become prevalent in academic or public discourse. In addition, there are ethical reasons why it is potentially useful to continue using the term *personalised* medicine, as the use of this term offers the possibility not only to assume the favoured aims as set by biomedicine, but also to critically question the practice regarding its personalisation and, thus, its patient-centredness and, furthermore, to add new objectives (SAMW, 2012; Deutscher Ethikrat, 2013).

This chapter refers to first results of an ongoing study. The purpose of our analysis is the development of biomarkers which should serve as new prognostic tests by means of gene expression profiling for rectal carcinoma, and are to be examined in a large-scale German research study (so-called KFO 179/2). First, the physician-researcher perspective was elicited (Heßling, 2012; Heßling

1   We want to thank all interviewees for their participation and colleagues of the University Medical Centre Göttingen (UMG) for their support. This study was funded by the DFG (Schi/631/4–1).

and Schicktanz, 2012) in a multistage process,[2] then the patient perspective was added in a second research phase.[3] In this chapter, we will focus on the latter.

In order to classify the results, an overview is needed to demonstrate to what extent oncology is a suitable area of investigation for the assessment and ethical implications of *personalised* medicine. We will present our approach in more detail in the section on methodology and react to the patient perspective. The focus is on the particularly relevant fields of informed consent, information and physician–patient communication from an ethical point of view.

The Relevance of Gene Expression Profiling for the Treatment of Rectal Carcinoma

Research in oncology on gene expression profiling and pharmacogenetic tests (summarised as 'biomarker' research in the following) attempts to examine and predict the cause of the patient's response to treatment and the reoccurrence of tumours. It has now become widely known that the response to treatment varies from patient to patient. Not all patients benefit equally from their treatment. This also applies to current treatment of rectal carcinoma, which is the second most common cancer and the second most common cause of death by cancer in Germany.

The current standard treatment consists of three successive steps: neoadjuvant radio-chemotherapy, surgical tumour removal and adjuvant chemotherapy (Schmiegel et al., 2008). Radio-chemotherapy can involve extremely significant side effects. This becomes an even larger burden for patients if they do not respond to neoadjuvant treatment. Thus, an ethical dilemma is associated with the attempt to prolong survival time, on the one hand (with the attempt of intensified treatment), and the preservation of life quality, on the other (with the omission of treatment and, thus, the avoidance of side effects). Currently, in practice, this conflict most commonly results in a decision in favour of intensified treatment.

More precise predictions whether patients will benefit from specific treatments should become possible on the basis of gene expression profiling; this could support the decision on the use or omission of intensified treatment

---

2   See also the results of the MD thesis by Heßling (2014).

3   This is a substantially revised version of Wöhlke et al., 'Wenn es persönlich wird in der "personalisierten Medizin": Aufklärung und Kommunikation aus klinischer Forscher- und Patientenperspektive im empirisch-ethischen Vergleich' ['When it gets personal in "personalised medicine": clinical researchers' and patients' perspectives on counseling and communication in an empirical–ethical comparison'] in: *Ethik in der Medizin* 2013, 25, 215–22. With kind permission of Springer Science+Business Media.

(Ghadimi et al., 2005). However, the application of pharmacogenetic tests and gene expression profiling is limited in the clinical context thus far (EGAPP, 2013; Johnson, 2013; Eckhardt et al., 2014).

Differences were found in the expression of various genes in rectal carcinoma patients, between those who responded to neoadjuvant radiochemotherapy (so-called responders) and those who did not respond (so-called non-responders) (Ghadimi et al., 2005). From the researchers' point of view, the aim of a *personalised* treatment would be the avoidance of an unsuccessful treatment with considerable side effects for non-responders by means of preselecting patients. Our empirical-ethical analysis of this research aims at contributing to the investigation and assessment of practice-oriented and clinical challenges, which are to be expected in the implementation of such testing procedures. At the same time, an important opportunity presents itself to learn considerably more about the clinical practice and patient expectations regarding *personalised* cancer treatment.

Previous problem areas in oncology as well as in *personalised* medicine must be considered in order to better localise the implications of such practice. These can be summarised as follows:

- Existing tradition of strong paternalism (Sandmann and Munthe, 2010; Miller and Joffe, 2013).
- Difficult assessment of treatment outcome and side effects (Oberthuer et al., 2010; Simon, 2010).
- Ethical challenges of non-treatment and non-response (Fierz, 2004; Meyer, 2004).
- Therapeutic misconception in clinical research (Brown et al., 2004; Hull et al., 2008; Wade et al., 2009, Pentz et al., 2012, Henderson et al., 2007).
- Uncertain effects of Big Data collection: will better diagnostics always result in better therapy and cure? (Hedgecoe, 2006; Hopkins et al., 2006; McKinnon et al., 2007; see also Chapter 12, this volume).

Material and Methods

The purpose of our investigation was to examine the research process of the KFO 179 from the patient perspective. Qualitative methods are especially suitable for understanding bioethically relevant values, personal opinions, experiences and context correlations (Chandros-Hull et al., 2001). Our methodological approach consists of two complementary perspectives; in a first step, the treatment and clinical trial consultation between the physician and patient was observed (August 2011 – February 2013; n = 54). In a second step, three interviews were conducted with each patient during the treatment and clinical trial process (September 2011 – October 2013; n = 93). Subsequently, the data was analysed using content analysis. Systematic qualitative empirical data collection was chosen for both research steps, as the research is in an explorative, hypothesis-generating stage (Green and Thorogood, 2009; Popay and Mallison, 2010).

The methodological setting of the interviewing[4] in this research step was complemented by the method of non-participatory (direct) observation (Schnell et al., 2005; Allen, 2010) of physician–patient interaction, due to our interest in the communicative interaction and self-awareness of a multidisciplinary treatment team. This should serve to provide better understanding of the extent to which not only information, but also expectations regarding the course and time of treatment are addressed, and how the process of understanding and, if necessary, consent is structured. Additionally, patients' assessment regarding their treatment was surveyed over the entire process, on average 24 weeks until the end of treatment, by means of semi-structured interviews (Sankar and Jones, 2008).

The non-participatory observation[5] of 50 physician–patient consultations in the surgical and radiotherapy wards took place when therapy options were discussed and the informed consent to undergo the treatment was addressed as well as the participation in the integrated clinical trial for research of biomarkers. During this consultation, *no* genetic test result was available. In order to make this study representative, this number of observed cases was based on the sample size/year/clinic: 50 per cent of approximately 100 cases. This estimated sample size corresponds to the principle of case saturation, with the result that no new aspects were observed after about 45 cases (compare with Table 10.1 on sample size and composition). By February 2013, 54 consultations with a total of 40 patients had been documented.[6]

Each patient was interviewed three times (see Figure 10.1).

The interviews were always conducted at the end of a treatment stage.[7] The first interview was conducted about six to eight weeks after the observation, the second interview during the fourteenth to sixteenth treatment week, and the

---

4   Identification code of the pseudonymised transcripts: M = male; F = female, 1, 2, 3 ... consecutive numbering. A, B or G refer to the respective form of treatment. I, II or III indicate the number of the interview. An additional (B) indicates a statement during the observation. Example: M1A (B) = male, subject no. 1, clinical trial A, observation; F1A, interview III = female, subject no. 1, clinical trial A, interview no. 3.

5   The colleague responsible for the documentation of the observations of the physician-patient consultations was Sabine Wöhlke.

6   The consultation was observed with a third of the patients included in the surgical and radiotherapy wards.

7   All interviews were conducted by Sabine Wöhlke and Julia Perry.

Table 10.1   Socio-demographic data of the observed or interviewed patients

Participants	Observations	Interviews
n = 40	n = 54	n = 93
Length (min.)	Ø 35 min.	Ø 25 min.
Termination of the clinical trial during treatment[a]		2 patients
Socio-demographic data of the included subject group		
Sex	Females	14
	Males	26
Age	18–40	3
	41–60	11
	61–70	17
	71–80	8
	Over 80	1
Educational background	No school-leaving qualification	1
	Elementary school	20
	Secondary school	12
	University degree	5
Family status	Single	2
	Long-term relationship	3
	Married	24
	Divorced	5
	Widowed	6
Religious affiliation	Protestant	25
	Catholic	8
	No religious affiliation	7

Note: [a] The patients' observation records are included in the evaluation, as the patients gave informed consent for the study at each observation or interview, in order not to further burden the patients during a treatment with significant side effects.

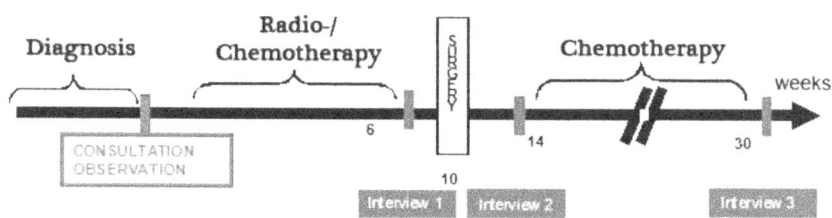

Figure 10.1   Treatment procedure and schedule of non-participatory observation and interviews

third at the end of treatment (approximately the twenty-first to twenty-fourth week after the observation). The central topics were:

- attitudes, evaluation and preferences in the physician–patient consultations;
- understanding of the illness and treatment;
- motivation to participate in oncological clinical trials; and
- assessment and evaluation of gene expression profiling.

The interview participants agreed to the digital recording, transcription and pseudonymisation for the purpose of publication. Participating physicians and patients gave their consent for the non-participatory observation.[8] These consultations were recorded in writing and edited for subsequent data analysis.

A qualitative content analysis (Mayring, 2000; Forman and Damschroder, 2008) was applied to the entire dataset with the programme Atlas.ti™ (Friese, 2011) in order to examine ethically relevant aspects and issues in everyday clinical practice. All of the interviews and observation records were systematically coded according to major topics and minor aspects. The interview guidelines provided the theoretical basis for the content analysis. In addition to the deductive coding, a peer-guided inductive coding was carried out.

Empirical Results

In most cases, patients are transferred to the university clinic treatment team by an external medical specialist with the diagnosis of rectal carcinoma, so that patients have already fundamentally dealt with the diagnosis 'cancer', thus we found aspects of denial (for example, Vos and de Haes, 2007) to not be relevant in this context. The evaluation of the physician–patient consultations observed indicates that informed consent took place orally at the same time as written information on the clinical trial was handed out. However, our detailed analysis of the comparison of informed consent consultations and the interviews conducted subsequently revealed three essential results which emphasise the limitations of informed consent to the biomarker research: (1) the patients are generally overburdened by the complexity of information; (2) the expectations concerning *personalised* medicine go beyond the scope of biomarkers; and (3) from the patients' perspective, 'pragmatic trust' authorises paternalistic informed consent.

---

8 Ethical approval was given for this study (No.1/6/2011) by the Ethics Committee of Göttingen on 12 July 2011.

Overburdening of Patients due to the Complexity of Information

The precarious situation in which the patients find themselves produces various interpretations of the meaning and aim of the biomarker trial, which is primarily characterised by the frequently uttered hope to survive:

> Interviewer: The biomarker trial, do you remember what kind of trial it is that you consented to?
>
> Ms. F: I understood the following: not everyone is asked to consent. And that the aim is to preferably save these patients. In my case the tumour has grown quite far. (P 9, F4B, interview I)

The observations of the consultations, in which informed consent for the locally running biomarker trial also took place, indicate recurring conversational patterns despite physicians maintaining their individual approach. The content of the consultation varies in its focus between the surgical and the radiotherapy ward (the two consultations take place within a few days), which is reasonable from a medical perspective. However, this is very difficult to comprehend for many patients. Confirming the diagnosis as well as the therapy regimen has priority in the surgical ward. The radiotherapy ward focuses especially on the comprehension of neoadjuvant treatment and the respective side effects.

It is especially striking that the actual aim of the clinical trial planned, that is to say stratification of responders/non-responders for neoadjuvant treatment, was not explicitly mentioned. Thus, detailed informed consent to the clinical trial did not take place. Instead, patients were merely asked to consent to specimen collection for scientific purposes, as the following sequence illustrates:

> Mr. E: Yes, sometimes you don't have questions until you're at home, but actually everything is clear. I can't change anything about it anyway (self-conscious laugh and glancing at the physician).
>
> Dr. V: I also need your signature for the specimen collection, with place and date.

The physician helps the patient orient himself in the document and shows where the patient should place his signature on the piece of paper. The patient signs the consent form unread (P 2, M2A (B), proceedings).

The very extensive forms that explain the clinical trial in more detail are frequently only handed to the subjects after the consent to the trial is given. For some patients, the reading posed practical (for example, due to poor eyesight) as well as intellectual challenges. On the part of the physicians, informed consent in the context of the clinical trial varied between efforts to keep expectations of the clinical trial low and highlighting the value of former treatment. Patients are to be motivated to consent to the clinical trial, which is better associated with an enhanced future treatment. Terms such as 'new treatment' and 'standard treatment' are often used in this context. The aim is to highlight that the standard treatment should be enhanced further. A content-related and even situational differentiation between informed consent to treatment and consent to the clinical trial is made in the radiotherapy ward by manually moving the pile of patient records aside and taking a new pile of patient records for the clinical trial.

Some patients interpreted the complex treatment and clinical trial information in a positive manner. Their personal interest in recovering or being cured had priority in the process:

> Mr. G: … first of all I, myself, want to recover … and then maybe also for the future in case it should come again so that they have better results. Well, you can participate and it won't hurt. My advantage is that I have direct contact people. Ms. P. for example or Ms. AB. and I do have the feeling that they could also make a difference. (P 83, M26A, interview I)

These patients perceived the clinical trial staff as having a positive effect by assuming that they were cared for more intensively. Nevertheless, many patients were disconcerted by the complexity of communication alternatives. Most commonly, it was difficult for them to distinguish between the parts belonging to the clinical trial and those belonging to the standard treatment, as the exemplified assertions of patients illustrate:

> Interviewer: Do you remember what the research of this clinical trial entails?

> Mr. V: I have no idea. I don't know. (P 20, M4A, interview I)

> Ms. H: When I was [done] … with it, I had chemo three more times after that. Whether that had something to do with the clinical trial, however, I don't know. (P 8, F3B, interview II)

Reasoning for the purpose of research participation varied on the part of the physicians. Thus, surgeons often used the argument for genetics that would especially become relevant in the future:

> Dr. F: The clinical trial is conducted within the clinical research group. The aim is to examine the tumour biology, not your genetics, but only that of the tumour, as this may have an effect on your children. (P 12, M7B (B), proceedings XII)

This line of argumentation turns out to be highly ambiguous, as patients, in later conversations, give the beneficial effect for their children as a main motive for their participation in research, as the following example indicates:

> Ms. M: Yes, Dr. F. told me that insights could possibly be gained later on that might be important for my relatives, so for my children, for example, to say, OK we maybe should go a bit sooner and have a colonoscopy done or something like that. So that's what I'm looking for in this. (P 12, F7A, interview I)

Being privileged as a clinical trial participant is understood in several conversations of patients with regard to their manner, for example, by referring to 'newer' methods and 'newest' research. Treatment and the aim of the clinical trial were difficult to differentiate for many patients due to research-oriented argumentation by physicians.

Physicians often used further lines of argumentation indirectly based on solidarity when introducing the clinical trial; they indicated that the patients were already profiting from research results of other clinical trial patients. The patients seized this directly and mentioned in interviews conducted subsequently that they also wanted to help others by their participation.

The majority of patients signed the informed consent forms despite initial concerns – in fact, unread, although initially encouraged by the physicians to take their time to read them. Concerns previously directly expressed by patients in most cases referred to organisational questions, such as the time course of the treatment. At the end of the informed consent consultations, it became evident that a number of patients had not understood the complexity of the treatment. Several patients also expressed this lack of understanding in the interviews conducted subsequently. They emphasised that they wanted to be treated without understanding the complexity of treatment rather than criticising the lack of informed consent. They trust the physicians, on the one hand, and do not see an option other than placing their trust in them, on the other hand. Only a few patients explicitly expressed critically, for example, that the amount of information was overwhelming or that they had to sign so much at the clinic in so little time that they did not remember what they had already signed.

Expectations towards Personalised Medicine

The interviews revealed that patients could not conceptualise differentiated treatment due to molecular genetic tests of *personalised* or of *individualised* medicine. By contrast, the term develops a form of dynamic which could actually change the expectations of patients. Thus, it entailed a rather psychosocial interpretation of the person, individual or individuality:

Mr. A: Oh dear, that's difficult. Personal? So referring to the person? Yes, meaning that each individual is catered to, and this data is then collected. (P 26, M7B, interview I)

The expectations went to the length that the term *personalised* medicine was intended as an extremely positive vision for medical care, an ideality:

Mr. G: Personalised? That means it would be directly tailored to a person, right? If I had a doctor who took care of me [and] a nurse who always took care of me. Yes, the ideal, right? (P 83, M26A, interview I)

The idea of what the content or research aim of the clinical trial was turned out to be equally positive. Almost none of the patients interviewed could reconstruct the objective/purpose of stratification of a 'prognostic' test.[9] Improvement of treatment or combination of active ingredients was always highlighted in the patients' explanations, even if they rudimentarily (which rarely occurred) understood the principle of stratification regarding pharmacogenetics.

Ms. F: That you could more precisely say: this and this person should take that and that remedy. Or get that potency for that. I think that's a good thing. ... That's how I understood this. Is that right? And that's exactly why I like this clinical trial. That the attempt is made to protect people from getting an overdose from which they suffer or precisely too little so that it cannot have an effect somehow, have a proper effect. (P 53, F4B, interview II)

The prognostic possibility of early diagnosis with a genetic test was, however, emphasised by some patients.

Mr. G: Of course it would be even better if it could be genetically excluded in advance, [you] will have this illness or [you] will not have this illness. (P 83, M26A, interview I)

The knowledge of the diagnosis 'cancer' as a deadly illness and the immediate bodily experience with treatment marked by numerous side effects does not give patients the option of refusing aggressive treatment, given their will to survive. The assessment of clinical trial participation was, thus, usually interpreted as

---

9   Research is currently directed at the development of an effective prognostic test with the help of biomarkers for the treatment of rectal carcinoma. The aim, in the future, is to classify the neoadjuvant treatment for a certain patient group. The idea is to spare patients who do not respond to neoadjuvant treatment from unnecessary side effects.

having a beneficial effect on one's own illness, especially with regard to the time course. The reference by physicians giving informed consent that future generations could benefit from clinical trial results was, thereby, not related to future generations by some patients, but to themselves.

> Mr. E: It could happen that I get this again. So it [treatment] should be improved and also improved for curing or what. And above all, if I participate in this clinical trial, I'll be doubly well provided for, the blood is tested again, right. I mean that also is [better] for my safety. Because he can see in my blood or so if it is getting worse or better. (P 46, M2B, interview I)

This indicates how complex a form of therapeutic misconception can be, especially as genetic, prognostic and oncological practice converge in this case.

Criticism of *personalised* medicine is expressed concerning special medical knowledge which could prevent the physician from regarding the patient holistically.

> F4B: [...] Personalised [...], then I would if someone said [that] to me spontaneously, then I would say that that is someone who specialises in this. In this area. In my colon cancer for example. And the person responsible for this, but I think it's important not to forget to regard the person as a whole. (P 9, F4B, interview I)

Only in a very few cases was the concept of a prognostic biomarker test understood in the context of *personalised* medicine. The possibility of stratification, however, was regarded very critically:

> Mr. D: Well, but it always is – like in my case – if you don't do it [treatment], you'd later maybe say, if I had done it and I would have gained something. If I'm then told, no nothing is responding, no treatment is, then you'd have drawn the short straw – then you'd be a B-patient. So along the lines of, well, we won't treat you at all, right. (P 24, M6A, interview II)

The wife of a patient who cared for her husband during treatment expressed herself similarly:

> Ms. C: But then you simply don't have the chance … to live longer. Because you simply don't get this treatment, right. (P 19, Wife of M3A, interview II)

'Pragmatic Trust' Authorises Paternalistic Practice in Informed Consent from the Patients' Perspective

The patients' assertions indicate trust as an essential element for consenting to complex medical treatment or trials as a patient. The special relationship to the treating physician is still very important to patients during cancer treatment; the physicians (should) have professional competence in communicating complex medical information. This relationship is embedded in a particular social practice of trust. The kind of trust patients express towards their physicians is, however, neither blind (in a sense of feeling totally dependent and having an emotional bond like a child trusts its parents), nor does it rest upon a mutual relationship based on shared experience and expectations showing each other good will (for example, Baier, 1986), such as that which might exist between equal partners or spouses. It is rather a form of institutional trust, in which patients see the physician in a particular role, but not as an individual person. According to this role, particular expectations of competence (especially with regard to communication) are expressed, including why patients trust their physicians. We call this 'pragmatic trust', as it is neither emotionally based nor dependent on the very personal inter-individual relationship. It is more based and restated in the social practice of physician–patient interaction expressed in the very situation of communication. It is also pragmatic, in the sense that the patient often has no alternative in this situation. Medical decisions based on trust are needed, especially if the decisions are too complex or, as in biomarker research, not all the information is available.

Many patients thus conform to the physician's paternalistic approach in this complex decision situation.

> Mr. E: I actually assumed that the doctors will do this correctly … I thought that if the doctor says that it will be done as such, then that will be correct, because I know nothing about medicine. For now I have to do what the doctor tells me, don't I? (P 17, M2B, interview III)

The professional competence represents an important criterion for the patients, as patients expect from their physicians that they (the physicians) will be able to communicate the complex medical interrelations in a comprehensive manner. They are aware that softer skills, such as empathy, go with this ability to communicate.

> Ms. F: So I think it is very good that there are doctors who specially focus on those kinds of things, who are specialists in that area, so that I have the feeling that he knows exactly what he is doing, what he is prescribing … There has to be a relationship of trust. I have [to be able] to say that that man is personable,

that woman is personable. I trust her and if there is something [between us], then you should look for someone else or place your trust in somebody else. (P 58, F4B, interview I)

Several patients defer to their physicians, others report of their strategy of going to other physicians to get necessary information.

Ms. B.: Yes, but I think that also depends on the people as doctors, the one was better at it and [with] another you didn't feel taken seriously. Then I didn't ask anything else in some cases, because I didn't get an answer. (P 7, F10G, interview I)

This does not only apply to the flow of information, but also to the respective amount of information requested by the patients. Highly complex medicine overburdens patients so that some of them want to make use of their right not to know. The physician's role and obligation is, however, to fully inform the patients. So some patients here see a conflict between their own wishes and the physician's professional duty. The patients must consent to treatment and a connected trial, which they do based on 'pragmatic trust' in the clinic as an institution without, however, being offered a guarantee. For the patients, the selection of information depends on the complexity of treatment; it is seen as part of the physician's duty to make such a selection. The 'pragmatic trust' encompasses an acceptable compromise from both sides with the obligation of informed consent, as the following statement illustrates:

Ms. M: The doctors ... have to explain all of the side-effects and complications ... that's too much for me, that rather scares me. I also said that to Dr. A. ... I told him, you don't have to explain that to me. Well yes, but you have to sign this and I need to inform you about this ... Well OK, is what I thought, say no more. Dr. A. back then said I do have to tell you the most important things, you also have to sign this, but if you don't want to know the rest, because – as I said that makes me frantic – well then you can read this, but I don't necessarily have to tell you, I mean if you don't want me to. So I did have the option back then and then I thought that was OK. (P 12, F7A, interview I)

Instead of a plethora of information, it is very important to the patients, in the oncological context, not to receive euphemistic assertions concerning their illness situation. Correspondingly, they expect honesty and sincerity in relation to critical diagnoses:

Ms. B.: What is important to me? Honesty. So that when I ask, I really get the answer to how it will go on or what it could be like. And that actually always

[was] good up until now, if a doctor did not know, that they did honestly say that it could be like this or like that, we also don't know this, we have to check ourselves. It was always the case that I got good answers, but you have to ask. They won't tell you that much on their own. (P 7, F10G, interview I)

Overall, it becomes apparent that patients frequently act defensively in daily clinical practice due to their illness situation, and develop strategies to deal with authoritarian communication situations. Thus, several patients report that they do not listen closely during the numerous consultations with the physicians, as they are overwhelmed. Instead they only selectively listen by absorbing the aspects important to them or, where applicable, check with the physicians again. The special thing about the 'pragmatic trust' of patients, therefore, lies within weighing and selecting information which leaves the decision process 'open' concerning 'evidence' coming from physicians they trust. This concept goes far beyond 'blind trust', where insufficient information is accompanied by critical thinking. 'Pragmatic trust', apart from the insight concerning complexity, is a product of experience, determination and obligation, as well as general trust in medicine and science for decision-making.

Final Considerations

The preliminary results of our study indicate that the relationship between physician and patient, from the patient's perspective, sways to and fro between the desire for control and self-determination and – rather pragmatic – trust. In their situation, it is often difficult to differentiate between current treatment and research. This behaviour is enhanced by the fact that the use and especially effort of the clinical trials are not always pointed out to the patients (Brown et al., 2011). In addition, the patients' assertions indicate that participation in the clinical trial more frequently originates from personal interest to receive possibly 'better' treatment in the future or to feel more 'secure'. Hence, therapeutic misconception is promoted by communicating the prognostic character of the biomarker trial. A way to avoid this is to be tested in practice with new communication strategies. Along with others (Henman et al., 2002; Sutrop, 2007), our results confirm the relevance for patients to possess medical knowledge; to have the feeling of being informed. This feeling conveys control even if they cannot use it for direct medical decisions. By selecting knowledge, patients fight against losing control, not only with respect to their bodies, but also for future prospects.

From an ethical point of view, it is especially interesting which social dynamic is triggered by the concept of *personalised* medicine. On the part of the medical staff, the concept of *personalised* medicine, thus far, only sporadically enters communication, but here triggers great expectation towards more evidence-based, molecular genetically 'verified' oncological treatment (Heßling and Schicktanz, 2012). On the part of the patients, the expectations are, to a lesser extent, evidence-based or molecular genetic, but much more holistic – whereas a successful physician–patient relationship still primarily requires honesty and empathy on the part of the physician. Interestingly, and contrary to other studies (Hillen et al., 2012), the patients interviewed do not mention the otherwise so important aspect of confidentiality. *Personalised* medicine from the patients' perspective gets personal when the person, as such, has priority, whereas they perceive their illness as multifactorial and not as purely molecular genetic (Gollust et al., 2012) – thus, communication is every bit as important as successful treatment.

With regard to communication and information, our results are similar to those in the study by Wäscher et al. (2013) (see also Chapter 11, this volume), implying that physicians in some cases conduct the conversation with fixed, ethically animated strategies (for example, informing intensively, although this is not desired by the patient). By doing this, they may not only direct decisions, but may also reduce the concept of self-determination to a content-related, cognitive-oriented form (Brown et al., 2004).

On the basis of the empirical observations of a procedure on eliciting so-called informed consent, we experience numerous problems and unresolved questions (Jenkins et al., 2011). There must be a critical discussion from an ethical standpoint whether the formal paradigm of information, for example, in the form of page-filling informed consent forms, really fulfils the strengthening of patient autonomy. We are concerned that it is instead just a process of juridification of the informed consent procedure. It is imperative that alternative models of information and communication are developed and empirically tested successively from an ethical point of view. The 'slippery slope' would be that the plethora of information of molecular biological tests would presumably push the already problematic situation further in the direction of a flood of information, and thus, towards more paternalistic behaviour in practice again, even if theoretically not wanted.

References

Allen, D., 2010. Fieldwork and participant observation. In: I. Bourgeault, R. Dingwall and R. De Vries, eds. *Qualitative methods in health research*. Los Angeles: Sage. pp.353–72.

Baier, A.C., 1986. Trust and antitrust. *Ethics*, 96, pp.231–60.

Brown, R.F., Bylund, C.L., Siminoff, L.A. and Slovin, S.F., 2011. Seeking informed consent to Phase I cancer clinical trials: identifiying oncologists' communication strategies. *Psycho-Oncology*, 20, pp.361–8.

Brown, R.F., Butow, P.N., Butt, D.G., Moore, A.R. and Tattersall, M.H.N., 2004. Developing ethical strategies to assist oncologists in seeking informed consent to cancer clinical trials. *Social Science & Medicine*, 58(2), pp.379–90.

Chandros-Hull, S., Taylor, H. and Kass, N., 2001. Qualitative methods. In: J. Sugarman and D. Sulmasy, eds. *Methods in medical ethics*. Washington, DC: Georgetown University Press. pp.146–68.

Deutscher Ethikrat 2013. *Die Zukunft der genetischen Diagnostik – von der Forschung in die klinische Anwendung – Stellungnahme [The future of genetic diagnostics – from research to clinical application – opinion]*. Berlin. [online] Available at: http://www.ethikrat.org/dateien/pdf/stellungnahme-zukunft-der-genetischen-diagnostik.pdf [Accessed 22 May 2014].

Eckhardt, A., Navarini, A.A., Recher, A., Rippe, K.P., Rütsche, B., Telset, H. and Marti, M., 2014. *Personalisierte Medizin [Personalised medicine]*. Zürich: TA-SWISS, Zentrum für Technologiefolgen-Abschätzung.

EGAPP (Evaluation of Genomic Applications in Practice and Prevention) Working Group, 2013. Recommendations from the EGAPP Working Group: can testing of tumor tissue for mutations in EGFR pathway downstream effector genes in patients with metastatic colorectal cancer improve health outcomes by guiding decisions regarding anti-EGFR therapy? [EGAPP Recommendation Statement]. *Genetics in Medicine*, 15(7), pp.517–27.

Fierz, W., 2004. Challenge of personalized health care: to what extent is medicine already individualized and what are the future trends? *Medical Science Monitor*, 10(5), pp.RA111–23.

Forman, J. and Damschroder, L., 2008. Qualitative content analysis. In: L. Jacoby and L.A. Siminoff, eds. *Empirical methods for bioethics: a primer*. Amsterdam: Elsevier. pp.39–63.

Friese, S., 2011. *Qualitative data analysis with Atlas.ti*. London: SAGE Publications Ltd.

Ghadimi, B.M., Grade, M., Difilippantonio, M.J., Varma, S., Simon, R., Montagna, C., Füzesi, L., Langer, C., Becker, H., Liersch, T. and Ried, T., 2005. Effectiveness of gene expression profiling for response prediction of rectal adenocarcinomas to preoperative chemoradiotherapy. *Journal of Clinical Oncology*, 23(9), pp.1826–38.

Gollust, S.E., Gordon, E.S., Zayak, C., Griffin, G., Christman, M.F., Pyeritz, R.E., Wawak, L. and Bernhardt, B.A., 2012. Motivations and perceptions of early adopters of personalized genomics: perspectives from research participants. *Public Health Genomics*, 15(1), pp.22–30.

Green, J. and Thorogood, N., 2009. *Qualitative methods for health research*. 2nd edn. London: Sage.

Hayes, D.F., 2010. Contribution of biomarkers to personalized medicine. *Breast Cancer Research*, 12(4), pp.1–2.

Hedgecoe, A.M., 2006. Context, ethics and pharmacogenetics. *Studies in History and Philosophy of Biological and Biomedical Sciences*, 37(3), pp.566–82.

Henderson, G.E., Churchill, L.R., Davis, A.M., Easter, M.M., Grady, C., Joffe, S., Kass, N., King, N.M.P., Lidz, C.W., Miller, F.G., Nelson, D.K., Peppercorn, J., Rothschild, B.B., Sankar, P., Wilfond, B.S., Zimmer, C.R., 2007 Clinical Trials and Medical Care: Defining the Therapeutic Misconception. *PLoS Medicine*, 4(11), pp.1735–38.

Henman, M.J., Butow, P.N., Brown, R.F., Boyle, F. and Tattersall, M.H., 2002. Lay constructions of decision-making in cancer. *Psycho-Oncology*, 11, pp.295–306.

Heßling, A., 2012. 'Everything better than 50% is better than now'. In: P. Dabrock, M. Braun and J. Ried, eds. *Individualized medicine between hype and hope*. Zürich and Berlin: Lit-Verlag. pp.111–35.

Heßling, A., 2014. *Exploration medizinethischer Implikationen individualisierter Diagnostik und Prognostik beim lokal fortgeschrittenen Rektumkarzinom aus Sicht von Ärzten und Forschern – eine empirisch-ethische Untersuchung [Exploration of physicians' and researchers' understanding of the implications of individualized medicine of the locally advanced colorectal cancer on medical ethics. An ethical–empirical study]*. M.D. Universitätsmedizin Göttingen, Göttingen.

Heßling, A. and Schicktanz, S., 2012. What German experts expect from individualized medicine: problems of uncertainty and future complication in physician–patient interaction. *Clinical Ethics*, 7, pp.86–93.

Hillen, M.A., Onderwater, A.T., van Zwieten, M.C., de Haes, H.C. and Smets, E.M., 2012. Disentangling cancer patients' trust in their oncologist: a qualitative study. *Psycho-Oncology*, 21(4), pp.392–9.

Hopkins, M.M., Ibarreta, D., Gaisser, S., Enzing, C.M., Ryan, J., Martin, P.A., Lewis, G., Detmar, S., van den Akker-van Marle, M.E., Hedgecoe, A.M., Nightingale, P., Dreiling, M., Hartig, K.J., Vullings, W. and Forde, T., 2006. Putting pharmacogenetics into practice. *Nature Biotechnology*, 24(4), pp.403–10.

Hull, S.C., Sharp, R.R., Botkin, J.R., Brown, M., Hughes, M., Sugarman, J., Schwinn, D., Sankar, P., Bolcic-Jankovic, D., Clarridge, B.R. and Wilfond, B.S., 2008. Patients' views on identifiability of samples and informed consent for genetic research. *American Journal of Bioethics*, 8(10), pp.62–70.

Hüsing, B., Hartig, J., Bührlen, B., Reiß, T. and Gaisser, S., 2008. *Individualisierte Medizin und Gesundheitssystem. Zukunftsreport [Personalised medicine and the health system. Future report]*. Arbeitsbericht Nr. 126. Berlin: Büro für Technikfolgen-Abschätzung beim deutschen Bundestag.

Jenkins, V., Solis-Trapala, I., Langridge, C., Catt, S., Talbot, D.C. and Fallowfield, L.J., 2011. What oncologists believe they said and what patients believe they heard: an analysis of phase I trial discussions. *Journal of Clinical Oncology*, 29(1), pp.61–8.

Johnson, J.A., 2013. Pharmacogenetics in clinical practice: how far have we come and where are we going? *Pharmacogenomics*, 14(7), pp.835–43.

Langanke, M., Lieb, W., Erdmann, P., Dörr, M., Fischer, T., Kroemer, H., Flessa, S. and Assel, H., 2012. Was ist individualisierte Medizin? – Zur terminologischen Justierung eines schillernden Begriffs [What is personalised medicine? – To a terminological adjustment of a dazzling concept]. *Zeitschrift für medizinische Ethik*, 58(4), pp.295–314.

Mayring, P., 2000. Qualitative content analysis. *Forum Qualitative Sozialforschung*, [online] 1(2). Available at: http://www.qualitative-research.net/index.php/fqs/article/view/1089/2385%3E [Accessed 13 June 2014].

McKinnon, R.A., Ward, M.B. and Sorich, M.J., 2007. A critical analysis of barriers to the clinical implementation of pharmacogenomics. *Journal of Therapeutics and Clinical Risk Management*, 3(5), pp.751–9.

Meyer, U.A., 2004. Pharmacogenetics – five decades of therapeutic lessons from genetic diversity. *Nature Reviews*, 5(9), pp.669–76.

Miller, F.G. and Joffe, S., 2013. Phase 1 oncology trials and informed consent. *Journal of Medical Ethics*, 39, pp.761–4.

Oberthuer, A., Hero, B., Berthold, F., Juraeva, D., Faldum, A., Kahlert, Y., Asgharzadeh, S., Seeger, R., Scaruffi, P., Tonini, G.P., Janoueix-Lerosey, I., Delattre, O., Schleiermacher, G., Vandesompele, J., Vermeulen, J., Speleman, F., Noguera, R., Piqueras, M., Bénard, J., Valent, A., Avigad, S., Yaniv, I., Weber, A., Christiansen, H., Grundy, R.G., Schardt, K., Schwab, M., Eils, R., Warnat, P., Kaderali, L., Simon, T., Decarolis, B., Theissen, J., Westermann, F., Brors, B. and Fischer, M., 2010. Prognostic impact of gene expression-based classification for neuroblastoma. *Journal of Clinical Oncology*, 28(21), pp.3506–15.

Pentz, R.D., White, M., Harvey, D.R., Farmer, L.Z., Liu, Y., Lewis, C., Dashevskaya, O., Owonikoko, T., Khuri, F.R., 2012. Therapeutic Misconception, Misestimation, and Optimism in Partcipants Enrolled in Phase I Trials. *Cancer*, 118(18), pp.4571–8.

Popay, J. and Mallison, S., 2010. Qualitative research. Review and synthesis. In: I. Bourgeault, R. Dingwall and R. de Vries, eds. *Qualitative methods in health research*. London: Sage. pp.289–307.

SAMW (Schweizerische Akademie der Medizinischen Wissenschaften), 2012. *Potenzial und Grenzen von 'Individualisierter Medizin' (personalized medicine) [Potential and limits of 'Individualized Medicine' (personalized medicine)]*. Basel: Schwabe AG.

Sandmann, L. and Munthe, C., 2010. Shared decision making, paternalism and patient choice. *Health Care Analysis*, 18(1), pp.60–84.

Sankar, P. and Jones, N.L., 2008. Semi-structured interviews in bioethics research. In: L. Jacoby and L.A. Siminoff, eds. *Empirical methods for bioethics: a primer*. Amsterdam: Elevesier. pp.117–39.

Schleidgen, S., Klingler, C., Bartram, T., Rogowski, W.H. and Marckmann, G., 2013. What is personalized medicine: sharpening a vague term based on a systematic literature review. *BMC Medical Ethics*, 14, p.55.

Schmiegel, W., Pox, C., Reinacher-Schick, A., Adler, G., Fleig, W., Fölsch, U.R., Frühmorgen, P., Graeven, U., Hohenberger, W., Holstege, A., Junginger, T., Kopp, I., Kühlbacher, T., Porschen, R., Propping, P., Riemann, J.-F., Rödel, C., Sauer, R., Sauerbach, T., Schmitt, W., Schmoll, H.-J., Zeitz, M. and Selbmann, H.-K., 2008. S3-Leitlinie 'Kolorektales Karzinom' Ergebnisse evidenzbasierter Konsensuskonferenzen am 6./7. Februar 2004 und am 8./9. Juni 2007 (für die Themenkomplexe IV, VI und VII) [S3-Guideline 'Colorectal Cancer' 2004/2008]. *Zeitschrift für Gastroenterologie*, 46, pp.1–73.

Schnell, R., Hill, P.B. and Esser, E., 2005. *Methoden der empirischen Sozialforschung [Methods of empirical social research]*. München: Oldenbourg.

Simon, R., 2010. Clinical trial designs for evaluating the medical utility of prognostic and predictive biomarkers in oncology. *Personalized Medicine*, 7(1), pp.33–47.

Sutrop, M., 2007. Trust. In: M. Sutrop, ed. *The ethics and governance of human genetic databases*. Cambridge: Cambridge University Press. pp.190–8.

Vos, M.S., de Haes, J.C.J.M, 2007. Denial in cancer patients, an explorative review. *Psycho-Oncology*, 16(1), pp.12-25.

Wade, J., Donovan, J.L., Lane, J.A., Neal, D.E. and Hamdy, F.C., 2009. It's not just what you say, it's also how you say it: opening the 'black box' of informed consent appointments in randomised controlled trials. *Social Science & Medicine*, 68(11), pp.2018–28.

Wäscher, S., Schildmann, J., Brall, C. and Vollmann, J., 2013. 'Personalisierte Medizin' in der Onkologie: Ärztliche Einschätzungen der aktuellen Entwicklung in der Krankenversorgung ['Personalised medicine' in oncology: physicians' perspectives concerning current developments in patient care. Results of a qualitative interview study]. *Ethik in der Medizin*, 25(3), pp.205–14.

Wöhlke, S., Heßling, A. and Schicktanz, S., 2013. Wenn es persönlich wird in der 'personalisierten Medizin': Aufklärung und Kommunikation aus klinischer Forscher- und Patientenperspektive im empirisch-ethischen Vergleich [When it gets personal in 'personalised medicine': clinical researchers' and patients' perspective on counseling and communication in an empirical-ethical comparison]. *Ethik in der Medizin*, 25, pp.215–22.

Chapter 11

'Personalised Medicine' in Oncology: Physicians' Perspectives on Contributions to and Challenges for Clinical Practice[1]

Sebastian Wäscher,* Jan Schildmann,* Caroline Brall and Jochen Vollmann[2]

Background

So-called 'personalised medicine' as a genomic-based stratification of patient groups[3] has been part of many controversies in the public and scientific sphere (Cascorbi, 2010). Within medicine, the phrase stands as a symbol for new developments and hopes for future progress in prevention, diagnostics and therapy (Hempel, 2009; Hamburg and Collins, 2010; Siegmund-Schultze, 2011). However, there are also critical remarks such as reference to the current scarcity of solid evidence for targeted therapy and questions regarding the financing of effective measures for often small patient groups within a public health-care system (Browman et al., 2011; Ludwig, 2012; Vollmann, 2013).

---

*   Shared first authorship.

1   This chapter was originally published in German in a slightly modified form, under the title '"Personalisierte Medizin" in der Onkologie: Ärztliche Einschätzungen der aktuellen Entwicklung in der Krankenversorgung Ergebnisse einer qualitativen Interviewstudie' in: *Ethik in der Medizin* 2013, 25, 205–14. With kind permission of Springer Science+Business Media.

2   This study was conducted in the research network Personalised Medicine in Oncology: An Interdisciplinary Study on Ethical, Medical, Economical and Legal Aspects (Grant project number: 01 GP 1001A-C), which is supported by the German Federal Ministry of Education and Research (Bundesministerium für Bildung und Forschung – BMBF). The authors declare no conflicts of interest.

3   For a discussion on the term, see Siegmund-Schultze (2011), Langanke et al. (2012) or Schleidgen et al. (2013).

The discussions in medical ethics are concerned with the conception of a 'personalised medicine' and the analysis of ethical implications for the health-care system (Gadebusch Bondio and Michl, 2010). On the conceptual level, the phrase 'personalised medicine' is in the centre of the criticism (for a discussion on the definition of 'personalised medicine', see Chapter 1, this volume). The use of the normative laden word 'person' in the context of a genetic make-up reduced medical approach is criticised among many contemporary articles (Dabrock et al., 2012; Maio, 2012; Vollmann, 2013; see also chapters 4 and 5, this volume). On the level of individual ethics, the right of informational self-determination of test participants and patients is the starting point of several normative discussions. In this context the frequent practice of 'broad' consent has been challenged and the application of standards of informed consent has been called for (Boniolo et al., 2012; Kohnen et al., 2012; for discussion on biobanking, see chapters 7 and 8, this volume). From a social ethics perspective, questions of allocation are in the centre of medical ethics analyses. The comparison of high-cost basic research required for 'personalised medicine' and the expensive targeted therapies (Meropol et al., 2009; Elkin and Bach, 2010), on the one hand, with the resources available for psychosocial and patient-centred measures deemed important by the public on the other hand (Bundesministerium für Bildung und Forschung, 2011), raises the question of a fair and justified distribution of financial means in the health-care system.

Ethical aspects of 'personalised medicine' from the perspective of relevant stakeholders has been researched only occasionally (Gollust et al., 2012; Heßling and Schicktanz, 2012; see also Chapter 10, this volume). In the present qualitative interview study, physicians active in research and clinical work in haematology and oncology have been asked to state their perceptions and judgments on 'personalised approaches' in oncology. The main aspect of this chapter addresses the assessments of physicians in terms of the relevance of 'personalised medicine' for an improved health care for patients with cancer. In addition, the clinical and professional challenges in the context of 'personalised medicine' will be explored. The research results will be discussed against the backdrop of theoretical and empirical papers dealing with medical and ethical aspects of 'personalised medicine'.

Research Participants and Methods

The physicians interviewed worked in the patient and/or outpatient clinic with a speciality in haematology and oncology. The first subset of interview partners was recruited through a convenience sampling of personally known physicians. After the first interview, more interview partners were recruited by recommendation following snowball sampling.[4]

The participants were informed about the study and gave their consent to the digital audio recording of the interviews. The research interviews were conducted on the basis of a semi-structured guideline. The guideline was structured into four parts. The first part asks for the meaning of 'personalised medicine' and is used to enter the interview. The other three parts dealt with the status quo of 'personalised medicine', the expectations of physicians on the future of 'personalised medicine' and anticipated problems of implementation. The transcribed and anonymised interviews were analysed on the basis of grounded theory principles (Strauss and Corbin, 1996).[5] The interviews have been coded by iterative analysis of data gathering and data analysis.

The next step of analysis was to summarise similar topics or interrelated concepts into general categories. On the basis of the first six interviews, preliminary categories were constructed and then discussed by the authors in several workshops. These categories served as a basis for further analysis of the remaining interviews. The results of the analysis were again discussed in an interdisciplinary research colloquium with researchers from the fields of medicine, medical ethics, philosophy and social sciences. Theoretical saturation has been reached which means that the discussions made clear that new evidence would probably not change the interpretation. This chapter focuses on the interview passages that address the current state-of-the-art and the future potential of so-called 'personalised medicine'.

Results

Eleven research interviews were conducted. The interviews took 49 minutes on average (from 17 to 66 minutes). Most (n = 9) of the physicians interviewed were clinicians and researchers in the field of medicine.

Table 11.1 gives an overview of the demographics of the interview participants.

---

4   The research project was approved by the ethics committee of the Ruhr-University Bochum on 1 July 2012 (4431–12).

5   A qualitative picture and literature analysis preceded the interview study. This analysis had an impact on the construction of the interview guideline, as well as on the categories derived from the interview data.

Table 11.1 Socio-demographic data

Interviewee	Age	Sex	Position	Setting	State
PM 01	42	m	consultant	Hospital	Lower Saxony
PM 02	45	f	consultant	Practice	Berlin
PM 03	35	m	consultant	Hospital	North Rhine-Westphalia
PM 04	43	m	attending	Hospital	Lower Saxony
PM 05	40	m	attending	Hospital	Berlin
PM 06	39	m	consultant	Hospital	Saxony
PM 07	30	f	physician	Hospital	Saxony
PM 08	41	m	attending	Hospital	Saxony
PM 09	45	f	attending	Hospital	North Rhine-Westphalia
PM 10	53	m	attending	Hospital	Bavaria
PM 11	45	m	attending	Hospital	Bavaria

State-of-the-Art of 'Personalised Medicine' and its Potential for Further Development in Oncology

The physicians interviewed generally take a positive perspective in terms of the new possibilities due to genetic, stratifying approaches. Contrary to the often high expectations from the public with regard to 'personalised medicine', physicians draw a more balanced picture. 'Personalised medicine' is viewed as a part of the medical progress which helps to improve the medical care for cancer patients. Regarding future advances of 'personalised medicine', the interviewees think that an improvement of medical care for subgroups due to genetic stratification is realistic. However, an individually tailored therapy is judged to be unrealistic. The physicians stress that the whole change in medicine labelled 'personalised medicine' is a continuous development rather than a new medical age from a clinical and practical point of view.

> I don't expect that something spectacular will happen but rather a refinement of medical indication and therapy options. Thus, a broader choice of therapeutic options. Without doubt, there will be smaller groups of patients which will be treated more specifically. But personalised medicine by its name would mean that everybody would get his or her tailored medicine and that is something I really don't see nowadays. (PM 10)

Increase of Information as the Basis for Challenges Emerging in the Context of 'Personalised Medicine'

The increase of information in the context of 'personalised medicine' is one central topic within the research interviews. There is a widely shared agreement about a huge information increase within a short period of time due to molecular findings.

> Due to the huge projects during the last few years, it is possible to generate information much faster and in much more detail than it was 20 years ago; also much more complex information, which we certainly understand only rudimentarily nowadays. (PM 01)

Taking into account all of these new aspects raises the complexity of decision-making and challenges oncological physicians in terms of understanding, overview and utilisation of genetically based information.

> It got extremely difficult to find, let's say, the really important information and to filter it. That's the one thing, that the mass of information has risen extremely and the other matter of fact is that the complexity of information has increased. (PM 08)

In addition to the general statements of the physicians interviewed on the increase in information and complexity, the interviews revealed several challenges and response strategies used in clinical practice.

Understanding and Making Use of Information for Clinical Practice

In light of the obvious increase of research data, one main challenge following the people interviewed is to understand the richness of information in terms of their thinking regarding diagnostics, prognostics and therapy for the individual/ single patient and, therefore, utilising these for clinical practice.

> I think that most of the job will be, first of all, the knowledge of data, and secondly, the estimation. If and for which patients – for me – may be reasonable … that means I have to keep in mind things I didn't have to keep in mind before. (PM 02)

For the physicians, this means that they have to use their resources in the first line to read the relevant studies in order to recognise the whole spectrum of possibilities. The broadened spectrum of possibilities makes the appropriate selection of information and afterwards the decision for a specific treatment more difficult.

> It is so complex that you can't really overview everything anymore. That's a bit the problem we have ... We have huge amounts of data and, like I said before, if you analyse a tumour, you may have 50 hits. Then the question arises, which of these 50 hits is now the one keeping the tumour alive. (PM 04)

Partially, the physicians speak of mental overload, due to the need to stay up to date with the scientific development, especially in view of an already high workload.

> I believe that this cannot be carried out with a regular activity of synapses. At least not with concerns of this amount. (PM08)

Differentiation of Expertise

One result of the challenges mentioned above from the physicians' perspective is the differentiation of additional medical expertise. This development is understandable, as the information flood has to be reduced to an amount which can be overviewed and handled by a single individual in order to make clinical use of the information. Expertise in this manner can be understood as a strategy to reduce complexity to a practicable amount.

> You have to imagine, you go from one branch or from the tree's trunk further and further to the branching, then you sit somewhere far to the left, but nobody knows the branch on the right or at least not as well anymore because he can't overview everything. And that's the problem – when you go from the trunk to the periphery, and that's the problem this personalised medicine bears, that you need more and more experts due to the new diagnostic possibilities. (PM 03)

The increased differentiation of expertise and division of labour leads to the challenge to gather the expertise needed for a specific treatment in clinical practice. Corresponding to this, it becomes more difficult for physicians to be a competent counterpart for the patient in terms of a broad overview of the patient's medical history.

> I think this development in medicine and also the specialisation maybe even in terms of this personalised medicine will result in many specialists who have knowledge in one medical field and that one person alone can't cover everything. Thus, this classic oncologist who knows everything, that's very hard to obtain anyway. (PM03)

'Personalised Medicine' and Standardisation

The respondents in several research interviews say that an increasing standardisation due to clinical guidelines and treatment decisions on the basis of biomarker findings may develop in the context of 'personalised medicine'.

> I worry that indeed physicians will become such administrators of markers. That the art of healing and – What is a human? What is the end of life? How to deal with the illness? – that this gets into the background. Instead, you build a follow-up of therapies thinking, that's the best for a group of patients with such and such features – like guideline appropriate, like pigeonholing. The human can't be pigeonholed. (PM 02)

Standardisation in clinical practice can be understood as an additional means to reduce complexity. Due to standards, not all coherences have to be taken into account. Instead, algorithms can be used to decide actions in a short period of time.

Albeit the respondents see this development not only in the context of 'personalised medicine', but also several interviews showed that guidelines and similar recommendations may lead to tension for the physicians concerning an individual treatment for patients.

> The matter is to find the right therapy for the individual patient. We have no cookbook medicine, especially not in oncology … With increasingly complex therapy options there is more than one right therapy for the patient. By now, I exaggerate, we have ten options. And to find the right therapy from the three, to eight, to ten, is just possible on behalf of the individual situation of the patient. (PM 09)

Discussion

On the basis of the interviews analysed, a nuanced picture of 'personalised medicine' can be drawn . Besides the reference to improvements which have occurred already in respect of medical treatment of some cancer patient subgroups and positive expectations regarding further progression due to the improved understanding of the whole genome, the interviews convey that the whole development in clinical practice is described as an evolution rather than a revolution, or even a paradigm shift (Hempel, 2009). The valuation of the physicians interviewed can inform the scientific and public debate insofar as they present a standpoint in between two extremes in medicine (Chin et al., 2011 versus Ludwig, 2012), as well as in medical ethics and other professional fields (Prainsack et al., 2008; Brand, 2009 versus Maio, 2012), of the chances and risks of 'personalised medicine'.

Following the interviews, one core problem in the context of 'personalised medicine' is the heavy increase of information (see p.153 for another discussion on challenges due to the data amount, see Chapter 12, this volume). Because of molecular genetic analysis, lots of new data pour into the medical daily routine which can be handled only with difficulty (Sledge, 2012). The physicians view this as a major challenge (see pp.153f.). Consequently, the physicians' professional self-perception is exposed to an almost paradoxical tension. On the one hand, the physicians want to meet the needs of their patients and see the potential due to the new options to provide a better individual treatment. On the other hand, the overwhelming information flood seems to force them to find solutions in the form of strategies to reduce complexity.

The procedures of solutions to handle the information flood identified (see pp.154f.) bear problems themselves, from which only two can be sketched here. First, due to the increased differentiation of expertise, it is likely that a holistic physician–patient relationship will be constantly eroded. Because of the numerous contacts with experts, it becomes increasingly difficult to preserve an overview for the treating physicians. Second, treatment could be constantly generalised due to increasing standardisation and usage of molecular biomarkers, with the result that the focus of the treatment lies on the specific parameter of the illness and body functions instead of on the patient.

On the basis of the interviews analysed, it seems possible that, due to a change in the physician–patient relationship and the upcoming new standards of therapy, a process may begin which can be framed with the phrase 'fragmentation of the person'. This thesis is also supported by other authors who realise the reduction of the patient to impersonal datasets as a 'depersonalisation' (Heßling and Schicktanz, 2012). Even though it does not mean the same phenomena, the findings could be interpreted in a similar direction. In view of this sketched development and the resulting consequences, one has to ask whether a 'personalised medicine' can serve the patient as a person, like the name suggests, or not. Based on the qualitative analysis of the research interviews, it can be summarised that a promotion of 'personalised medicine' is in general supported by oncological physicians. However, a one-sided orientation on genetic stratification and a corresponding priority setting of resources in research and practice is not reasonable from a medical practical point of view. Besides this, the focus on genetic information for diagnostics and therapy may lead to conflicts within the clinical practice in terms of patient-centred medicine.

It can be stated principally that the development of new technologies and the information generated by this are not in contradiction on a principal level to patient-centred medicine (Dabrock et al., 2012). The tension mentioned can be interpreted as a conflict of priority setting of the physician's resources (Vollmann, 2013). The statements of the respondents in the context of information increase and increase of complexity indicate that a professional and competent utilisation and judgement of genetic information requires an expertise which cannot be taken for granted. This more or less critical appraisal is especially interesting because of the homogeneity of the physicians interviewed, who work largely clinically and do research at university hospitals. From a medical ethics perspective, it is questionable whether priority setting should lay weight on education in genetic knowledge or not (Konstantinopoulos et al., 2009), and keep in mind the time-consuming aspects in daily clinical practice in terms of ideal medical care (Burke and Psaty, 2007). Furthermore, the amount and the growing complexity of information have to be discussed as a challenge for an appropriate procedure of informed consent.

Limitation

Qualitative studies offer the opportunity to explore complex matters of fact, such as the perceptions and judgements on 'personalised medicine'. In this way, profound expert knowledge can be utilised for medical and ethical discussion. The research results cannot be generalised for all oncologists due to the methodological design. The fact that the (sub-)categories are contingent, that means plausible and well-funded, but not 'objective', should also be taken into account.

References

Boniolo, G., di Fiore, P.P. and Pece, S., 2012. Trusted consent and research biobanks: towards a 'new alliance' between researchers and donors. *Bioethics*, 26, pp.93–100.

Brand, A., 2009. Integrative genomics, personal-genome tests and personalised healthcare: the future is being built today. *European Journal of Human Genetics*, 17, pp.977–8.

Browman, G., Hébert, P.C. and Coutts, J., 2011. Personalised medicine: a windfall for science, but what about patients? *Canadian Medical Association Journal*, 183, p.E1277.

Bundesministerium für Bildung und Forschung, 2011. *Bürgerreport Hightech-Medizin – Welche Gesundheit wollen wir? [Citizens report: high-tech medicine – what health do we want?]*. Berlin: Bundesministerium für Bildung und Forschung.

Burke, W. and Psaty, B.M., 2007. Personalised medicine in the era of genomics. *Journal of the American Medical Association*, 298, pp.1682–4.

Cascorbi, I., 2010. The promises of personalised medicine. *European Journal of Clinical Pharmacology*, 66, pp.749–54.

Chin, L., Andersen, J.N. and Futreal, P.A., 2011. Cancer genomics: from discovery science to personalised medicine. *Nature Medicine*, 17, pp.297–303.

Dabrock, P., Braun, M. and Ried, J., 2012. Individualisierte Medizin [Individualised medicine]. *Forum*, 27, pp.209–13.

Elkin, E.B. and Bach, P.B., 2010. Cancer's next frontier: addressing high and increasing costs. *Journal of the American Medical Association*, 303, pp.1086–7.

Gadebusch Bondio, M. and Michl, S., 2010. Individualisierte Medizin. Die neue Medizin und ihre Versprechen [Individualised medicine. The new medicine and its promise]. *Deutsches Ärzteblatt*, 107, pp.A1062–4.

Gollust, S.E., Gordon, E.S., Zayac, C., Griffin, G., Christman, M.F., Pyeritz, R.E., Wawak, L. and Bernhardt, B.A., 2012. Motivations and perceptions of early adopters of personalised genomics: perspectives from research participants. *Public Health Genomics*, 15, pp.22–30.

Hamburg, M.A. and Collins, F.S., 2010. The path to personalised medicine. *New England Journal of Medicine*, 363, pp.301–4.

Hempel, U., 2009. Personalisierte Medizin I. Keine Heilkunst mehr, sondern rationale, molekulare Wissenschaft [Personalised medicine I. No more medicine, but rational, molecular science]. *Deutsches Ärzteblatt*, 106, pp.A2068–70.

Heßling, A. and Schicktanz, S., 2012. What German experts expect from individualized medicine: problems of uncertainty and future complication in physician-patient interaction. *Clinical Ethics*, 7, pp.86–93.

Kohnen, T., Schildmann, J. and Vollmann, J., 2012. Patients' self-determination in 'personalised medicine': the case of whole genome sequencing and tissue banking in oncology. In: P. Dabrock, M. Braum and J. Ried, eds. *Individualised medicine between hype and hope*. Münster: LIT. pp.97–110.

Konstantinopoulos, P.A., Karamouzis, M.V. and Papavassiliou, A.G., 2009. Educational and social-ethical issues in the pursuit of molecular medicine. *Molecular Medicine*, 15, pp.60–3.

Langanke, M., Lieb, W., Erdmann, P., Dörr, M., Fischer, T., Kroemer, H., Fleßa, S. and Assel, H., 2012. Was ist Individualisierte Medizin? – Zur terminologischen Justierung eines schillernden Begriffs [What is individualised medicine? – to a terminological adjustment of a dazzling concept]. *Zeitschrift für medizinische Ethik*, 58, pp.295–314.

Ludwig, W.D., 2012. Möglichkeiten und Grenzen der stratifizierenden Medizin am Beispiel von prädiktiven Biomarkern und 'zielgerichteten' medikamentösen Therapien in der Onkologie [Possibilities and limitations of stratifying medicine using the example of predictive biomarkers and 'targeted' drug therapies in oncology]. *Zeitschrift für Evidenz, Fortbildung und Qualität im Gesundheitswesen*, 106, pp.11–22.

Maio, V.G., 2012. Chancen und Grenzen der personalisierten Medizin – eine ethische Betrachtung [Opportunities and limitations of personalised medicine – an ethical consideration]. *Gesundheit und Gesellschaft Wissenschaft*, 12(1), pp.15–19.

Meropol, N.J., Schrag, D., Smith, T.J., Mulvey, T.M., Langdon, R.M., Jr., Blum, D., Ubel, P.A. and Schnipper, L.E., 2009. American Society of Clinical Oncology guidance statement: the cost of cancer care. *Journal of Clinical Oncology*, 27, pp.3868–74.

Prainsack, B., Reardon, J., Hindmarsh, R., Gottweis, H., Naue, U. and Lunshof, J.E., 2008. Misdirected precaution. *Nature*, 456, pp.34–5.

Schleidgen, S., Klingler, C., Bertram, T., Rogowski, W.H. and Marckmann, G., 2013. What is personalized medicine: sharpening a vague term based on a systematic literature review. *BMC Medical Ethics*, 21, p.55.

Siegmund-Schultze, N., 2011. Personalisierte Medizin in der Onkologie. Fortschritt oder falsches Versprechen? [Personalised medicine in oncology. Progress or false promise?]. *Deutsches Ärzteblatt*, 108, pp.A1904–9.

Sledge, G.W., 2012. The challenge and promise of the genomic era. *Journal of Clinical Oncology*, 30, pp.203–9.

Strauss, A. and Corbin, J., 1996. *Grounded Theory: Grundlagen qualitativer Sozialforschung [Basics of qualitative research]*. Weinheim: Psychologie Verlags Union.

Vollmann, J., 2013. Persönlicher – besser – kostengünstiger? Kritische medizinethische Anfragen an die 'personalisierte Medizin' [Personal – better – cost-effective? Critical medical ethics questions regarding 'personalised medicine']. *Ethik in der Medizin*, 25(3), Themenheft 'Personalisierte Medizin. Medizinische, ethische, rechtliche und ökonomische Analysen' [Special issue 'Personalised medicine. Medical, ethical, legal and economic analyses'], pp.233–41.

Chapter 12

Through Thick and Big: Data-Rich Medicine in the Era of Personalisation

Barbara Prainsack

Introduction

A decade ago, the term 'personalised medicine' was largely synonymous with the matching of drug therapies to the genomes of individual patients (for example, Hedgecoe, 2004; see also Jones, 2013). Since then, the concept has started to become more inclusive, often referring to the consideration of individual characteristics – both molecular and otherwise – in medical research and practice (for example, Pokorska-Bocci et al., 2014).[1] A recent report of the European Science Foundation (ESF, 2013), for example, defined personalised medicine as considering individual characteristics at every stage of medical practice, from prevention, diagnosis and therapy to monitoring. Other policy papers and reports – some of which use different notions, such as stratified medicine[2] or precision medicine (for example, NAS, 2011; Eckhart et al., 2014) – also discuss the phenomenon of personalisation in medicine in similar terms. In this broader vision of personalised medicine, medical decision-making increasingly relies on the analysis and interpretation of data on the patient's genome and gene-expression, lifestyle, or other relevant clinical and personal information.[3] The idea is that these datasets will be stored in a place where they are accessible for

---

1   For a discussion of the concept of personalised medicine from a different perspective, see Chapter 1, this volume.

2   The term 'stratified medicine' is also often used to refer to existing practices of assigning patients to different diagnostic or treatment groups (on the basis of their gender, age, the particularity of their symptoms within a disease group, or their genetic or other molecular characteristics). See also Pokorska-Bocci et al. (2014).

3   The author of this chapter was involved in this ESF Forward Look as one of its co-chairs. The argument in this chapter owes much to discussions and explorations with academics, practitioners and patients from various disciplines and contexts that took place as part of, or in the margins of, the Forward Look.

whatever clinical decisions need to be made. They could be stored in the clinic, or elsewhere as determined by the patient (Steinbrook, 2008; Hafen et al., 2014).

A person consulting their doctor because of a persistent cough, for example, would not only be able to share access to all their previous health-care records with their doctor, but also their genome data and information on lifestyle, on family histories, on diet and on the use of prescription drugs. If the patient had a chest X-ray done, these imaging data, together with relevant annotations, diagnoses and treatment decisions made in that instance could be added to the repository. In this way – and with the help of algorithm-based decision aids[4] – diagnosis could take place on the basis of a variety of datasets considered in conjunction. The choice of treatment would be based on what drugs or treatments the person is likely to respond well to. Ultimately, such 'big data' approaches, it is hoped, will also enable the stratification of patients into groups with different likelihood of treatment success (for example, Pizzagalli, 2011; Kelloff and Sigman, 2012).

While this broadening of the notion of personalised medicine, marking a move away from a narrow focus on high-tech genomic medicine, is, overall, a welcome development (Burki, 2015), two aspects have been neglected in dominant articulations of this vision. The first is the large extent to which such data-intense personalisation relies on the contributions from patients. A report, for example, by the US National Academies of Science envisages a future of 'precision medicine' underpinned by multilayered sets of data, ranging from stable datasets, such as a patient's genome, to dynamic data, such as gene expression, lifestyle, medical histories, use of prescription drugs and side effects, changes in levels of pain, or wellbeing (NAS, 2011; see also Weber et al., 2014).

One problem with this vision is that we do not know yet how to integrate these datasets in meaningful and feasible ways. Moreover, many of these datasets are not even available through the health-care system at present. If patients want to benefit from the personalisation of diagnosis, treatment and monitoring on the basis of their own data, they need to be willing to contribute data actively. These contributions can range from the willingness to undergo genetic or genome-wide testing, to the willingness to collect data about their diet and lifestyle, to

---

4   The paradigmatic example of an algorithm-based decision aid is 'Dr Watson', a computer software developed by IBM. 'Dr Watson' will be designed to compare patient data against information from medical journals, protocols and treatment guidelines available on the Internet. A blog on *The Economist* website featuring the software recently assured doctors that 'Dr Watson' would not compete with them but support them, and that 'human doctors' would remain the boss: 'the human doctor can tell the computer to show how it arrived at the conclusion, linking back to the original data. If the doctor disagrees, or wishes to add any constraints, he can tell the program by speaking into a microphone' (T.C., 2013).

monitor their glucose level, blood pressure or other relevant biomarkers remotely from their homes, to contributing information about the medical histories of their relatives. The question of what happens to those who cannot or are not willing to do so, remains largely unanswered. Questions about the consequences that this vision has for those who need to overcome technological, social, economical, language-related or other barriers in order to contribute such data and information for the 'personalisation' of their health care also still need to be addressed. While I discuss these questions elsewhere (Prainsack, 2013, 2014b), this chapter foregrounds the challenges that accompany personalised medicine insofar it relies on datasets with unclear meaning and utility.

Data-Rich Medicine: From a Solution to a Problem?

If we had to choose one term to represent the way in which many people in the rich world think about core challenges of our society – in domains as diverse as politics, economics and medicine – then it is 'big data'. 'Big data' is more than a noun – it describes both a paradigm and an approach to making predictions. Internet governance experts Viktor Mayer-Schönberger and Kenneth Cukier (2013, p.14) describe the key tenet of the 'big data' paradigm as a shift away from the 'age-old search for causality':

> As humans we have been conditioned to look for causes ... In a big-data world, by contrast, we won't have to be fixated on causality; instead we can discover patterns and correlations in the data that offer us novel and invaluable insights. The correlations may not tell us precisely why something is happening, but they alert us *that* it is happening. (Mayer-Schönberger and Cukier, 2013, p.14)

In other words, what sets 'big data' apart from 'small data', according to these authors, is the following: in the context of 'small data', it is important for every single data point to be correct; in the context of 'big data', by contrast, the larger scale makes up for the inaccuracies in single data points. If, for example, a person measured their temperature once a day, it would be important for this measurement to be accurate if we wanted to obtain a reliable fever curve over the course of the week. If they measured their temperature every three seconds, then it would be practically irrelevant if a few of these measurements were wrong. While this example pertains to data taken from a single person, the principle, so Mayer-Schönberger and Cukier (2013, p.14) argue, is also applicable to population-level data: 'If millions of electronic medical records reveal that cancer sufferers who take a certain combination of aspirin and orange juice see their disease go into remission, then the exact cause for the improvement in health may be less important than the fact that they lived.'

But this is not the full picture. What Mayer-Schönberger and Cukier miss mentioning here is that data mining typically provides probabilistic predictions. To stick with the example of aspirin and orange juice: if an analysis of data from 200,000 cancer patients who consumed aspirin and drank orange juice on a daily basis showed that 80 per cent of them went into remission, Peter's doctor would not know whether Peter would personally benefit from aspirin and orange juice. Peter could be like one of the 20 per cent of people in the study who did not benefit from this combination. If we do not understand what causes a particular effect, we cannot tell whether something will work for a particular patient or not, regardless of the size of the dataset.

Nor is it true that scale can always compensate for inaccuracies. David Spiegelhalter, Professor of Public Understanding of Risk at Cambridge University, put it this way: 'There are a lot of small data problems that occur in big data … They don't disappear because you've got lots of the stuff. They get worse' (Harford, 2014, p.29). In the words of communication studies scholar Gina Neff (2013), 'big data won't cure us': in order to overcome the trap of collecting data merely for the sake of collecting data, we also need to pay more attention to the 'social interoperability' of different types of data. This means that we need to try to make the different meanings and utilities of different data for different actors in the medical domain more explicit, and to obtain a better understanding of the 'differences in how people generate, use and even talk about data' (Neff, 2013, p.119). We also need to find other ways to make 'big data' meaningful. Integrating different datasets can go a long way, but integration challenges have only started to be addressed.

In sum, while the supposedly great problem-solving power of 'big data' dominates debates in public discourse, in the lives of many in the health domain, 'big data' have become as much a problem as a solution. Information overload (Toffler, 1970), which for a long time has been seen as a problem of individual people unable to deal with large amounts of information being presented to them, has become a condition characterising our society (Weinberger, 2011).

The challenge of rendering 'big data' in the health domain meaningful and actionable is notoriously difficult. Several factors contribute to this difficulty: first of all, many large datasets that medical research and the clinic are producing at the moment have not been validated, which means that their accuracy is unclear. Sometimes it is even known to be low. This is the case with high-throughput genetic data, or with many kinds of data that are collected in a non-standardised manner (for example, Janssens, 2014; see also Kallinikos and Tempini, 2014). In addition to problems with the analytic validity of many large datasets, their clinical utility – that is, their usefulness for clinical decision-making – is also often unclear. Authors, including myself, have called for greater acknowledgement that the information can lead to positive health benefits even if it is not *clinically* useful in the strict sense of the word: for example, when people learn about their genetic predisposition to a disease for which there is no cure or treatment, having this information can be useful for them by enabling them to plan ahead. Another example of non-clinical utility would be the increase in scientific and medical literacy when engaging with health information (see also Prainsack and Vayena, 2013). Such an acknowledgement of other, more personal and social forms of utility of health data is a very important consideration when we have to decide who should have access to health data (for example, Lunshof et al., 2014). It does not, however, provide a solution for how to deal with data entering the realm of clinical decision-making when the predictive power of the data is unclear, or when the condition that it refers to cannot be prevented or effectively treated. The recent discussion about the return of 'incidental findings' – that is, findings that arise as a 'by-product' of a diagnostic test or procedure that aimed at finding out something else[5] – are but one illustration of this challenge (Wolf et al., 2012; Green et al., 2013; Presidential Commission for the Study of Bioethical Issues, 2013; see also Chapter 7, this volume).

Not All Data are Created Equal

All these factors contribute to a situation where patients and their families, doctors and other medical professionals are faced with increasing quantities of data that are not clearly meaningful or actionable (Heßling and Schicktanz, 2012; Wäscher et al., 2013; see also chapters 10 and 11, this volume). The meaning of these data – in the sense that actionable inferences can be made from these data for the diagnosis, the best course of treatment or the most effective way of monitoring for a specific patient – can be improved by linking them with other datasets and by improving their quality. A proteome profile of a patient with a heart condition, for example, becomes more meaningful if it is linked with information about relevant aspects of this person's lifestyle. We should note here that there is nothing radically new about this process: doctors have always connected one set of data (for example, a fever curve) with other datasets (for example, information about when the fever started, in what body parts the patient experiences pain, whether the patient has been in any areas or engaged in any practices that would have posed a high risk of exposure to viruses causing the fever). In this sense, medicine has always been 'personalised'. Physicians and other health professionals have always taken into consideration individual characteristics of their patients when diagnosing,

---

5   An example for an 'incidental finding' would be if the chest X-ray performed on a patient suspected of suffering from pneumonia showed a tumour, or if a clinical genetic test disclosed a case of non-paternity (in the biological sense).

treating and caring for them (see also Hunter, 1991). What has changed within the renewed focus on personalisation in medicine is our understanding of what counts as 'evidence'. The notion of evidence-based medicine has contributed to an understanding of 'evidence' that foregrounds information that is available in a quantitative format. In addition, the 'data' of data-rich personalised medicine are typically those that are quantified, structured and computable.

This is, however, not inevitable. Projects are already under way that seek to include the ways that patients talk about their pain, the way that they perceive and describe mood or functional changes and changes in their quality of life, in the kinds of 'evidence' that can be used for the personalisation of medicine (for example, Banerjee et al., 2013; Okun, 2012; Frost et al., 2011). Such initiatives are sometimes discussed under the label of patient-centred medicine, which Charles Bardes (2012, p.782) defined as 'focus[ing] medical attention on the individual patient's needs and concerns, rather than the doctor's'. When Bardes speaks of 'the doctor's concerns' in this respect, he does not refer the doctor's personal preferences or benefits, of course. Instead, he points to the concerns that doctors may act upon that stem from their textbook-based training. Their understanding of relevant functional changes, for example, may differ from their patient's. Patient-centred care would mean, in such a situation, that the doctor listens to the patient, but also that categories and nomenclatures that are meaningful to patients are included in the sets of data that are used to base medical decisions on. Recent commentators have highlighted the need for 'thick data' that capture *why* and *how* people do things, rather than merely recording what they do. 'Thick data' is also meant to show what emotional value and what meanings certain practices and technologies have for people (for example, Madsbjerg and Rasmussen, 2014). Ironically, what these authors call 'thick data' has been around for a long time: it has been known as findings from qualitative research.

Protecting Health Data in the Era of Personalisation

An additional challenge inherent in data-rich medicine lies in adequate data protection. We cannot merely transpose the concepts and solutions from the paper age to the digital age. Digital data can be transferred, copied or shared much more easily. Computerised data mining also greatly increases the possibility of reidentifying anonymised or even anonymous data. Moreover, some studies have found that attitudes towards privacy are changing, particularly in the younger generation (see, for example, Rainie and Wellman, 2012). All of these developments suggest that our control-based understanding of privacy – that is, one that defines privacy as the possibility to exercise control over information about ourselves – may not be very helpful when we try to solve contemporary data protection challenges.

For this reason, Los Angeles-based legal scholar Jerry Kang and colleagues (2012) suggest the concept of 'flow' as a potential alternative to a control-based understanding of privacy. As the authors explain:

> for any particular type of information (e.g., public-record data, medical data, or e-mail contents), we could ask where, how quickly, and with what bandwidth does such information flow … Under such a flow conception, public-record data about ourselves, such as whether we voted, flows faster than medical data, which is treated confidentially by law and custom. (Kang et al., 2012, p.821; see also Prainsack, 2014a)

Using the concept of data 'flow' instead of a control-based understanding of privacy, the authors argue, we are better equipped to address questions of non-deliberate disclosure (that is, when people share data about themselves without being aware of it, or because they cannot refuse to do so; see also Peppet, 2012, p.83). Moreover, the notion of 'flow' may also better able to accommodate changing cultural norms:

> The flow conception is less focused on a particular individual's exercise of control and more on the data type's flow – how it generally tends to move, as gauged in probabilistic and macro terms, within some information environment. Accordingly, the flow metric can, for example, come to a sharply different measure of privacy for webcam images. If we as a society become sufficiently exhibitionist such that most of us regularly and voluntarily broadcast naked pictures of ourselves on the Internet, our privacy may not have decreased under a control metric. By contrast, the flow of such information will have increased and, conversely, privacy (in the flow sense) will have decreased under the flow metric. (Kang et al., 2012, pp.821–2)

A disadvantage of the flow metrics is, however, that the metaphor suggests that the entity in question is constantly in flux, like a river, the blood in our body or electricity (see Leonelli, under review). Although any 'flow' can be temporarily interrupted, the assumption is that flux is the default state. Applying this assumption to data or information is problematic, as the point of privacy protection is often specifically to *prevent or restrict* the movement of data. Leonelli (under review) uses the term 'data travel' to accommodate this. Internet and society scholar Sara Watson (2013) goes a step further by arguing that concepts such as 'ownership' and 'privacy' are unsuitable to capture the realities and concerns in an era when we, ourselves, 'are becoming data'. Watson argues that the key to developing more adequate ways of framing and addressing contemporary data challenges lies in ceasing to draw analogies to the physical world when we are discussing data. 'We instinctively say, "I should own my data". But "ownership" over data suggests that we prevent others from it – and that doesn't align with the realities of how easily data is copied and transferred.' Watson suggests that instead of talking about ownership, we should talk about the 'right to use' personal data (Watson, 2013). One of the big challenges in the context of data-rich personalised medicine lies in translating these insights into workable legal and regulatory frameworks (see also Taylor, 2012), and in creating room for patients to have a say in what data and information about and from them are collected in the first place.

Conclusion

This chapter started with the observation that the notion of personalised medicine has been broadening in recent years. While it had been used to signify the matching of drug therapies to genetic and genomic markers up until the last decade, the early 2010s have marked a shift towards understanding the term more broadly as considering individual characteristics of every kind, molecular and otherwise.

Some of the most prominent position papers and publications on this topic articulate visions of personalised medicine that are underpinned by the integration of dynamic and non-dynamic datasets pertaining to individual patients. In this vision, data at the personal level would be used for two purposes: the first purpose is to inform diagnosis, treatment and monitoring of individual patients (in the form of individual health data repositories bringing together data and information on a person's genome, genome expression, diet, lifestyle, use of prescription drugs, mood curves, weight changes, family histories, etc.). The second purpose is to be aggregated and integrated with data from other patients and being mined for relevant patterns (which, in turn, aim at allowing inferences that apply to individual patients). This vision entails that the ongoing convergence between clinic and research continues to increase, and that medicine becomes ever more data-rich.

Such visions bear tangible challenges. First of all, a lot of the data that such understandings of data-rich personalised medicine include are not available in our health-care system, and thus require that patients and other actors collect or contribute them. It is, at the moment, unclear what structural consequences those who cannot, or will not, contribute personal data for the purpose of personalisation of their own care will face. Moreover, a lot of the data that patients and physicians encounter – for example, when patients access information online, or when oncologists are required to interpret gene expression data – do not have clear utility. If such data enter the domain of clinical decision-making, they can become a source for uncertainty for all actors.

Last but not least, the challenges pertaining to data protection in the era of digital health data are different from those in the paper age. Digital data can easily be copied, shared and sometimes also leaked; in the context of changing notions of privacy, we also require novel approaches to their protection.

References

Banerjee, A.K., Okun, S., Edwards, I.R., Wicks, P., Smith, M.Y., Mayall, S.J., Flamion, B., Cleeland, C. and Basch, E., 2013. Patient-reported outcome measures in safety event reporting: PROSPER consortium guidance. *Drug Safety*, 36(12), pp.1129–49.

Bardes, C.L., 2012. Defining 'patient-centered medicine'. *New England Journal of Medicine*, 366(9), pp.782–3.

Burki, T.K. 2015. UK and US governments to fund personalised medicine. *Lancet Oncology* [online first: http://dx.doi.org/10.1016/ S1470-2045(14)71204-5].

Eckhart, A., Navarini, A.A., Recher, A., Rippe, K.P., Rütsche, B., Telser, H. and Marti, M., 2014. *Personalisierte Medizin (Eine Studie des Zentrums für Technologiefolgen-Abschätzung) [Personalised medicine (a study by the Centre for Technology Assessment)]*. Zürich: Hochschulverlag.

European Science Foundation (ESF), 2013. *Personalised medicine for the European citizen – towards more precise medicine for the diagnosis, treatment and prevention of disease*. Strasbourg: ESF. Available at: http://www.esf.org/coordinating-research/forward-looks/biomedical-sciences-med/current-forward-looks-in-biomedical-sciences/personalised-medicine-for-the-european-citizen. html [Accessed 1 April 2014].

Frost, J., Okun, S., Vaughan, T., Heywood, J. and Wicks, P., 2011. Patient-reported outcomes as a source of evidence in off-label prescribing: analysis of data from PatientsLikeMe. *Journal of Medical Internet Research*, 13(1), p.e6.

Green, R.C., Berg, J.S., Grody, W.W., Kalia, S.S., Korf, B.R., Martin, C.L., McGuire, A.L., Nussbaum, R.L., O'Daniel, J.M., Ormond, K.E., Rehm, H.L., Watson, M.S., Williams, M.S. and Biesecker, L.G., 2013. ACMG recommendations for reporting of incidental findings in clinical exome and genome sequencing. *Genetics in Medicine*, 15(7), pp.565–74.

Hafen, E., Kossmann, D., and Brand, A. (2014). Health Data Cooperatives–Citizen Empowerment. *Methods of Information in Medicine* 53(2), 82-86.

Harford, T., 2014. Big data: are we making a big mistake? *Financial Times Weekend Magazine*, 29/30 March, pp.28–31.

Hedgecoe, A., 2004. *The politics of personalised medicine: pharmacogenetics in the clinic.* Cambridge: Cambridge University Press.

Heßling, A. and Schicktanz, S., 2012. What German experts expect from individualized medicine: problems of uncertainty and future complication in physician–patient interaction. *Clinical Ethics*, 7(2), pp.86–93.

Hunter, K.M., 1991. *Doctors' stories: the narrative structure of medical knowledge*. Princeton: Princeton University Press.

Janssens, C.J.W., 2014. Raw data: access to inaccuracy. *Science*, 343(6174), p.968.

Jones, D.S., 2013. How personalized medicine became genetic, and racial: Werner Kalow and the formations of pharmacogenomics. *Journal of the History of Medicine and Allied Sciences*, 68(1), pp.1–48.

Kallinikos, J. and Tempini, N., 2014. Patient data as medical facts: Social media practices as a foundation for medical knowledge creation. *Information Systems Research*, 25(4), pp.817–33.

Kang, J., Shilton, K., Estrin, D., Burke, J. and Hansen, M., 2012. Self-surveillance privacy. *Iowa Law Review*, 97, pp.809–47.

Kelloff, G.J. and Sigman, C.C., 2012. Cancer biomarkers: selecting the right drug for the right patient. *Nature Reviews Drug Discovery*, 11(3), pp.201–14.

Leonelli, S., *Researching life in the digital age: a philosophical study of data-centric biology*. Chicago University Press (under review).

Lunshof, J.E., Church, G.M. and Prainsack, B., 2014. Raw personal data: providing access. *Science*, 343(6169), pp.373–4.

Madsbjerg, C. and Rasmussen, M.B., 2014. The power of 'thick' data. *The Wall Street Journal*, [online] 21 March. Available at: http://online.wsj.com/news/articles/SB10001424052702304256404579449254114659882 [Accessed 30 March 2014].

Mayer-Schönberger, V. and Cukier, K., 2013. *Big data*. London: John Murray Publishers.

[US] National Academy of Sciences (NAS), 2011. *Toward precision medicine: building a knowledge network for biomedical research and a new taxonomy of disease*. Washington, DC: NAS.

Neff, G., 2013. Why big data won't cure us. *Big Data*, 1(3), pp.117–23.

Okun, S., 2012. Patient voices: the power of shared knowledge. *Medicine 2.0*, [online], 10 September. Available at: http://www.medicine20congress.com/ocs/index.php/med/med2012/paper/view/1129 [Accessed 31 March 2014].

Peppet, S.R., 2012. Privacy & the personal prospectus: should we introduce privacy agents or regulate privacy intermediaries? *Iowa Law Review Bulletin*, 97, pp.77–93.

Pizzagalli, D.A., 2011. Frontocingulate dysfunction in depression: toward biomarkers of treatment response. *Neuropsychopharmacology*, 36(1), pp.183–206.

Pokorska-Bocci, A., Stewart, A., Sagoo, G.S., Hall, A., Kroese, M. and Burton, H., 2014. 'Personalised medicine': what's in a name? *Personalized Medicine*, 11(2), pp.197–220.

Prainsack, B., 2013. Let's get real about virtual: online health is here to stay. *Genetics Research*, 95(4), pp.111–13.

Prainsack, B., 2014a. Review of M. Taylor, genetic data and the law: a critical perspective on privacy protection (Cambridge, UK: Cambridge University Press, 2012). *Medial Law Review*, 22(2), pp.291–5.

Prainsack, B., 2014b. The powers of participatory medicine. *PLoS Biology*, 12(4), p.e1001837.

Prainsack, B. and Vayena, E., 2013. Beyond the clinic: 'direct-to-consumer' genomic profiling services and pharmacogenomics. *Pharmacogenomics*, 14(4), pp.403–12.

[US] Presidential Commission for the Study of Bioethical Issues, 2013. *Anticipate and communicate. Ethical management of incidental and secondary findings in the clinical, research, and direct-to-consumer contexts*. Washington, DC [online] Available at: http://www.bioethics.gov [Accessed 30 March 2014].

Rainie, L. and Wellman, B., 2012. *Networked*. Cambridge, MA: MIT Press.

Steinbrook, R., 2008. Personally controlled online health data – the next big thing in medical care? *New England Journal of Medicine*, 358(16), pp.1653–6.

Taylor, M., 2012. *Genetic data and the law: a critical perspective on privacy protection*. Cambridge: Cambridge University Press.

T.C. 2013. Doctor Watson. *The Economist*, [online] 14 February. Available at: http://www.economist.com/blogs/babbage/2013/02/computer-aided-medicine [Accessed 2 May 2014].

Tempini, N., 2013. 'The paradox of context flexibility: balancing user engagement and semantic context in distributed data collection'. 29 EGOS Colloquium – European Group of Organizational Studies, HEC, Montreal, 4–6 July. Available at: https://www.academia.edu/5164963/The_paradox_of_context_flexibility_balancing_user_engagement_and_semantic_context_in_distributed_data_collection [Accessed 29 June 2014].

Toffler, A., 1970. *Future shock*. New York: Amereon Ltd.

Wäscher, S., Schildmann, J., Brall, C. and Vollmann, J., 2013. 'Personalisierte Medizin' in der Onkologie: Ärztliche Einschätzungen der aktuellen Entwicklung in der Krankenversorgung ['Personalised medicine' in oncology: medical assessments of developments in health care]. *Ethik in der Medizin*, 25(3), pp.205–14.

Watson, S.M., 2013. You are your data. *Slate*, [online] 12 November. Available at: http://www.slate.com/articles/technology/future_tense/2013/11/quantified_self_self_tracking_data_we_need_a_right_to_use_it.html [Accessed 13 January 2014].

Weber, G.M., Mandl, K.D. and Kohane, I.S., 2014. Finding the missing link for big biomedical data. *The Journal of the American Medical Association*, [online first: doi:10.1001/jama.2014.4228].

Weinberger, D., 2011. *Too big to know*. New York: Basic Books.

Wolf, S.M., Crock, B.N., Van Ness, B., Lawrenz, F., Kahn, J.P., Beskow, L.M., Cho, M.K., Christman, M.F., Green, R.C., Hall, R., Illes, J., Keane, M., Knoppers, B.M., Koenig, B.A., Kohane, I.S., Leroy, B., Maschke, K.J., McGeveran, W., Ossorio, P., Parker, L.S., Petersen, G.M., Richardson, H.S., Scott, J.A., Terry, S.F., Wilfond, B.S. and Wolf, W.A., 2012. Managing incidental findings and research results in genomic research involving biobanks and archived data sets. *Genetics in Medicine*, 14(4), pp.361–84.

PART III
Personalised Medicine in Health-Care Systems

Chapter 13

Benefit Assessment of Personalised Interventions: Methodological Challenges and Approaches to a Solution[1]

Jürgen Windeler and Stefan Lange[2]

Introduction

The keyword 'personalised medicine' refers to a concept that is supposed to lead to new, improved management options through classification of patients into subgroups, largely by means of 'novel' biomarkers. This approach is also called 'individualised medicine', or more recently, 'precision medicine'. The term 'stratified medicine' has also been proposed as a neutral and suitable term (Windeler, 2012). However, classification into subgroups (for example, by age, sex or individual characteristics) and subsequent adaptation of patient management have always been components of medical thinking and action (for a detailed discussion on the definition of personalised medicine see Chapter 1, this volume).

If one looks at the two main aspects of personalised medicine, these can be specified, on the one hand, as the question of the correct classification of patients, and on the other, as the question of the patient-relevant medical benefit or added benefit of an intervention. Neither question is new.

Example of Stratified Medicine

One of the common risk classifications for people from the general population, the Systematic Coronary Risk Evaluation Project (SCORE) European High

1   This chapter was originally published in German in a slightly modified form, under the title 'Nutzenbewertung personalisierter Interventionen: Methodische Herausforderungen und Lösungsansätze' in: *Ethik in der Medizin* 2013, 25, 173–82. With kind permission of Springer Science+Business Media.

2   The authors thank Natalie McGauran for the translation of the manuscript.

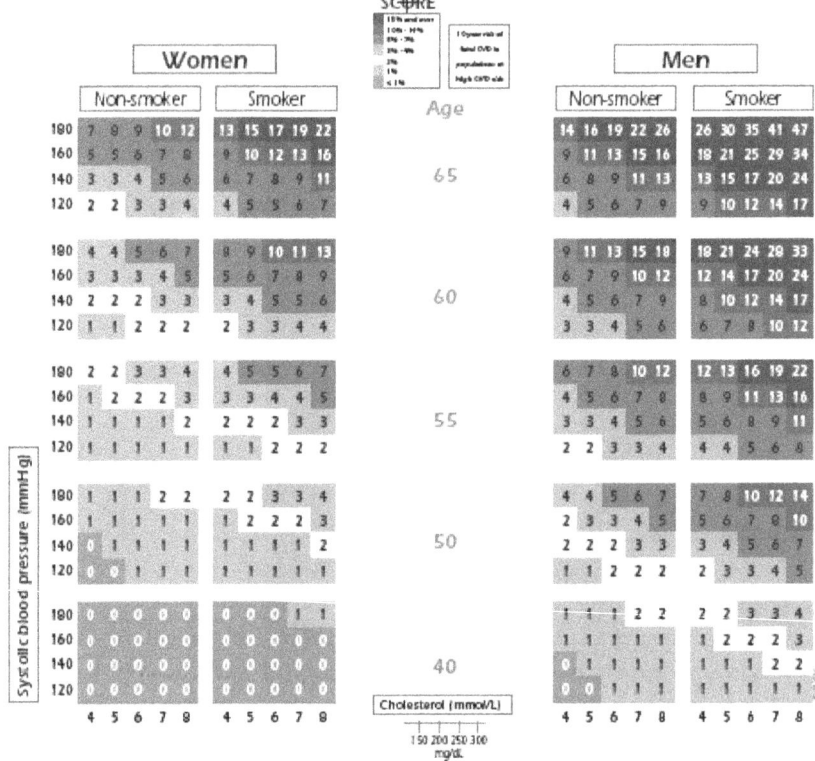

Figure 13.1 Cardiovascular risk score (SCORE) to illustrate the principle of personalised medicine

Source: Perk et al. (2012, p.1648), with permission of Oxford University Press (UK), © European Society of Cardiology, www.escardio.org/guidelines.

Risk Chart, used five patient characteristics (markers) to estimate the 10-year risk of fatal cardiovascular disease: age, sex, smoking, systolic blood pressure and total cholesterol (Perk et al., 2012). The continuous characteristics were divided into four or five classes, leading to a 2x2x5x5x4 matrix with 400 cells. People in whom the cardiovascular risk is of interest can thus be classified into 400 different groups on the basis of these risk markers (Figure 13.1).

The following questions now arise: is this classification correct? Does the classification of a certain person reliably describe his or her risk? How high is the error rate? This is a typical problem of diagnostic or prognostic tests. If a larger number of separate pieces of information is examined in parallel or sequentially, then the question can become complex, but basically, it concerns the quality of a classification. This question can be examined and answered using methods of evidence-based medicine (EbM).

For the people in the seven different risk strata (shades of grey in the figure) derived from the total of 400 cells, one can now argue that they must receive different therapeutic or preventive interventions or recommendations, as results will differ depending on whether people are managed in the same way, or differently according to the seven classes. Methodologically, such a situation is termed an 'interaction' – different intervention effects are present in the different risk classes.

Methodological Approach

The crucial question of whether there is an interaction means that the measurement of a marker is only meaningful if people will be treated differently depending on the test result (or, more generally, if they will experience different consequences) *and* if they will have different advantages from these different treatments. The interaction between the result of the biomarker measurement and an intervention effect should be examined in prospective, comparative studies, ideally in randomised controlled trials (Sargent et al., 2005). Such interactions can generally not be examined in prognosis studies, where only the course of patients' state of health is followed within the different risk strata, without comparison of treatment options. Unfortunately, the literature on biomarkers mainly concerns prognosis studies (Ioannidis and Tzoulaki, 2010), whilst prospective, comparative studies that can also investigate interactions are still an exception.

We describe the main scenarios in the following text to illustrate the potential consequences of classifying patients by means of biomarkers and we interpret these scenarios. The letter 'P' refers to a population of patients or healthy people (in the case of preventive measures). 'M' refers to a marker or a combination of markers. There are two categories here – the marker is either positive or negative, a simple situation. The effect of an intervention is described by the difference between application and non-application of the intervention, namely, 'T' for treatment and 'C' for control.

Scenario 1

The first scenario (Figure 13.2) is a clear, positive effect in the marker-positive group and a clear treatment-related inferiority (harm) in the marker-negative group. Methodologically, this is a qualitative interaction, as the effect goes in opposite directions.

If one only considers this result and initially disregards other aspects of the assessment, one can conclude that a measurement of the marker is meaningful, as the following can be stated: M+ patients should be treated as they will probably experience an advantage, but M– patients should not be treated as

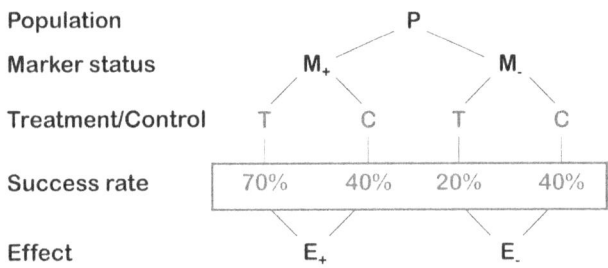

Figure 13.2   Potential results in an interaction design: Scenario 1

they will probably suffer a disadvantage. For this conclusion, adverse effects and other aspects of treatment are initially disregarded. Basically, such an analysis is also feasible and interpretable for more aggregated outcomes (for example, quality-adjusted life years).

This situation is easy to interpret, but presumably rarely occurs. A fairly recent and real-life example is the choice of first-line therapy in patients with non-small-cell lung cancer: in the subgroup of patients who were positive for the epidermal growth factor receptor (EGFR) gene mutation, progression-free survival (PFS) was significantly longer among those who received the tyrosine kinase inhibitor gefitinib than among those who received the standard chemotherapy of carboplatin and paclitaxel (hazard ratio [HR]: 0.48; 95 per cent confidence interval [CI]: 0.36–0.64). The opposite effect was shown in patients who were negative for the mutation (HR: 2.85; 95 per cent CI: 2.05–3.98) (Mok et al., 2009). With this example in mind, one could discuss the patient relevance of the outcome PFS. It should also be critically noted that only about a third of the patients originally randomised were considered in the analysis. Nevertheless, this qualitative interaction is impressive, and gefitinib is only approved for treatment of non-small-cell lung cancer in patients with a confirmed EGFR mutation.

Scenario 2

In the second scenario (Figure 13.3) the effects, namely, the differences between T and C, are the same in the marker-positive and marker-negative groups. The interpretation is also simple; there is no interaction. The result of the marker measurement provides no information on which patient groups experience especially large effects and which do not. The marker is not needed for a treatment decision and should therefore not be measured. To come to such a conclusion, it is essential to have information on the treatment effect in the marker-negative group (see below for further details).

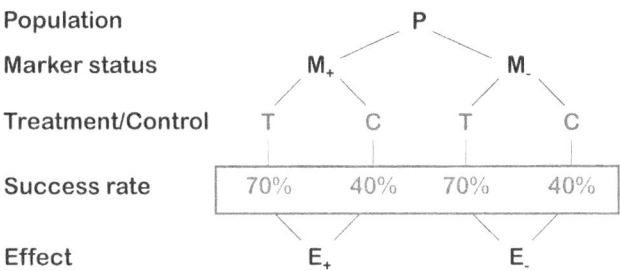

Figure 13.3   Potential results in an interaction design: Scenario 2

It should also be considered that exact equivalence of treatment effects cannot be demonstrated. One relies rather on the result of a statistical test to determine the (non-)existence of any interaction; if this is not significant (usually at a significance level of α = 5 per cent), then it is mostly assumed that such an interaction does not exist. This can be a problem, as the statement: 'Absence of evidence is not evidence of absence' (Altman and Bland, 1995, p.485) also applies here; this particularly concerns a statistical interaction test, as it usually has low statistical power. From a methodological point of view it would be more appropriate to define a 'more than irrelevant' interaction and to exclude its existence by means of a statistical hypothesis test (with the usual significance level). The fact that this has hardly ever been implemented (or perhaps not at all) may also be due to the fact that such an interaction and the corresponding measures are rather abstract. In addition, if minor interactions are present, the power problem may increase, but in the opposite direction. An – albeit methodologically weaker – alternative is to test for the non-existence of any interaction, with a higher significance level (for example, α = 20 per cent) (Institute for Quality and Efficiency in Health Care, 2013).

Scenario 3

In the third scenario (Figure 13.4), the clear effect already described is shown in marker-positive patients, but no difference is shown between the treatment and control group in marker-negative ones – treatment has no effect. The effect is different in the M + and M− groups; an interaction is present that is, in principle, also a 'qualitative' one.

According to the usual approach, one should refrain from treating patients in the M− group due to a lack of benefit, that is, a lack of prospect of success. However, in contrast to Scenario 1, where the harm caused by treatment is already directly evident, the consideration of additional aspects of harm is particularly important so as to allow for a conclusive interpretation of the situation.

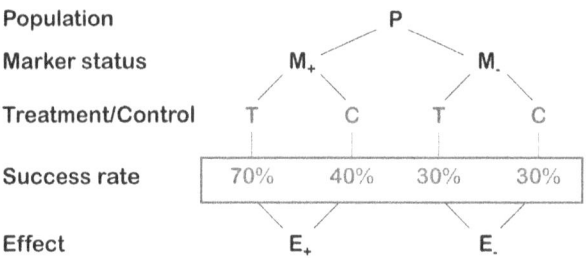

Figure 13.4   Potential results in an interaction design: Scenario 3

One of the most prominent examples of personalised medicine on the basis of the scenario above is tamoxifen for (early-stage) breast cancer in women with oestrogen-receptor (ER) positive tumours: a large meta-analysis showed that the risk of breast cancer-related death was reduced by about a third in ER-positive patients who received adjuvant tamoxifen therapy for about five years (Early Breast Cancer Trialists' Collaborative Group, 2005). No such effect was shown in ER-negative patients. According to the summary of product characteristics, the precondition for use of tamoxifen is the prior confirmation of ER-positive breast cancer.

In connection with the biological principles of personalised medicine, this scenario is of particular relevance. It is widely believed that on the basis of the underlying (molecular) biological knowledge, or more exactly, the biological model, this is the biological standard scenario, a type of default. On the other hand, the basis of this default, the theory derived from the biological model that no effect can occur or is to be expected in the M− group, leads to the exclusion of this group from studies.

Such a (commonly used) approach is termed 'enrichment design' (Simon, 2010). The biomarker is measured but only marker-positive patients are included in the treatment study. The other patients are not treated and not followed up on the basis of the biological model that 'there can be no effect'. The opposite situation of only patients with a marker-negative result being included in the study is also conceivable, for instance, to examine deescalation strategies (for example, as in Picardi et al., 2007).

From the perspective of EbM, which in the past decades has repeatedly shown that biological models fail to provide a basis for conclusions on the benefit of interventions, a naive belief in such models can pose a serious problem (see also Chapter 14, this volume). Not for the development of hypotheses – biological models are required for this purpose – but for drawing conclusions on benefit. Although examples are available showing that conclusions based on such models are possible (Mallal et al., 2008; Simon, 2010), these are exceptions based on simple relationships. Biological models are usually so complex that they are almost inevitably incomplete and insufficient to be used for drawing conclusions on the benefit of interventions. For instance, a recent article described an enormous genetic variety of renal cell cancers and the authors concluded that 'Intratumour heterogeneity can lead to underestimation of the tumour genomics landscape portrayed from single tumour-biopsy samples and may present major challenges to personalised-medicine and biomarker development' (Gerlinger et al., 2012, p.883).

The 'blind spot' systematically generated by enrichment designs means that the situation described in Scenarios 1 to 3 cannot be recognised. For Scenarios 1 and 3 this may not be too problematic, as patients who should not be treated on the basis of the information gained from these scenarios would, without this information, not be treated either. However, this blind spot is of major relevance for Scenario 2, as enrichment designs do not allow answers to the questions as to whether the marker is required for the treatment decision at all, and whether the biological model is correct.

Scenario 4

The challenge involved and the necessity of comprehensive information is particularly pronounced in Scenario 4 (Figure 13.5). There is a clear treatment effect in the marker-positive group, but there is also an effect in the marker-negative group, albeit to a smaller extent – a quantitative interaction.

Only if one concluded, without taking further factors into account, that marker-negative patients should not be treated because of the smaller effect, as in Scenarios 1 and 3, decisions made with the information obtained would be the same as decisions without it. However, the questions immediately arises as to how large the distance between the effects in M+ and M- should or is allowed to be to justify such a direct decision, and at the latest it becomes clear here that a decision on treatment (or non-treatment) of the marker-negative

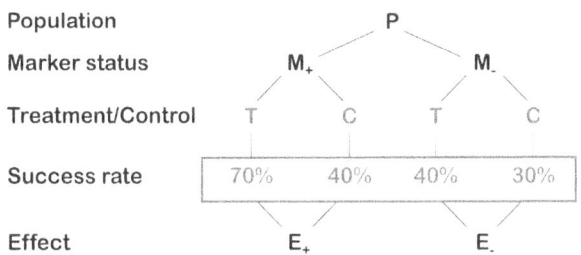

Figure 13.5   Potential results in an interaction design: Scenario 4

group can generally be made only on the basis of empirical evidence of the effects in this group.

The situation becomes even more problematic, but not basically different, if by using a biomarker, a decision is to be made not on the use of a new treatment, but on the use (or non-use) of a standard treatment for the whole group (both marker-positive and marker-negative patients). This means that for one of the groups, the measurement of the biomarker would potentially result in dispensing with or modifying this standard treatment.

Of course, the question of the classification of the treatment effect also immediately concerns the question of the use of the marker. If all patients are to receive treatment, even if effects on certain subgroups may be smaller or larger than on others – a completely normal constellation – then the marker is not required for a treatment decision. However, if patient groups with a smaller treatment effect are not to receive treatment because of this smaller effect, the marker would have a direct influence on decision making. If the biomarker is only one of several pieces of information on which the treatment decision is based, the logical question that arises is whether this marker should be measured in all patients, as in some or many patients, the decision on a certain treatment option could already have been made (or could be made) on the basis of other information.

However, the crucial point of these remarks is that the above situations potentially exist if one does not blindly believe in a biological model that may be unacceptable. A study on trastuzumab plus adjuvant chemotherapy for breast cancer included only human epidermal growth factor receptor HER2-positive patients; HER2-negative patients were not considered. The results showed a marked improvement in disease-free survival and a less marked improvement in overall survival (Romond et al., 2005). However, follow-up studies showed that improvements could also be achieved in patients with a HER2-negative primary tumour (Georgoulias et al., 2012; Mandrekar and Sargent, 2009). The biological model is thus obviously incomplete. A more complete picture is created if not only the primary tumour is considered, but also tumour cells circulating in the blood. Again, this shows the genetic variety of the same type of cancer (see above); even if the primary tumour is HER2-negative, affected patients apparently may have circulating HER2-positive tumour cells that are susceptible to trastuzumab (Georgoulias et al., 2012). Complete information on a topic is required as a basis to decide whether a biomarker is needed for making a treatment decision and how potential larger and smaller effects are to be taken into account (for a discussion on possible problems resulting of 'big data' see Chapter 12, this volume).

In the informative studies outlined here it is therefore essential to determine which of the four scenarios is present and how large the difference in effects actually is. Ultimately, decisions on the benefit of the combination of the diagnostic test and therapeutic intervention can only be made on this basis, enabling the adequate management of patients.

The type of studies outlined here should and can be conducted, as the examples above show. Even what is seemingly evident should be (and is being) investigated for good reason: abacavir, a nucleosid reverse transcriptase inhibitor, is used in combination with other anti-retroviral agents in patients with human immunodeficiency virus infection. However, within the first six weeks of treatment, about 5–8 per cent of patients receiving abacavir had previously experienced an immunologically mediated hypersensitivity reaction, which can be accompanied by serious symptoms (Mallal et al., 2008). In addition, an association between the occurrence of this reaction and the presence of a genetic characteristic, the human leukocyte antigen (HLA)-B*5701 allele, has been shown. A randomised study examined whether prospective HLA-B*5701 screening before planned treatment with abacavir, with exclusion of HLA-B*5701 positive-patients from abacavir treatment, could prevent such a hypersensitivity reaction. This was impressively accomplished. No immunologically confirmed hypersensitivity reaction occurred in the prospective-screening group versus nearly 3 per cent in the control group (Mallal et al., 2008). The screening test used to detect this type of hypersensitivity reaction showed a sensitivity of 100 per cent, with a specificity of nearly 97 per cent (Mallal et al., 2008). Despite an almost 'perfect' test (based on diagnostic quality), the authors deemed it appropriate to test the biological model in a randomised study.

The fact that this model does not always work is suggested by a study on 'individualised' antiplatelet therapy in patients scheduled for coronary stenting. Platelet function monitoring and subsequent treatment adjustment showed no advantage over standard therapy (Collet et al., 2012). Furthermore, this study illustrates an additional point: Even a qualitative interaction may sometimes be insufficient to examine the benefit of a diagnostic or prognostic test. Beyond mere information gain, such tests may also cause physical (adverse) effects, as well as psychological ones triggered by informing the test participant about the test result; such effects can only be determined by a direct randomised comparison of test application versus non-application (Bossuyt and McCaffery, 2009).

Conclusion

The aim of personalised medicine – as of any form of medicine – is to provide better health care for patients. The means used mainly include specifically defined biomarker-supported therapeutic interventions, which vary depending on the marker status. The question is: does one achieve the aim with these means?

An appropriate method to answer this question is a prospective, comparative intervention study, in which, and this is the crucial difference to the studies commonly conducted, the interaction of the intervention with the biomarker is of primary interest. Such questions and studies belong to the standard spectrum of EbM. New methods are not required.

References

Altman, D.G. and Bland, J.M., 1995. Absence of evidence is not evidence of absence. *BMJ*, 311(7003), p.485.

Bossuyt, P.M. and McCaffery, K., 2009. Additional patient outcomes and pathways in evaluations of testing. *Medical Decision Making*, 29(5), pp.E30–8.

Collet, J.P., Cuisset, T., Range, G., Cayla, G., Elhadad, S., Pouillot, C., Henry, P., Motreff, P., Carrie, D., Boueri, Z., Belle, L., Van Belle, E., Rousseau, H., Aubry, P., Monsegu, J., Sabouret, P., O'Connor, S.A., Abtan, J., Kerneis, M., Saint-Etienne, C., Barthelemy, O., Beygui, F., Silvain, J., Vicaut, E. and Montalescot, G., 2012. Bedside monitoring to adjust antiplatelet therapy for coronary stenting. *New England Journal of Medicine*, 367(22), pp.2100–9.

Early Breast Cancer Trialists' Collaborative Group, 2005. Effects of chemotherapy and hormonal therapy for early breast cancer on recurrence and 15-year survival: an overview of the randomised trials. *Lancet*, 365(9472), pp.1687–717.

Georgoulias, V., Bozionelou, V., Agelaki, S., Perraki, M., Apostolaki, S., Kallergi, G., Kalbakis, K., Xyrafas, A. and Mavroudis, D., 2012. Trastuzumab decreases the incidence of clinical relapses in patients with early breast cancer presenting chemotherapy-resistant CK-19mRNA-positive circulating tumor cells: results of a randomized phase II study. *Annals of Oncology*, 23(7), pp.1744–50.

Gerlinger, M., Rowan, A.J., Horswell, S., Larkin, J., Endesfelder, D., Gronroos, E., Martinez, P., Matthews, N., Stewart, A., Tarpey, P., Varela, I., Phillimore, B., Begum, S., McDonald, N.Q., Butler, A., Jones, D., Raine, K., Latimer, C., Santos, C.R., Nohadani, M., Eklund, A.C., Spencer-Dene, B., Clark, G., Pickering, L., Stamp, G., Gore, M., Szallasi, Z., Downward, J., Futreal, P.A. and Swanton, C., 2012. Intratumor heterogeneity and branched evolution revealed by multiregion sequencing. *New England Journal of Medicine*, 366(10), pp.883–92.

Institute for Quality and Efficiency in Health Care. 2013. General methods: version 4.1 [pdf]. Cologne: IQWiG. Available at: https://www.iqwig.de/download/IQWiG_General_Methods_Version_%204–1.pdf [Accessed 20 March 2014].

Ioannidis, J.P. and Tzoulaki, I., 2010. What makes a good predictor? The evidence applied to coronary artery calcium score. *JAMA*, 303(16), pp.1646–7.

Mallal, S., Phillips, E., Carosi, G., Molina, J.M., Workman, C., Tomazic, J., Jagel-Guedes, E., Rugina, S., Kozyrev, O., Cid, J.F., Hay, P., Nolan, D., Hughes,

S., Hughes, A., Ryan, S., Fitch, N., Thorborn, D. and Benbow, A., 2008. HLA-B*5701 screening for hypersensitivity to abacavir. *New England Journal of Medicine*, 358(6), pp.568–79.

Mandrekar, S.J. and Sargent, D.J., 2009. Clinical trial designs for predictive biomarker validation: theoretical considerations and practical challenges. *Journal of Clinical Oncology*, 27(24), pp.4027–34.

Mok, T.S., Wu, Y.L., Thongprasert, S., Yang, C.H., Chu, D.T., Saijo, N., Sunpaweravong, P., Han, B., Margono, B., Ichinose, Y., Nishiwaki, Y., Ohe, Y., Yang, J.J., Chewaskulyong, B., Jiang, H., Duffield, E.L., Watkins, C.L., Armour, A.A. and Fukuoka, M., 2009. Gefitinib or carboplatin-paclitaxel in pulmonary adenocarcinoma. *New England Journal of Medicine*, 361(10), pp.947–57.

Perk, J., De Backer, G., Gohlke, H., Graham, I., Reiner, Z., Verschuren, M., Albus, C., Benlian, P., Boysen, G., Cifkova, R., Deaton, C., Ebrahim, S., Fisher, M., Germano, G., Hobbs, R., Hoes, A., Karadeniz, S., Mezzani, A., Prescott, E., Ryden, L., Scherer, M., Syvanne, M., Scholte op. Reimer, W.J., Vrints, C., Wood, D., Zamorano, J.L. and Zannad, F., 2012. European Guidelines on cardiovascular disease prevention in clinical practice (version 2012): the Fifth Joint Task Force of the European Society of Cardiology and Other Societies on Cardiovascular Disease Prevention in Clinical Practice (constituted by representatives of nine societies and by invited experts); developed with the special contribution of the European Association for Cardiovascular Prevention & Rehabilitation (EACPR). *European Heart Journal*, 33(13), pp.1635–701.

Picardi, M., De Renzo, A., Pane, F., Nicolai, E., Pacelli, R., Salvatore, M. and Rotoli, B., 2007. Randomized comparison of consolidation radiation versus observation in bulky Hodgkin's lymphoma with post-chemotherapy negative positron emission tomography scans. *Leukemia & Lymphoma*, 48(9), pp.1721–7.

Romond, E.H., Perez, E.A., Bryant, J., Suman, V.J., Geyer CE Jr, Davidson, N.E., Tan-Chiu, E., Martino, S., Paik, S., Kaufman, P.A., Swain, S.M., Pisansky, T.M., Fehrenbacher, L., Kutteh, L.A. and Vogel, V.G., 2005. Trastuzumab plus adjuvant chemotherapy for operable HER2-positive breast cancer. *New England Journal of Medicine*, 353(16), pp.1673–84.

Sargent, D.J., Conley, B.A., Allegra, C. and Collette, L., 2005. Clinical trial designs for predictive marker validation in cancer treatment trials. *Journal of Clinical Oncology*, 23(9), pp.2020–7.

Simon, R., 2010. Clinical trials for predictive medicine: new challenges and paradigms. *Clinical Trials*, 7(5), pp.516–24.

Windeler, J., 2012. Individualized medicine: our (lack of) understanding. *Zeitschrift für Evidenz, Fortbildung und Qualität im Gesundheitswesen*, 106(1), pp.5–10.

Chapter 14

The Relevance of the Analytic Validity of Genetic Biomarker Tests in Personalised Medicine in Oncology

Franz Hessel[1]

Introduction

A crucial attribute of genetically stratifying personalised medicine technologies is the combination of a biomarker test (or a set of more than one) and a therapeutic decision which is made according to the test results. The biomarker test – often called a 'companion diagnostic' – is an essential part of the personalised medicine treatment strategy. The US FDA (Food and Drug Administration) approval agency even stated in a recent reflection paper that it would not approve a new drug without the companion biomarker test if a marker is known (FDA, 2011).

Biomarker tests for personalised medicine are classified as *in vitro* diagnostics (IVD) belonging to the macro-group of medical devices. In general, IVD tests have been influencing therapy decisions for a long time, and traditionally, they are often seen either as a commodity or, in some cases, as a scientific playground for specialised laboratory physicians without practical relevance to routine care. This has changed towards a greater attentiveness of IVDs since the development of genetic markers. Some stakeholders, for example, some European payers and reimbursement decision-making bodies, seem to be afraid that the era of drug blockbusters will be replaced by a new era of biomarkers and personalised medicine 'niche busters'. Looking at the number of new drugs approved by the FDA and the European Medicines Agency (EMA), we can say

1   This study was conducted in the research network Personalised Medicine in Oncology: An Interdisciplinary Study on Ethical, Medical, Economical and Legal Aspects (Grant project number: 01 GP 1001A-C), which is supported by the German Federal Ministry of Education and Research (Bundesministerium für Bildung und Forschung – BMBF).

that personalised medicine technologies are on the increase, although the drug landscape has not changed dramatically.

With regards to market access and benefit evaluations of new health-care technologies, IVD tests are not evaluated as a stand-alone technology, but as so-called complex interventions in combination with the therapy component. Therefore, the value of the diagnostic test always relies on the subsequent therapeutic consequences, whether it is a blood glucose measurement or a genetic tumour marker in oncology. However, there is another side of the coin. The value of a pharmaceutical also relies on the quality of the diagnostic test. Looking at the aspect of the two companions from the other side seems to be under discussion and in the focus of health-care decision-making bodies to a much smaller extent. (For further reflections on this topic, see Chapter 15, this volume.)

Compared to pharmaceuticals which must demonstrate their clinical efficacy and their safety in extensive studies before they are approved for marketing, with the exception of companion diagnostic tests of a specific brand which are approved with the drug, there is no comparable regulatory approval process required for IVD tests. The quality of the test itself and the accuracy of the test results are seen as 'given' by the majority of the health-care decision-making bodies. The companion diagnostic test for personalised medicine drugs must be performed before the drug can be given to the patient, however, at least in European countries, there are only general recommendations that 'a validated, high-quality test' should be used.

The objective of this chapter is to discuss the impact of the analytic validity of biomarker tests in personalised medicine technologies on therapy decisions and the gap between existing recommendations for the evaluation of the analytical validity of diagnostic tests and the extent of consideration in health-care decision-making processes.

The Value of Biomarker Tests

Genetic biomarker test results seem to transport the image that they represent the 'absolute truth' and pure causal inferences can be made on the basis of test results. In reality, they rarely offer a clear yes or no result concerning long-term clinical outcomes. They often just classify the risk and, in many cases, they are only one piece of the diagnostic puzzle. The clinical validity of biomarker tests in routine care is always massively influenced by other factors, such as compliance or comorbidity. It is obvious that a change of the test strategy – for example, adding a second-line test or replacing a generic test by a more specific new test – is influencing the number of correctly identified patients and, consequently, the overall long-term outcomes. A recent example is the refining of the V-Ki-ras2 Kirsten rat sarcoma viral oncogene homolog (short KRAS) test strategy for patients with colorectal cancer treated with epidermal growth factor receptor (EGFR) inhibitors (PRIME Study) with the consequence of a clear improvement of the patients' survival rate (Douillard et al., 2013).

However, despite the various factors influencing the clinical consequences of a test result, the basis of a successful personalised medicine strategy is a correct test result of the test itself. In any case, all diagnostic tests should be accurate and, as with any other diagnostic test, modern genetic biomarker tests should show a high analytic performance.

There are three basic aspects to be considered in the evaluation of biomarkers: the analytical validity of the marker, the clinical validity and the clinical utility. The analytic validity can be summarised with the question: can I trust the results of the test? The clinical validity is the degree to which a test result can be used to correctly identify patients with the target condition. Finally, the clinical utility describes the actual consequences of the whole treatment strategy on patients' clinical outcomes.

The main components of the validation of genetic tests are summarised by the US Center for Disease Control (CDC) in the so-called ACCE wheel. The name ACCE is derived from (1) **A**nalytic validity, (2) **C**linical validity, (3) **C**linical utility, and (4) **E**thical, legal and social implications (Haddow and Palomaki, 2003).

The quality of the biomarker test – or, in technical terms, the test performance – consists of the clinical validity and the analytic validity. The analytic validity answers the question how accurately and reliably the test measures the genotype of interest, and it consists of the sensitivity (how many patients are correctly classified as test positive?) and the specificity (how many healthy patients are correctly classified as test negative = healthy?) (Loong, 2003). There are a number of factors influencing sensitivity and specificity, such as the technical aspects of the test itself, of the platform or of the sample, and also the experience of the laboratory personnel, respectively the pathologist. Even if these aspects are perfectly standardised, there are a number of factors leading to heterogeneous results of IVD assays: there are variations in specimen composition and tissue processing, as well as concerning the statistics used for analysing the data. In the analytic stages of performing the assay, differences in molecular forms of the biomarker are present. The sampling procedure itself (for example, fine-needle aspirate or biopsy obtained during surgery, biomarker concentration in serum or plasma), the source of tissue (fresh or frozen), storage conditions (time, temperature, etc.), and tissue processing steps may also severely influence the final assay results (Benraad et al., 1996). Further variations are caused by the use of different standards and reference materials and different statistical techniques to derive clinical recommendations from test results.

Using a simple mathematical example concerning sensitivity and specificity, it can be demonstrated that the analytic validity of a genetic biomarker test is an important factor in the care of cancer patients: improving the sensitivity of a biomarker test means improving the rate of test positive individuals in the group of all individuals with the genetic marker. Therefore, improving sensitivity by 5 per cent means that five additional patients out of 100 patients with the genetic marker are treated with an effective therapy who might not have been treated otherwise. Due to the often higher percentage of marker-negative compared to marker-positive individuals, sensitivity is possibly even more relevant but more often neglected in personalised medicine in oncology. Sensitivity is defined as the number of test-negative individuals in the population of all individuals who do not have the genetic marker. In this case, improving the specificity of a biomarker test by 5 per cent means that an additional five out of 100 individuals without the marker – and, therefore, healthy or not responding to the therapy – are treated with a less effective or ineffective therapy which might have severe adverse events.

The Analytic Validity of Biomarker Tests in Routine Care

There is a considerable degree of heterogeneity concerning the results of biomarker tests. This problem has mainly been discussed in the context of the validity of clinical studies of biomarkers and the companion therapy. The complexity of the – often new – assays and independent protocol development between laboratories result in relatively high data variability and poor reproducibility of the results (van der Burg et al., 2011). Quality control through harmonisation of laboratory protocols and the introduction of standard operating procedures and assay performance benchmarks are widely used measurements to overcome these limitations. The main challenge remaining is to minimise the heterogeneity in routine patient care. The phases of biomarker development and the corresponding instruments and changes of bias are summarised in a recent review from Marchio et al. (2011). The main sources of bias for the analytic validity of biomarker test results in routine care are the following: the marker tests are often technically developed using clinical samples which are not comparable to the later routine care analyses; the lack of reliable positive and negative controls; technical challenges, such as a poor fixation of the sample; training and competencies of the staff; and a relative reluctance of some pathologists and laboratories concerning quality assurance programmes. These factors can be divided into technical issues and human issues, such as the competencies of professionals and compliance of patients. Recommendations for the development and validation of biomarker assays for use in patients' routine health care to minimise bias and to standardise process steps are available, although it has to be kept in mind that the technical challenges and the evaluation of the routine care context of the assay are considerable (Marchio et al., 2011).

A further step to demonstrate the patient-relevant impact of the analytic validity of biomarker tests in oncology is to look at the range of real-life sensitivity and specificity of genetic biomarker tests for personalised medicine technologies in oncology. The number of studies investigating real-life routine care settings is small compared to the number of studies on the development of new biomarkers. Routine care studies are limited to widespread well-established technologies, such as KRAS testing for colorectal or pancreatic cancer or human epidermal growth factor receptor 2 (HER2) testing in women with breast cancer. Weichert et al. (2010) compared different methods of analysis in a German laboratory centre and concluded that different commercially available standard methods for detecting KRAS mutations show sufficiently concordant results and were equally effective. A very recent study from de Biase et al. (2014) reported promising improvements of the accuracy of KRAS mutation analysis by next generation sequencing compared to the standard methods of Allele Specific Locked Nucleic Acid Quantitative PCR (ASLNA) and Sanger sequencing. The analyses showed improvements in sensitivity by more than 20 per cent. Again, the improved results for next generation sequencing have to be confirmed in other routine care settings, but the study shows the enormous potential for improvement in the analytic validity of well-established biomarker tests.

Another widely used genetic biomarker test in oncology, HER2 (human epidermal growth factor receptor 2) testing in breast cancer therapy stratification, is chosen as a second example. The accuracy of HER2 testing in breast cancer is of enormous importance to the patients, as the decision for or against chemotherapy and Herceptin therapy is directly affected by the HER2 status (Wolff et al., 2007). The gold standard of HER2 status assessment in breast cancer still seems to be under debate (Hicks and Schiffhauer, 2011). The most widespread technology used to detect HER2 mutations is immunohistochemistry (IHC), although for some years, clinical recommendations such as the ASCO (American Society of Clinical Oncology) Guidelines and German recommendations prefer fluorescence *in-situ* hybridization (FISH) as a testing method. In a recent literature review, Lee and colleagues (2011) detected 72 studies comparing different HER2 test methods, 46 of them comparing IHC and FISH. Only seven studies met the ASCO/CAP (College of American Pathologists) guidelines of 95 per cent concordance, leaving the impression of an enormous potential for quality improvement. In a preceding systematic review, Dendukuri et al. (2007) had chosen the same approach. Their meta-analysis of a total of 18 studies comparing seven different HER2 test strategies yielded a variation between none and 9 per cent false positive results and none and 6 per cent false negative results due to the analytic performance of the biomarker tests. In other words, because of the insufficient quality of the test, 9 out of 100 women with breast cancer are treated with chemotherapy without adequate clinical benefit but considerable adverse events, and 6 out of 100 women are denied a helpful therapy.

Both standard approaches – IHC and FISH – can be influenced by pre-analytical factors, assay conditions and interpretation of test results. A study by Varga et al. (2013) analysed biopsies over a period of 12 years and detected a considerable variation of IHC results over time due to changes in the analytic standards. Comparing the periods from 2001–2004 and from 2011–2012, the overall concordance rate between IHC and FISH HER2 status in breast cancer improved significantly from 84 per cent to 97 per cent. Other preceding studies also reported relevant changes of more than 10 per cent of the rate of HER2 test-positive women from 2003 to 2012 using only one diagnostic approach (Middleton et al., 2009; Vergara-Lluri et al., 2012). From these studies and the continuous improvements of the analytical validity of HER2 tests over the last 15 years presented, it is concluded that a strict guideline adherence is essential.

Furthermore, IHC and FISH HER2 assays are subjected to inter-observer variability, the number of assays one pathologist analyses per year, and the number of pathologists who are involved (Reddy et al., 2006; Tubbs et al., 2007; Atkinson et al., 2011; Moelans et al., 2011). A number of further studies support the considerable variation of real-world performance of HER2 testing, especially between local, small laboratories and central, respectively reference, laboratories. The studies showed that small local laboratories classified up to 25 per cent of additional women as test-positive who were classified as negative in reference laboratories (Paik et al., 2002; Dowsett et al., 2003, 2007; Perez et al., 2006). The concordance rates between different test technologies were described as sufficient when ASCO/CAP quality standards were fulfilled (Arnould et al., 2012; Vergara-Lluri et al., 2012).

In summary, it can be concluded from the large number of studies on HER2 testing that the main factor influencing the real-life analytic validity is not the choice of the technical approach (IHC or FISH), but the adherence to quality standards and, as a surrogate, the size of the laboratory.

Concluding Remarks

Due to the development of drug therapy towards genetically stratifying approaches, companion diagnostic biomarker tests are gaining more and more relevance. If biomarker tests directly affect therapy decisions in life-threatening diseases, the tests are no longer seen as a commodity, but as an essential part of the therapeutic strategies.

The test strategies and characteristics are improving and quality standards for laboratories and pathologists are being established. The performance of the tests is being increasingly standardised.

It should be kept in mind that there is a natural limit to the clinical validity of genetic tests concerning the ability to predict the development of a disease. Dreyfuss et al. (2012) demonstrated in a statistical model that genetic biomarker tests can never be perfect in the sense of reaching 100 per cent sensitivity and specificity to predict the development of a disease. It is important to be aware of these limitations, but they are not an excuse to lower one's sights with regard to the analytic validity, respectively the technical quality, of the test. The accuracy of the test might matter even more if the clinical validity is low or if the consequences of the test results are medically severe, for example, because the drug might also induce severe adverse events in patients who are falsely classified as having the specific genetic marker.

Health care has always been tailored to the individual patient and, for example, in traditional Chinese medicine, this is a fundamental principle. It seems that evidence-based medicine (EbM) and health technology assessment (HTA) has evolved, over the last few decades, to the fundamental principle of health care in industrialised Western countries. The use of specific medical technologies is only recommended after the benefit of the use of the technology has been demonstrated with statistical significance in scientific clinical studies of the highest evidence levels, preferably randomised clinical trials within specific patient populations. EbM, therefore, leads to a different way of thinking concerning the individuality of patients. The differentiation of subgroups is an essential part of EbM, however, relying on statistical significance is connected to sample size and, therefore, EbM has its limitations when smaller subgroups are looked at and more than one part of a health-care strategy is influencing the outcomes. It is, by definition, the case in personalised medicine that we are facing multicomponent complex health-care interventions and a stratification in more and more, as well as smaller and smaller subgroups of patients. Therefore, the established algorithms of EbM might face some limitations when personalised medicine strategies and genetic biomarker tests in combination with specific pharmaceutical interventions are evaluated. (For a more comprehensive elaboration on the methods for evaluation of biomarker tests and personalised medicine drugs, see Chapter 13, this volume.)

The analytical validity of genetically stratifying biomarker tests is one important factor influencing the effectiveness of personalised medicine strategies. There are established methodological standards for studies on the analytic validity of biomarker tests, such as the STARD (Standards for the Reporting of Diagnostic accuracy studies) initiative on accurate and transparent reporting (Bossuyt et al., 2003) and the quality assessment tool for diagnostic accuracy studies (QUADAS) checklist for systematic reviews (Whiting et al., 2003). Clear standards for the evaluation of genetic tests have been in place in the United States since ACCE, and in the United Kingdom, a guidance for the health economic evaluation of diagnostic tests was developed within the Diagnostic Assessment Programme

(DAP) of the National Institute for Health and Clinical Excellence (NICE). Specific position papers for approval purposes have also been released by the US and European regulatory agencies, FDA and EMA, respectively.

The basics of how to handle genetically stratifying biomarker tests and how to include the analytic validity of the tests in Germany is somehow intransparent and has not yet been fully clarified (for more details, see Chapter 15, this volume). Briefly summarising, the Federal Joint Committee (G-BA) and the Institute for Quality and Efficiency in Healthcare (IQWiG) so far exclude diagnostic tests from the evaluation of personalised medicine technologies, with the argument that the current, legally binding process of evaluation of new pharmaceuticals (AMNOG: *Arzneimittelmarkt-Neuordnungsgesetz* – Pharmaceuticals Market Reorganisation Act) is a process to evaluate drugs, but not diagnostic tests. The analytic validity of the companion diagnostics is assumed to be given by the relatively weak requirements for approval of diagnostics in Europe, without taking into consideration the real-life variations.

It has been demonstrated that the analytic validity of genetic biomarker tests might have a considerable influence on the therapeutic outcome of the patients. The patients have the right to be treated in the best way. For the sake of the medical benefit of the patients, the legal framework for health-care decision-making processes and the consequent methodological approaches of decision-making bodies, such as the G-BA, should be adapted towards an inclusion of the quality of biomarker tests in the evaluation process of personalised medicine technologies.

References

Arnould, L., Roger, P., MacGrogan, G., Chenard, M.P., Balaton, A., Beauclair, S. and Penault-Llorca, F., 2012. Accuracy of HER2 status determination on breast core-needle biopsies (immunohistochemistry, FISH, CISH and SISH vs FISH). *Modern Pathology*, 25, pp.675–82.

Atkinson, R., Mollerup, J., Laenkholm, A.V., Verardo, M., Hawes, D., Commins, D., Engvad, B., Correa, A., Ehlers, C.C. and Nielsen, K.V., 2011. Effects of the change in cutoff values for human epidermal growth factor receptor 2 status by immunohistochemistry and fluorescence in situ hybridization: a study comparing conventional brightfield microscopy, image analysis-assisted microscopy, and interobserver variation. *Archives in Pathology and Laboratory Medicine*, 135(8), pp.1010–16.

Benraad, T.J., Geurts-Moespot, J. and Grondahl-Hansen, J., 1996. Immunoassays (ELISA) of urokinase-type plasminogen activator (uPA): report of an EORTC/BIOMED-1 workshop. *European Journal of Cancer*, 32A, pp.1371–81.

Bossuyt, P.M., Reitsma, J.B., Bruns, D.E., Gatsonis, C.A., Glasziou, P.P., Irwig, L.M., Lijmer, J.G., Moher, D., Rennie, D. and de Vet, H.C.W., 2003. Towards complete and accurate reporting of studies of diagnostic accuracy: the STARD initiative. *British Medical Journal*, 326(4), pp.41–4.

de Biase, D., Visani, M., Baccarini, P., Polifemo, A.M., Maimone, A., Fornelli, A., Giuliani, A., Zanini, N., Fabbri, C., Pession, A. and Tallini, G., 2014. Next generation sequencing improves the accuracy of KRAS mutation analysis in endoscopic ultrasound fine needle aspiration pancreatic lesions. *PLoS One*, 9(2), p.e87651.

Dendukuri, N., Khetani, K., McIsaac, M. and Brophy, J., 2007. Testing for HER2-positive breast cancer: a systematic review and cost-effectiveness analysis. *Canadian Medical Association Journal*, 176(10), pp.1429–34.

Douillard, J.Y., Oliner, K.S., Siena, S., Tabernero, J., Burkes, R., Barugel, M., Humblet, Y., Bodoky, G., Cunningham, D., Jassem, J., Rivera, F., Kocákova, I., Ruff, P., Błasińska-Morawiec, M., Šmakal, M., Canon, J.L., Rother, M., Williams, R., Rong, A., Wiezorek, J., Sidhu, R. and Patterson, S.D., 2013. Panitumumab-FOLFOX4 treatment and RAS mutations in colorectal cancer. *New England Journal of Medicine*, 369(11), pp.1023–34.

Dowsett, M., Bartlett, J., Ellis, I.O., Salter, J., Hills, M., Mallon, E., Watters, A.D., Cooke, T., Paish, C, Wencyk, P.M. and Pinder, S.E., 2003. Correlation between immunohistochemistry (HercepTest) and fluorescence in situ hybridization (FISH) for HER-2 in 426 breast carcinomas from 37 centres. *Journal of Pathology*, 199(4), pp.418–23.

Dowsett, M., Hanna, W.M., Kockx, M., Penault-Llorca, F., Rüschoff, J., Gurjahr, T., Habben, K. and van de Vijver, M.J., 2007. Standardization of HER2 testing: results of an international proficiency-testing ring study. *Modern Pathology*, 20, pp.584–91.

Dreyfuss, J.M., Levner, D., Galagan, J.E., Church, G.M. and Ramoni, M.F., 2012. How accurate can genetic predictions be? *BMC Genomics*, 13, p.340.

FDA (Food and Drug Administration), 2011. *Draft guidance for industry and food and drug administration staff. In vitro companion diagnostic devices.* Rockville, MD: Food and Drug Administration.

Haddow, J.E. and Palomaki, G.E, 2003. ACCE: A model process for evaluating data on emerging genetic tests. In: M. Khoury, J. Little and W. Burke, eds. *Human genome epidemiology: a scientific foundation for using genetic information to improve health and prevent disease.* Oxford: Oxford University Press. pp.217–33.

Hicks, D.G. and Schiffhauer, L., 2011. Standardized assessment of the HER2 status in breast cancer by immunohistochemistry. *Labmedicine*, 42(8), pp.459–67.

Lee, J.A., Shaheen, M., Walke, T. and Daly, M., 2011. Clinical and health economic outcomes of alternative HER2 test strategies for guiding adjuvant trastuzumab therapy. *Expert Reviews in Pharmacoeconomics and Outcomes Research*, 11(3), pp.325–41.

Loong, T.W., 2003. Understanding sensitivity and specificity with the right side of the brain. *British Medical Journal*, 327(7417), pp.716–19.

Marchio, C., Dowsett, M. and Reis-Filho, J.S., 2011. Revisiting the technical validation of tumour biomarker assays: how to open a Pandora's box. *BMC Medicine*, 9(41), pp.1–6.

Middleton, L.P., Price, K.M., Puig, P., Heydon, L.J., Tarco, E., Sneige, N., Barr, K. and Deavers, M.T., 2009. Implementation of American Society of Clinical Oncology/College of American Pathologists HER2 Guideline Recommendations in a tertiary care facility increases HER2 immunohistochemistry and fluorescence in situ hybridization concordance and decreases the number of inconclusive cases. *Archives in Pathology and Laboratory Medicine*, 133(5), pp.775–80.

Moelans, C.B., de Weger, R.A., Van der Wall, E. and van Diest, P.J., 2011. Current technologies for HER2 testing in breast cancer. *Critical Reviews in Oncology and Hematology*, 80(3), pp.380–92.

Paik, S., Bryant, J., Tan-Chiu, E., Romond, E., Hiller, W., Park, K., Brown, A., Yothers, G., Anderson, S., Smith, R., Wickerham, D.L. and Wolmark, N., 2002. Real world performance of HER2 testing – National Surgical Adjuvant Breast and Bowel Project experience. *Journal of the National Cancer Institute*, 94, pp.852–4.

Perez, E.A., Suman, V.J., Davidson, N.E., Martino, S., Kaufman, P.A., Lingle, W.L., Flynn, P.J., Ingle, J.N., Visscher, D. and Jenkins, R.B., 2006. HER2 testing by local, central, and reference laboratories in specimens from the North Central Cancer Treatment Group N9831 intergroup adjuvant trial. *Journal of Clinical Oncology*, 24(19), pp.3032–8.

Reddy, J.C., Reimann, J.D., Anderson, S.M. and Klein, P.M., 2006. Concordance between central and local laboratory HER2 testing from a community-based clinical study. *Clinical Breast Cancer*, 7(2), pp.153–7.

Tubbs, R.R., Hicks, D.G., Cook, J., Downs-Kelly, E., Pettay, J., Hartke, M.B., Hood, L., Neelon, R., Myles, J. and Budd, G.T., 2007. Fluorescence in situ hybridization (FISH) as primary methodology for the assessment of HER2 Status in adenocarcinoma of the breast: a single institution experience. *Diagnostic Molecular Pathology*, 16(4), pp.207–10.

van der Burg, S.H., Kalos, M., Gouttefangeas, C., Janetzki, S., Ottensmeier, C., Welters, M.J., Romero, P., Britten, C.M. and Hoos, A., 2011. Harmonization of immune biomarker assays for clinical studies. *Science in Translational Medicine*, 3(108), pp.108–44.

Varga, Z., Noske, A., Ramach, C., Padberg, B. and Moch, H., 2013. Assessment of HER2 status in breast cancer: overall positivity rate and accuracy by fluorescence in situ hybridization and immunohistochemistry in a single institution over 12 years: a quality control study. *BMC Cancer*, 13, p.615.

Vergara-Lluri, M.E., Moatamed, N.A., Hong, E. and Apple, S.K., 2012. High concordance between HercepTest immunohistochemistry and ERBB2 fluorescence in situ hybridization before and after implementation of American Society of Clinical Oncology/College of American Pathology 2007 guidelines. *Modern Pathology*, 25(10), pp.1326–32.

Weichert, W., Schewe, C., Lehmann, A., Sers, C., Denkert, C., Budczies, J., Stenzinger, A., Joos, H., Landt, O., Heiser, V., Röcken, C. and Dietel, M., 2010. KRAS genotyping of paraffin-embedded colorectal cancer tissue in routine diagnostics comparison of methods and impact of histology. *Journal of Molecular Diagnostics*, 12(1), pp.35–42.

Whiting, P., Rutjes, A.W.S., Reitsma, J.B., Bossuyt, P.M.M. and Kleijnen, J., 2003. The development of QUADAS: a tool for the quality assessment of studies of diagnostic accuracy included in systematic reviews. *BMC Medical Research Methodology*, 3(25), pp.1–13.

Wolff, A.C., Hammond, M.E., Schwartz, J.N., Hagerty, K.L., Allred, D.C., Cote, R.J., Dowsett, M., Fitzgibbons, P.L., Hanna, W.M. and Langer, A., 2007. American Society of Clinical Oncology/College of American Pathologists guideline recommendations for human epidermal growth factor receptor 2 testing in breast cancer. *Journal of Clinical Oncology*, 25(1), pp.118–45.

Zono, K.D., Terry, P.F. and Terry, S.F., 2009. A measure of truth in genetic testing. *Genetic Testing and Molecular Biomarkers*, 13(3), pp.285–6.

Chapter 15

Approval and Reimbursement of Personalised Drugs: Interim Results of the Adjustment Process

Michael Noweski, Anke Walendzik, Franz Hessel,
Rebecca Jahn and Jürgen Wasem[1]

Introduction

According to drug manufacturers, the pharmaceutical industry is suffering from an 'innovation crisis'. Nowadays, the development of new products requires significantly more investment than in the past. Most of the simple but useful chemical entities seem to have been discovered already. Moreover, many top-selling drugs lose their patent protection ('patent cliff') and, subsequently, prices and sales of the original drug are undermined by competing generics. Producers try to compensate for the loss of sales by launches of new molecular entities (Jimenez, 2012). However, the new compounds generate fewer sales. As market observers calculated, new products launched in the period from 2001 to 2005 achieved annual average sales of USD 208 million after three years. New products of the period from 2006 to 2010 reached only USD 143 million (Rockoff and Winslow, 2013). Development of a drug which yields more than a billion USD per year ('blockbuster') succeeds less often. Drugs combined with biomarker-based diagnostic tests, stratifying patients into groups characterised by different drug reactions, appear to be one way out of trouble, because a new generation of patented products seems attainable (Scollen and Phelan, 2014).

The biotechnology industry has announced that stratifying potential patients will make drug therapy safer, more successful and more cost-effective (Hawkins, 2013). From the perspective of clinicians, such innovations are welcomed. An adequate regulatory framework appears to be one precondition of companies'

1   This study was conducted in the research network Personalised Medicine in Oncology: An Interdisciplinary Study on Ethical, Medical, Economical and Legal Aspects (Grant project number: 01 GP 1001A-C), which is supported by the German Federal Ministry of Education and Research (Bundesministerium für Bildung und Forschung – BMBF).

willingness to develop these new products. Possibly existing unnecessary hurdles concerning the approval and reimbursement process, not tolerably discouraging the development of stratifying products, should be removed.

Approval in the United States

The jurisdictions to approve drugs and diagnostic tests in the United States are located at the US Food and Drug Administration (FDA). Within the FDA, competencies are separated. Drugs are assessed by the Center for Drug Evaluation and Research (CDER) and tests by the Center for Devices and Radiological Health (CDRH). The ACCE model, which verifies the analytical validity, clinical validity, clinical utility, and ethical, legal and social impacts is the basis of the latter examination. The procedure is based on the classification of the test in risk class I, II or III. Genetic tests are often classified with stage III. In these cases, the 'Premarket Notification', also called '510(k)', which compares candidates with already approved products, is not sufficient. Instead, the 'Premarket Approval (PMA)' is necessary; only this requires randomised and controlled trials.

Almost all pretests in drug therapy are *in vitro* diagnostic medical devices (IVDs). These are examined by the Office of *In Vitro* Diagnostics and Radiological Health (OIR) at the CDRH (Day, 2013). A subunit of the OIR is the Personalised Medicine Staff which analyses the specific problems of stratifying pretesting in drug therapy and assists several offices. Pursuant to Section 862.9 of the *Code of Federal Regulations Title 21* (21 CFR), the exception to the PMA relying on Section 510(k) is not possible if the application of the test can lead to misdiagnosis and, subsequently, to high mortality and morbidity risk. Therefore, if the test is classified under class I or II, because of low risks in application, PMA is, nevertheless, required because the consideration of the results may lead to harm.

The FDA has expanded its guidance significantly in recent years. In 2003, it released an exposition, the *Draft Guidance for Industry on Pharmacogenomic Data Submission*, calling on drug manufacturers to use genetic tests in their development projects and to submit the data collected, allowing the authority to improve procedures and methods of data analysis. The Voluntary Exploratory Data Submissions (VXDS) are evaluated by the Institutional Pharmacogenomics Review Group (IPRG). The European Medicines Agency (EMA), the European equivalent of the FDA, is connected to the programme as a partner. The draft of 2003 made a perceptible statement that stratifying genetic testing is desirable and should be incorporated into the product development. It was the first guide for manufacturers showing in which way the results of testing and stratification would affect the appraisal of the clinical studies and also clarifying what kind of data increases the chances of market authorisation. Since 2004, the FDA has called its campaign to promote genetic testing the 'Critical Path Initiative' (Kim et al., 2012). The final guideline, *Guidance for Industry: Pharmacogenomic Data Submissions*, was published in 2005. In 2007, another draft guideline, *Guidance for Industry: Pharmacogenomic Data Submissions – Companion Guidance*, with further specifications concerning the application of tests, followed.

Since 2007, the FDA has also specified necessary information regarding the assessment of pharmacogenomic tests. The draft guideline *Pharmacogenetic Tests and Genetic Tests for Heritable Markers* defines requirements for data used for the 510(k) and the PMA. The applicant shall disclose the clinical purpose, the biomarker and the group of patients addressed. The paper includes specifications for comparative studies using already approved products, for the use of software, for the design of clinical trials and for labelling. In 2011, the FDA published the guideline *In Vitro Companion Diagnostic Devices*, which categorises biomarker-based tests, distinguishing three possible uses: the stratification of patients according to probable success of treatment, the stratification according to expectable adverse reactions and the monitoring of the course of therapy. The guideline states that pretests should be validated by manufacturers in the examination of drug effectiveness during phase II and III. The FDA announced that pretests will be evaluated in the context of their application in conjunction with a specific drug. Whether the OIR initiates the 510(k) or the PMA depends on the application risks. The offices of drug approval and of test approval act together. If a manufacturer intends to market an already approved test as part of another medication, this represents a new application and a new approval procedure is required. If a manufacturer intends to market a test as a competitor to an already marketed test, it requires their own approval.

The FDA supports companies in the development of drugs for rare diseases ('orphan drugs'). Here, it grants up to USD 150,000 for phase I studies and up to USD 300,000 for studies in phase II and III. Accelerated approval procedures with reduced demands on the significance of the study results are possible. Not surprisingly, companies having invested millions of dollars in the development of pretests also demand support for drugs addressing small patient groups with rare genotypes and divergent drug reactions. However, according to the FDA, the *Orphan Drug Act* (ODA) of 1983 offers no legal basis for granting such privileges (Gutmann Koch, 2012).

Approval in Europe

The EMA welcomes the use of stratifying tests in drug development. The department responsible is the Committee for Medicinal Products for Human

Use (CHMP). The guideline *Reflection paper on the use of pharmacogenetics in the pharmacokinetic evaluation of medicinal products* from 2007 states:

> When the genotype is predicted or known to markedly affect the pharmacokinetics of pharmacologically active compounds contributing to in vivo efficacy and/or safety of a medicinal product, genotyping is encouraged in as many of the phase I, II and III clinical studies as possible to increase the amount of data that will support the recommendations for use in the genetic subpopulation(s). (EMA, 2007, p.4)

Two draft guidelines followed in 2010, discussing the use of biomarker-based tests in drug development. The first relates to the general methods of stratification of patient populations. The second gives advice for the simultaneous development of pretest and drug. The *Guideline on the use of pharmacogenetic methodologies in the pharmacokinetic evaluation of medicinal products*, published in 2012, provides more details on the requirements of the study designs and the expedient preparation of trial results for the application dossier.

There are no specific fast-tracks for the approval of genetically stratifying drugs so far in the United States and in Europe. A facilitated marketing authorisation is possible only in special circumstances by taking advantage of two different procedures occasionally used for drugs without test. The 'marketing authorisation under exceptional circumstances', mostly granted in cases of orphan drugs, is reviewed by the EMA every year. This option is highly interesting for drug manufacturers. It promises a permanent relief from a part of the costs caused by clinical trials. Since 2006, new drugs that promise therapeutic advantages in life-threatening diseases may get a 'conditional approval' for a year, which can be renewed if the company credibly assures that the required study results will be submitted.

In contrast to the FDA, the EMA does not approve the test. The assessment of the test as a medical device can be provided by 'Notified Bodies' selectable in any member state of the European Union (EU). The EU has adopted a guideline on the harmonisation of the procedure. It requires a certification according to European safety standards, as laid down in the *Directive 98/79/EC of the European Parliament and of the Council of 27 October 1998 on in vitro diagnostic medical devices*. Four groups of products are defined in the annexes of the guideline. Each group requires its own version of the conformity assessment procedure. The several versions are combinations of modules containing different means (Table 15.1). Sometimes the applicant can choose from two or more combinations of modules.

In Germany, the *Medical Devices Act* (*Medizinproduktegesetz*, MPG) and the *Medical Devices Regulation* (*Medizinprodukte-Verordnung*, MPV) are the legal basis for marketing and use of medical devices. They demand that the products have

Table 15.1   Modules of the conformity assessment procedure

Module A	internal production control
Module Aa	extended internal production control
Module B	EC type-examination
Module C	conformity to type
Module D	production quality assurance
Module E	product quality assurance
Module F	product verification
Module G	unit verification
Module H	full quality assurance

Source: Directive 98/79/EC of the European Parliament and of the Council of 27 October 1998 on in vitro diagnostic medical devices.

to show the 'CE mark', which confirms the conformity with European safety standards. The *Central Authority of the Federal States for Health Protection with regard to Medicinal Products and Medical Devices* (*Zentralstelle der Länder für Gesundheitsschutz bei Arzneimitteln und Medizinprodukten*, ZLG) designates specific laboratories operating product certification for IVDs. Health experts are often critical that IVDs which have received the CE mark have been inadequately reviewed in terms of their intended diagnostic use (Ieven et al., 2013). In the case of pretests in drug therapy, the certification without verification of functional benefit may be a risk for the patients because the results of testing may cause misdirected drug prescription. Thus, it is questionable whether the procedure is sufficient. A detailed examination of the benefit–risk ratio of the test-drug combination requires the inclusion of the clinical trials of the drug. However, an assessment of the test after the approval of the drug would delay the launch of the drug significantly. Therefore, concurrent procedures are desirable. However, closer co-operation between the EMA and Notified Bodies would be beneficial. A corresponding model already exists. In 2007, the EMA founded the Committee for Advanced Therapies (CAT). Its function is to assess genetically engineered pharmaceuticals and medicines for cell therapy. The examinations include medical devices as far as they are integral part of the products. Therefore, the CAT utilises data generated by the Notified Bodies. The EMA/CAT-NB Collaboration Group is the interface of this exchange.

The industry benefits from the fact that the assessment of tests is less strict and delays are very unusual. The requirements, however, were increased in the past in small steps and will be raised significantly by a proposed amendment of the EU In Vitro Directive (*Proposal for a regulation of the European Parliament and of the Council on in vitro diagnostic medical devices COM (2012) 541 final*).

Pursuant to Annex VII of the draft, tests for the stratification of patients shall be classified in the second highest risk category 'C'. Manufacturers of class C products are subjected to a conformity assessment based on a complete review of quality assurance in accordance with Annex VIII. Pursuant to paragraph 6.2 of the annex, the Notified Body shall evaluate the suitability of the product in conjunction with the related drug. The body has to consult the national drug regulatory authority or the EMA, which has to deliver a statement within 60 days, or at the latest, after 120 days. The documents for the product design in the technical documentation must be checked on a representative basis. Alternatively, the manufacturer may choose a conformity assessment on the basis of a pattern examination, which is set out in Annex IX, in combination with a conformity assessment based on the production quality assurance in Annex X. Again, the suitability in conjunction with the drug has to be assessed (Annex IX Paragraph 3.6). The implementation of the draft would be a further step towards an integrated approval process for test and drug. The most consistent solution would be the sole responsibility of the EMA.

Reimbursement in the United States

The United States is the most important market due to its size, but it is quite challenging for the industry to comprehend the decentralised decision-making processes concerning scope of coverage and modalities of reimbursement. The willingness to pay differs between the various insurers. Private payers finance drug therapy and genetic testing more frequently than public funding agencies. Large insurance companies have extensive analytical resources to assess new products. Their considerations are not uniform, but scientific reviews are an important part (Trosman et al., 2010). The firms have comprehensive internal guidelines on the requirements a product has to meet to be reimbursed. Therefore, the industry can foresee the market potential of their products relatively well. In the case of stratifying medicines, the quality of data is often problematic (Meckley and Neumann, 2010). The inclusion in the benefits package is repeatedly delayed, because the additional benefit compared to existing therapies (comparative effectiveness) is insufficiently demonstrated.

In the jurisdiction of the public payers Medicare and Medicaid, the health economic assessment and the decision to reimburse are made by the Centers for Medicare and Medicaid Services (CMS). This review body aims to align methods with the FDA and to make its judgment immediately after approval (Messner and Tunis, 2012). From the perspective of the industry, the co-operation of the CMS and FDA may create early feedbacks whether a product will be reimbursed. The CMS has the authority to make coverage decisions for all of its beneficiaries, but in the case of diagnostic tests, the agency has relied upon its regional contractors to set local coverage policies (Health Advances, 2010).

The manufacturers of diagnostic tests criticise the reimbursement system of Medicare. The fee coding system for billing the services seems too complex. The insurers reluctantly accept new products because the coding behaviour of physicians is difficult to predict. Instead of the current system with a code for each step of testing, the whole procedure should be remunerated by one code (Health Advances, 2010). Each test should have its own code according to indication, biomarker and product. The physicians would cease 'code stacking'. All insurers should use the same code system. The manufacturers of test kits would save marketing expenditures because they promote just one code. Another demand of the industry is the standardisation of health economic evaluation by payers. More transparency about criteria and thresholds would allow manufacturers to forecast whether a development project has the potential to achieve a positive rating.

Reimbursement in Germany

In the EU, the member states are responsible for benefit assessment and reimbursement. No integrated procedure to assess the benefit of drug-test combinations exists in Germany. Drugs and medical devices are evaluated by different organisations. The additional benefit of a new drug is regularly assessed six months after market introduction in an early benefit assessment processed by the Federal Joint Committee (*Gemeinsamer Bundesausschuss*, G-BA), which is the main negotiating body between funding agencies and service providers. In the case of an additional benefit in comparison to a comparator therapy, rebates on the manufacturer's prices are negotiated between the National Association of Statutory Health Insurance Funds (*Spitzenverband Bund der Krankenkassen*, GKV-SV) and the manufacturer. If there is no additional benefit, pharmaceuticals are integrated into reference price groups. If no agreement is reached in the central price negotiations, the rebates are usually determined by an arbitration board. This method ensures immediate market access and reimbursement of the drug shortly after approval, unless the manufacturer stops the marketing process in response to the arbitration award.

One advantage for the industry in Germany is that there are no restrictive central price negotiations for medical devices. If the device is reimbursed by the Social Health Insurance (*Gesetzliche Krankenversicherung*, GKV), the amount of reimbursement is based on the price of comparable products. The amount may be higher in private health insurance. The private insurance companies reimburse all pretests of drug therapy, as long as there are no known safety constraints. In the GKV, the reimbursement of mandatory companion diagnostics, which are specified on the label, is not problematic. However, for other products, the chances of being reimbursed are difficult to predict. The decision-making depends on the sector of the health system where the test is applied. In outpatient care, the tests can be billed by the performing physician if there is a suitable fee code in the reimbursement scheme called the Uniform Value Scale (*Einheitlicher Bewertungsmaßstab*, EBM). The updating of the EBM is the responsibility of the Evaluation Committee (*Bewertungsausschuss*), which is the federal negotiating body between statutory health insurance funds and physicians concerning the remuneration of outpatient service in the GKV. In the case of a test representing a new method, an assessment of the new medical procedure by the G-BA regarding medical benefit and cost-effectiveness is required. After a positive result, the G-BA instructs the Evaluation Committee to adapt the EBM. Installation of new codes for testing methods already medically used and only addressing other targets is within the power of decision of the Evaluation Committee without preceding assessment by the G-BA. Both the G-BA and the Evaluation Committee contain an equal number of representatives of providers and statutory health insurance funds. The difference between the two procedures is that in the case of a positive statement of the G-BA, the representatives of the funds mostly agree to an increase of the total reimbursement budget for outpatient physicians to avoid a decrease of the remuneration for other services. Without an assessment of the G-BA in the case of expected patient benefit, the representatives of the funds mostly allow a new code, but without additional money to raise the reimbursement budget. Hence, the new test would burden the physicians' budget for ambulatory care. As a rule, the representatives of the physicians in the Evaluation Committee reject such a concession because those groups of medical practitioners that do not benefit would protest strongly. Therefore, there might be considerable time lags in reimbursement decisions.

Inclusion of new tests in the remuneration system of hospitals is less demanding because it requires no examination by the G-BA. Individual hospitals and health insurance funds can agree on a provisional compensation. After a probation period, these tests are included into the regular reimbursement scheme for inpatient care. Because most patients get their test by outpatient service, the new code in the EBM remains the decisive prerequisite for market success. In some cases, a new section in the Fifth Book of the Social Security Code (*Sozialgesetzbuch V*, SGB V), the main legal source of the GKV, could be beneficial.

In the case of an assessment of the test by the G-BA, according to paragraph 137e SGB V, the manufacturer may submit a formal request for 'Potential Assessment' to the G-BA. Then, in co-operation with this committee, new clinical studies are commissioned. The additional evidence may influence the decision on the eligibility positively. Currently, the G-BA only has a small budget for Potential Assessments concerning new diagnostic or therapeutic procedures: only five analyses per year are provided.

The German Association of Research-Based Pharmaceutical Companies (*Verband Forschender Arzneimittelhersteller*, VFA) has criticised that there have been significant delays in decision-making procedures concerning reimbursement of tests. Approved drugs, therefore, were not prescribed to the full extent (Fischer, 2012). The manufacturers of tests have similarly complained about delays in reimbursement decisions (Schatz, 2013). Nonetheless, a study of the interest association Personalised Medicine Coalition rated Germany as the most attractive market for products of personalised medicine in Europe (Garfield, 2011). In summary, when drug and test are seen together, the opportunities of reimbursement and the level of amounts are considered to be comparatively high.

Conclusion

The approval of drug and test in the United States is carried out within the FDA and will become an integrated process in the future. In Europe, the procedures are separate and co-ordination between the EMA and Notified Bodies is a hope for the future. An integrated one-stop process requires a radical overhaul of the EU's In Vitro Directive. In the United States, the decision about reimbursement of drug and test by Medicare and Medicaid is carried out by the CMS. More collaboration between the FDA and CMS is under construction. In Germany, the question of refunding is more complicated. More co-operation and integration within the different institutions and procedures is an essential precondition to co-ordinate and speed up approval and reimbursement decisions. A link between the EMA and Notified Bodies is lacking as well as co-operation between the EMA and the G-BA. More communication between the G-BA and Notified Bodies is needed. It is a fundamental problem that the Notified Bodies are scattered throughout the member states of the EU. Despite the high institutional fragmentation, Germany is a relatively favourable market for stratifying drugs. All drugs with additional benefit are reimbursed a few months after approval at comparatively high prices. Despite increasing requirements, the approval of the tests is still unproblematic. There are also low hurdles for new tests in hospitals. If the additional benefits in comparison to established treatment options are not obvious, the reimbursement in ambulatory care can be delayed for years or it may never be achieved. In essence, there are no unreasonable barriers for innovative test-drug combinations. Given the regulatory conditions, restraint conversion to products of personalised medicine would not be justified. Whether a new generation of drugs would financially overwhelm the GKV in Germany is not clear. Nowadays, strict rationing of access is not needed and not expected over the next few years. However, it might be necessary to observe in which way the GKV-SV responds to an increase in drug expenditure, and to clear up the implications for the price negotiations of drugs and the reimbursement decisions with respect to testing.

References

Day, J., 2013. Introduction to in vitro diagnostic device regulatory requirements. In: G. Jenkins and C.D. Mansfield, eds. *Methods in molecular biology*. New York: Springer. pp.103–12.

EMA (European Medicines Agency), 2007. Reflection paper on the use of pharmacogenetics in the pharmacokinetic evaluation of medicinal products. [pdf] Available at: http://www.ema.europa.eu/docs/en_GB/document_library/Scientific_guideline/2009/09/WC500003890.pdf [Accessed 13 March 2014].

Fischer, B., 2012. 'Deutschland ist ein Top-Standort': interview with Birgit Fischer, Hauptgeschäftsführerin, vfa. *VentureCapital Magazin*, 2012(6), Special Supplement, Personalized Medicine, pp.14–15.

Garfield, S., 2011. Advancing access to personalized medicine: a comparative assessment of European reimbursement systems. [pdf] Available at: http://www.personalizedmedicinecoalition.org/sites/default/files/files/PMC_Europe_Reimbursement_Paper_Final.pdf [Accessed 13 March 2014].

Gutmann Koch, V., 2012. Incentivizing the utilization of pharmacogenomics in drug development. *Journal of Health Care Law & Policy*, 15(1), pp.263–302.

Hawkins, T., 2013. Companion diagnostics: an interview with Trevor Hawkins, SVP, Strategy Innovation and Business Development for Siemens Healthcare Diagnostics. *News-Medical.Net*, [online] Available at: http://www.news-medical.net/news/20130827/Companion-diagnostics-an-interview-with-Trevor-Hawkins-SVP-Strategy-Innovation-and-Business-Development-for-Siemens-Healthcare-Diagnostics.aspx [Accessed 13 March 2014].

Health Advances, 2010. The reimbursement landscape for novel diagnostics. [pdf] Available at: http://www.healthadvances.com/pdf/novel_diag_reimbursement.pdf [Accessed 13 March 2014].

Ieven, M., Finch, R. and van Belkum, A., 2013. European quality clearance of new microbiological diagnostics. *Clinical Microbiology and Infection*, 19(1), pp.29–38.

Jimenez, J., 2012. The CEO of Novartis on growing after a patent cliff. *Harvard Business Review*, 90(12), pp.39–42.

Kim, M.-J., Zineh, I., Huang, S.-M. and Lesko, L.J., 2012. Role of pharmacogenetics in registration processes. In: A.-H. Maitland-van der Zee and A.K. Daly, eds. *Pharmacogenetics and individualized therapy*. Hoboken: John Wiley & Sons. pp.461–75.

Meckley, L. and Neumann, P.J., 2010. Personalized medicine: factors influencing reimbursement. *Health Policy*, 94(2), pp.91–100.

Messner, D.A. and Tunis, S.R., 2012. Current and future state of FDA-CMS parallel reviews. *Clinical Pharmacology and Therapeutics*, 91(3), pp.383–5.

Rockoff, J.D. and Winslow, R., 2013. New medicines emerge, but few blockbusters: drug makers find it hard to elbow aside established, often cheaper, products. *Wall Street Journal*, [online] Available at: http://online.wsj.com/news/articles/SB10001424052702304281004579222362098933226 [Accessed 13 March 2014].

Schatz, P., 2013. 'Unsere Akquisitionsstrategie stützt die Gesamtstrategie': interview mit Peer Schatz, CEO, Qiagen N.V. *VentureCapital Magazin*, 2013(2), pp.22–3.

Scollen, S. and Phelan, A., 2014. Enabling next-generation pain therapeutics through precision medicine. In: C.H. Allerton, ed. *Pain therapeutics*. Cambridge: Royal Society of Chemistry. pp.326–48.

Trosman, J.R., Van Bebber, S.L. and Phillips, K.A., 2010. Coverage policy development for personalized medicine: private payer perspectives on developing policy for the 21-gene assay. *Journal of Oncology Practice*, 6(5), pp.238–42.

Chapter 16

Criteria for Fairly Allocating Scarce Health-Care Resources to Genetic Tests: Which Matter Most?[1]

Wolf H. Rogowski, Scott D. Grosse, Jörg Schmidtke and Georg Marckmann[2]

Introduction

The availability of new genetic tests and their use in health care is expanding rapidly (Schmidtke et al., 2005; Javaher et al., 2008). In spite of technical improvements leading to steadily lowering laboratory costs per test (Rogowski, 2006), the costs of bioinformatic evaluation, counselling and follow-up testing could easily outweigh the potential savings from early prevention and lead to an overall increase in health-care expenditures (Rogowski, 2007; Mardis, 2010). It has been demonstrated, for example, that it is not economically feasible to conduct cascade testing for all monogenic disorders for which tests are available (Krawczak et al., 2007). A recent survey of Canadian health-care providers also reported insufficient resources to fund all genetic tests that were considered desirable (Adair et al., 2009).

If resources for health services are limited, there is a large risk that limits are set unfairly. It is well-known that individuals with higher socioeconomic status

1   This paper was originally published in the European Journal of Human Genetics under the title 'Criteria for Fairly Allocating Scarce Health-care Resources to Genetic Tests: Which Matter Most?', 2013, 1–7, doi:10.1038/ejhg.2013.172. With kind permission of Nature Publishing Group.

2   We acknowledge the comments from various colleagues, especially Per Carlsson, Jürgen John, Helena Kääriäinen, Alastair Kent, Michael Krawczak, Ulf Kristofferson, and Irma Nippert. All errors of omission and commission remain our own. The study was partly supported by EuroGentest, an EU FP6 supported NoE contract number 512148 (EuroGentest Unit 3: Clinical genetics, community genetics and public health, Workpackage 3.2 (J. Schmidtke)) and its successor EuroGentest2 (contract number 261469).

The findings and conclusions in this chapter are those of the authors and do not necessarily represent the official position of the Centers for Disease Control and Prevention. The authors declare no conflict of interest.

experience longer lives and better health-related quality of life across Europe, and have better access to specialist health care (van Doorslaer et al., 2004). It is also likely that individuals with higher socioeconomic status are better informed about options for genetic testing, better at arguing their case with their general practitioner or when seeking a geneticist appointment, and more able to fund tests out of pocket. Although for many things in life, such as expensive cars or other luxury goods, it is widely accepted that societal allocation differs by income, for important health-care services this is frequently considered unfair.

Fair allocation of health-care resources requires that tests are allocated according to ethically reflected criteria (Huster, 2011). If resources are not sufficient to fund all desirable tests, there is a need to determine which tests are most important to provide. This is referred to as explicit 'prioritisation', that is, ranking genetic tests based on their perceived importance (Giacomini et al., 2003).

Frequently, decisions about health-care coverage and priority setting are associated with formal processes of national decision-making bodies. The UK National Institute of Health and Clinical Excellence (NICE), for example, recently implemented a 'Diagnostics Assessment Programme'. However, most health-care funding decisions are made in a less formalised manner at lower decision levels, such as health-care organisations (Rogowski et al., 2008). Adair and colleagues (2009) report that most Canadian decisions on which genetic tests would be covered were local level *ad hoc* decisions and concluded that a more coordinated approach would be desirable. The development of standards for prioritisation on a local and regional level could also be beneficial in Europe.

The appropriate criteria for prioritisation of genetic tests may differ by clinical condition or application. The successful prioritisation activities in Sweden include 'Defining the area of prioritization' (Broqvist et al., 2011). Prioritisation activities have been more successful in Sweden within clinical specialties than across clinical areas (Carlsson, 2012). An approach specifically targeted at genetic tests may, therefore, be particularly promising.

The challenge for prioritising genetic tests is to develop criteria that have a firm ethical basis, are sufficiently specific for genetic tests and that can be operationalised, measured and consistently applied across a variety of genetic tests and clinical applications.

This study provides an overview of ethical and economic concepts for prioritising scarce health-care resources towards genetic tests (for a detailed discussion on the analytic validity of biomarker tests in oncology, see Chapter 14, this volume). The study focuses on human genetics services which can be provided in potentially different local organisational contexts. The long-term aim is to develop structured prioritisation information which could be used to complement standardised information sources about genetic tests, such as the Clinical Utility Gene Cards published by the *European Journal of Human Genetics*

(Schmidtke and Cassiman, 2010) or the Gene Dossiers developed by the UK Genetic Testing Network (UKGTN).

Concepts and Methods

A wide range of definitions of genetic testing appear in international recommendations, guidelines and reports (Sequeiros et al., 2012). Genetic testing is defined here as the application of a laboratory test or assay (the analysis of human DNA, RNA, chromosomes, proteins or certain metabolites in order to detect alterations related to a heritable disorder or to specific reactions to medical treatments[3]) to a defined clinical context. A given genetic assay may have multiple applications, including diagnosis, population screening, or cascade testing of family members. The prioritisation of coverage of a given laboratory assay may differ depending on the specific type of clinical application.

The provision of genetic tests involves a range of ethical aspects, such as questions of privacy, unnecessary worry, or under what conditions a termination of pregnancy is ethically acceptable. Ethical considerations can provide important constraints to the practice and organisation of genetics services. These issues cannot be addressed here. This chapter is restricted to established genetics services that are considered by most observers to be ethically acceptable and to provide more good than harm. In particular, we exclude from this study carrier-, pre-implantation and prenatal testing for the purpose of family planning as well as population screening. These tests involve a range of very specific ethical issues which have been discussed elsewhere (Eisenberg and Schenker, 1997; West, 1988; Johnson and Elkins, 1988; Grosse et al., 2010).

The study is based on a large number of exploratory literature searches, complemented by a systematic search for existing prioritisation frameworks (appendix available on request).

Criteria for Allocating Health-Care Resources to Genetic Tests

Prioritisation of scarce health-care resources has been addressed by the health economic and ethical scientific communities for many years. Persad et al. (2009) classify normative criteria for allocating medical interventions into four categories: need-based allocation, benefit maximisation, equity, and

---

3   See http://www.genetests.org/servlet/access?id=8888891&key=Wt-CocgvbZ Fre&fcn=y&fw=FNL-&filename=/concepts/primer/primerwhatistest.html [accessed on 22 December 2009; pharmacogenetics included].

promotion and reward of social usefulness. The following sections discuss different normative frameworks for health-care prioritisation that account for these criteria and their application to the use of available genetic tests. Table 16.1 provides an overview of the most relevant criteria, their rationales, and examples for illustration.

Need-Based Allocation

As illustrated by the proverb 'A healthy person has many wishes, but the sick person has only one', 'health' is a good of specific importance. It is a prerequisite for the pursuit of happiness rather than one among a multitude of options to choose from. Therefore, medical need in terms of severity of disease and need for medical services to alleviate diseases are key criteria for decision making in the face of scarce health-care resources. However, the term 'need' in the context of prioritising health services requires further specification. 'Need' can be defined as the gap between an actual state experienced by an individual and a norm that prescribes something desirable. Different attributes of need can be used to illustrate this gap in genetics.

Health-related need

A 'health-related need' constitutes a gap between actual and desirable health states and is independent of whether there is anything that can be done to reduce the gap. In the 'fair innings' approach, measuring this gap involves a comparison of the total health individuals experience over their life span with an average amount they could have expected. This can relate to the life expectancy at birth, or to life expectancy adjusted by a weight for health-related quality of life (Williams, 1997).

A second example of health need, which is likely to be relevant independent from whether effective treatment is available, is the *a priori* probability of having the disease. According to this dimension of need, first-degree relatives of a known mutation carrier may be considered to have a higher need for genetic testing than individuals in an average population. High-risk individuals from population groups where a hereditary condition is relatively common may also be considered to have a higher need than do individuals from the average population.

Intervention need

Different from the health-related need, the concept of 'intervention need' requires that an intervention is available for which there is scientific evidence that it can reduce the gap between an actual and the desirable health state (PrioriteringsCentrum, 2008, pp.131ff.). In a situation in which no effective medical treatment exists, no intervention need exists according to this definition.

Given that different notions of 'need' can lead to different orders of priority, the question arises of what type of benefit has it to be in order to be considered as meeting an intervention need. If need is defined in terms of 'degree of ill health', for example, it can be argued that a threat to life is the most severe form of ill health and that life-saving or life-prolonging interventions should, therefore, take priority over life-enhancing ones (Cookson and Dolan, 2000). Huntington's disease (HD), for example, is a hereditary condition where virtually all mutation carriers develop the lethal neurodegenerative disorder for which there is no effective cure available. According to this definition, there would be no intervention need for HD testing (more precisely, some of the HD symptoms can be alleviated by medical treatment, so that there is some intervention need).

Need can also be interpreted in terms of 'immediacy of ill health', which includes reduced health-related quality of life. Untreatable disorders may incur substantial emotional distress and mental health challenges. In case these can be ameliorated effectively by psychosocial care, an intervention need may exist for mutation carriers even in the absence of a life-extending medical treatment. Intervention need can also be defined broadly as the 'potential to benefit from health care' (Cookson and Dolan, 2000). The latter definition is of particular relevance for the use of genetic tests because, like in the case of HD, the perceived benefits of genetic tests can extend beyond health outcomes: a patient at risk of HD can benefit in terms of information for making choices, such as whether to start a family or not. Such non-health benefits can contribute a lot to the value patients derive from genetic testing (Grosse et al., 2008). Currently, a range of instruments are in development to demonstrate such other benefit and, thus, intervention need, within clinical studies (Payne et al., 2008).

The role of 'need' in decision making

Generally, the proven ability of a medical technology to ameliorate intervention needs is likely to be the key criterion in explicit decision making about medical technology: most agencies for health technology assessment and for coverage decision making assess the scientific evidence of a technology's effectiveness if explicit coverage decisions are made (Rogowski et al., 2008).

Scientific evidence of intervention need also appears to be the most frequently addressed criterion for genetic testing. A number of groups have developed evidence-based approaches to evaluating the benefits of specific genetic tests and weighing them against potential harms, for example, the Evaluation of Genomic Applications in Practice and Prevention (EGAPP) initiative in the United States (Rogowski et al., 2009). Additionally, a survey about decision making about scarce resources for the use of genetic tests in the Canadian health-care system reported that 'evidential basis' and 'availability of preventative strategies' were among the criteria for decision making (Adair et al., 2009).

Apparently following the concept of intervention need, the Department of Health of New South Wales, Australia, distinguishes genetic tests of high and low priority based on their expected benefit. Diagnostic testing, for example, is assigned high priority 'When confirmation of a clinical diagnosis will lead to changes in management of an affected person', and low priority 'where the clinical diagnosis is confirmed by other means and genetic testing will not alter the patient's management or options'.[4] A similar guidance has been adopted by the Human Genetics Society of Australia.

However, approaches that assess genetic tests for one disorder at a time have limitations for prioritising all genetic tests. First, they typically only determine whether or not a test is needed, but do not prioritise among recommended tests. In addition, this approach has limitations to address the problem of escalating health-care costs, for example, because 'no evidence of effectiveness' does not necessarily imply 'evidence of no effectiveness', and funding may not be sufficient to establish effectiveness of all available technologies (Garber, 2004) – particularly in the field of genetic testing (Rogowski et al., 2009). Currently, a widespread application of this criterion would exclude by far most of the genetic tests available and used in clinical practice because only a few have been covered by evidence reviews.

Apart from intervention need/evidence of effectiveness, different notions of health-care need have been used as criteria for prioritisation across Europe, alongside further criteria (Kenny and Joffres, 2008). In Norway, for example, the first report of the Lønning-Komitee gave highest priority to acute life-saving technologies and low priority to technologies that are likely to improve health and quality of life, but do not incur serious damage if they are withheld (Marckmann, 2009). According to the prioritisation guidelines of the Danish Ethics Council, 'need' should be taken into account, which was defined as the gravity and prognosis of the disease, urgency, and capacity to benefit (Kenny and Joffres, 2008). However, these additional criteria have hardly been operationalised and used in a structured, evidence-based manner and no such framework could be identified for genetic tests. Therefore, there is a need for methodological work before such a needs-based approach can be used in prioritisation practice.

Benefit Maximisation

Purely need-based decision making can lead to counter-intuitive results. Although many would agree that a patient at immediate risk of death should be treated before a second patient who is suffering from a non-lethal disease,

---

4   http://www.health.nsw.gov.au/policies/gl/2007/pdf/GL2007_013.pdf [accessed on 19 January 2010].

for example, few would agree that all available health-care resources should be devoted to emergency rescue medical services. The important question is how many resources should be allocated to different health and intervention needs and to what extent higher needs justify higher resource spending. The two major health economic schools of thought provide different points of orientation for answering this question.

Welfare economics

Welfare economics corresponds with a view of patients as autonomous citizens and consumers whose welfare is to be maximised. The best judges of how much genetic tests contribute to welfare are assumed to be consumers who assess the expected value from accessing different types of tests. Consumers care about many things, not just health, and may be willing to trade off lower health gains for higher satisfaction of other desires. Whether scarce resources should be spent for a genetic test depends on whether the consumers' willingness to pay (WTP) exceeds the cost of the test. In theory, consumers choose a bundle of products that maximise their expected utility. The WTP for a genetic test measures the expected benefit relative to alternative choices. If adding another good to the bundle than a genetic test would provide more benefit for the same cost, the consumer should prefer buying that bundle (Hurley, 2000).

If microeconomic assumptions for perfectly competitive markets held, for example, perfect information, market sale of genetic tests would lead to an efficient and optimal provision of those genetic tests where WTP exceeds the cost. In the absence of well-functioning markets, as is the case in health care (Arrow, 1963), economists seek to simulate market outcomes by assessing consumer WTP values from stated preference questionnaires. The WTP values can then be compared in a cost–benefit analysis (CBA) to the costs associated with providing the tests (Boadway and Bruce, 1984, pp.292ff.).

It has been suggested that CBA may be of particular relevance for the economic evaluation of genetic tests because a lot of the utility a patient derives from testing is personal rather than clinical: the purpose of many genetic tests is to assist patients in making decisions about how to plan their life, rather than to guide clinical interventions (Rogowski et al., 2010; Grosse et al., 2008). According to the welfarist perspective, focusing just on health outcomes will likely understate the economic benefits of genetic testing.

Extra-welfarist economics

Critics of the welfarist perspective argue that normative principles other than individual preferences should be the starting point for assessing public resource spending (Sen, 1999). Many health-care decision makers base their decisions on aggregate health outcomes (Rogowski et al., 2008) and may explicitly reject the idea that WTP should guide the allocation of scarce health-care resources

(Brouwer et al., 2008). Those frameworks that include benefit measures other than individual welfare are labelled 'extra-welfarist' (Brouwer et al., 2008).

One particularly influential approach is the model of a societal decision maker who spends scarce health-care resources to maximise health gains for the covered population. If the overall health-care budget is fixed, the opportunity cost of adding a new technology consists of the health foregone from reductions in other services that are displaced because of the need to reallocate scarce resources currently spent on their provision. The health gain per additional euro spent of these services forgone can be used as a threshold to decide whether a new service should be funded (Claxton et al., 2008). Health economic evaluation provides a tool to assess the value of novel health technologies through a comparison of the incremental cost-effectiveness ratio with the threshold value.

In order to simultaneously consider quality of life and mortality, outcomes can be expressed in terms of quality-adjusted life-years (QALYs) (Brazier et al., 2007). In the calculation of QALYs, life-years are weighted by an index between one (representing full health) and zero (representing death). Methods of multi-criteria decision making are available which can establish a priority score across various dimensions simultaneously to assist decision makers in making rational decisions incorporating other criteria than health outcomes (Baltussen and Niessen, 2006). It should be noted that the benefits and harms of genetic testing include not just the impact on the individual being tested, but the health effects for family members as a result of cascade screening (Rogowski et al., 2010).

The more severe a disease, the higher the QALY gains theoretically possible in case the disease can be cured completely. However, the concern for severity independent of potential health gains is not incorporated in QALY maximisation models, even if tests for severe diseases without effective treatment are of particular importance for genetics. Finally, there are ethical concerns about benefit maximisation for the allocation of scarce health resources because individual claims rather than measures of (aggregate) benefit may be a more adequate basis for priority setting in health care (Klonschinski and Lübbe, 2011).

The role of benefit maximisation in decision making

Extra-welfarist economic evaluation is applied in decision-making procedures by the English National Institute of Health and Clinical Excellence (NICE), including the recently implemented 'Diagnostics Assessment Programme'. Health technologies are considered for inclusion or exclusion of the services provided by the United Kingdom's National Health Service, based on their cost-effectiveness (National Institute for Health and Clinical Excellence, 2008) (with a 'weak' threshold area of between £20,000 and £30,000 per QALY). Recently, NICE issued a clinical guideline supporting genetic cascade screening for familial hypercholesterolemia, which concluded that genetic testing was the most cost-effective strategy, with an incremental cost-effectiveness ratio of £2,700 per QALY (Minhas et al., 2009).

A framework for prioritising genetic tests by Kroese et al. (2010) for the United Kingdom appeared to be based on a benefit maximisation approach, although it did not explicitly account for costs. A work group for the UKGTN successfully developed and piloted a multi-criteria decision-making framework. Aiming to maximise the gains from limited resources, it was based on five dimensions of clinical utility: 'Reduction in morbidity and mortality', 'Information to provide reproductive choice', 'Improvement in the process of care', 'Deliverability of pathway of care' and 'Providing additional information not relevant to other criteria'. The criteria were measured for a set of genetic tests, weighted, and a rank order measuring overall benefit was established (Kroese et al., 2010).

Evidence of cost-effectiveness is also considered by the respondents of the Canadian survey (Adair et al., 2009) as well as a range of other decision bodies, but typically not as a sole criterion but alongside with other criteria (Anell, 2004).

Benefit maximisation in terms of individual WTP takes place when a customer acquires a genetic test out of their own pocket in the direct-to-consumer testing market or if patients seek private appointments with geneticists. However, it is unclear whether test users and potentially affected relatives are sufficiently informed about the potential harms that can arise from genetic testing (Kaye, 2008; Wasson et al., 2006). Additionally, it is unclear whether direct-to-consumer testing may result in high follow-up costs for health-care systems as individuals seek additional medical advice and further potentially unnecessary testing (McGuire and Burke, 2008).

Equity

Besides medical need and benefit maximisation, equity is also a widely acknowledged criterion of fair prioritisation.

Equity as a positive aim

Equity can be formulated as a positive aim, in the sense that some kind of equality is desired. However, it is not only difficult to define 'need'; establishing a universally agreed definition of desirable 'equality' which should guide fair allocation of resources is also an unresolved challenge.[5] This is, on the one hand, because not all types of inequality are necessary unfair: for example, if an

---

5   See *Justice and Access to Health Care, Stanford Encyclopedia of Philosophy*, available online at: http://plato.stanford.edu/entries/justice-healthcareaccess/#WheAccCarEqu [accessed on 27 September 2011].

individual has lower income because they chose to devote more time to leisure activity than to earning money.

Equity can also relate to different concepts, for example, equal health-care spending per capita (across regions), equal health, equal access to health care, or equitable allocation according to medical need (Culyer and Wagstaff, 1993). In addition, the World Health Organization's (WHO) concepts of horizontal equity (health care to all individuals with the same medical need) and vertical equity (preferential health care for those with greatest need) (Guindo et al., 2012) illustrates that using equity as a prioritisation criterion involves determining an ethically justified dimension of equality, like medical need.

One approach to account for equity concerns in resource allocation is to address trade-offs between resource allocations which maximise benefit and those which prioritise certain health needs. This could be done, for example, by assigning special weight to health gains that accrue to more severely ill patients. In genetics, special weight could be assigned to interventions with higher health need according to the concepts described above (for example, to diagnostic rather than predictive tests). However, equity weights are still subject to a range of methodological deficiencies (Wailoo et al., 2009).

Avoiding specific kinds of inequity
According to the WHO:

> *Equity* is the absence of avoidable or remediable differences among groups of people, whether those groups are defined socially, economically, demographically, or geographically. *Health inequities* therefore involve more than inequality with respect to health determinants, access to the resources needed to improve and maintain health or health outcomes. They also entail a failure to avoid or overcome inequalities that infringe on fairness and human rights norms.[6]

There are different ways in which concerns about avoiding inequities can arise in genetics. The expected benefit and cost-effectiveness of genetic tests, for instance, may depend on characteristics of the target group, for example, prevalence of the mutation (which depends on ethnic or family background) or gender (if disease expression differs according to sex, as in the case of hereditary haemochromatosis) (Rogowski, 2007). Stratifying patients by these criteria may raise both ethical and legal concerns – for example, if genetic testing for hereditary haemochromatosis in Northern European countries were to be limited to males or to people of European ancestry because cost-effectiveness

---

6   See http://www.who.int/healthsystems/topics/equity/en/ [accessed on 4 May 2013].

is better in these groups. As a consequence, limits may be defined for using the risk of disease as a criterion in decision making.

The role of equity in decision making

If resources are not sufficient to provide all genetic tests, equity as a prioritisation criterion can be implemented in terms of lotteries or first-come, first-served (Persad et al., 2009). Both of these principles are blind to additionally relevant factors; and particularly the latter in practice favours those who are wealthier, more powerful and better connected (Persad et al., 2009). While no use of lottery could be found in the genetics literature, the criterion 'length of waiting time' and, thus, 'first-come, first-served' was mentioned in the survey of Adair and colleagues (Adair et al., 2009).

Equity is likely to play a much larger role in the form of applying certain criteria (such as scientific evidence of health benefit) and procedures (such as rules for stakeholder participation) consistently across decisions. Furthermore, the concern about specific kinds of inequity appears to play a role in decision practice, which is illustrated by a range of legal regulations to avoid genetic discrimination (Otlowski et al., 2012).

Promotion and reward of social usefulness

The fourth category of principles for allocating scarce resources mentioned by Persad et al. (2009) is 'promoting and rewarding social usefulness'. Promoting social usefulness implies prioritising services to specific individuals to facilitate future usefulness, for example, by giving priority to the health-care staff in the allocation of scarce influenza vaccine. This may include allocation to individuals who use fewer resources, for example, by agreeing to improve their health. Rewarding social usefulness implies prioritising specific individuals who have promoted important values or have undergone specific sacrifice in the past. This may include allocation to individuals who reduced their need for health-care resources due to healthy lifestyle choices (Persad et al., 2009).

Denying care based on the principle of rewarding and promoting social usefulness involves a range of ethical concerns. Use of this principle, for example, might require intrusive and humiliating enquiries about whether or not an individual adhered to a healthy lifestyle (Persad et al., 2009). Currently, the principle of promoting and rewarding social usefulness does not seem to play an important role in prioritisation decisions in general, nor to be of high relevance for prioritising the use of genetic tests.

Table 16.1 provides an overview of prioritisation criteria. The criterion related to social usefulness is omitted because it is unlikely to be relevant for prioritising genetic tests.

Table 16.1 Substantive principles for prioritising genetic tests

Category	Criterion for prioritisation	Rationale for the criterion	Example of priority order if criterion is applied	Methods	Comments
Allocation according to greatest need	Health need, e.g. fair innings	Those at risk of a severe disease if left untreated are worse off than those at risk of a mild condition, and thus, have a stronger claim on scarce health-care resources.	FDR screening test for HNPCC ranked above FDR screening test for hereditary periodontal disease because the health loss associated with HNPCC is larger.	• Tools for describing and ranking different types of health and intervention need (few available) • Well-developed tools of evidence appraisal to establish intervention need	• Most important ethical claim • Evidence appraisal widely accepted • Limited possibilities to rank
	Intervention need	Claims on scarce health-care resources depend on, additional to health need, a medical intervention which can decrease the health need. Different types of benefit can be distinguished: reduction of mortality and morbidity or potential to benefit without tangible impact on health.	FDR screening test for HNPCC ranked above FDR screening test for HD because for HNPCC, health can be improved by increased colonoscopic surveillance.		
Allocation to maximise benefit	Maximise health	A new genetic test consumes health-care resources which alternatively would have been spent for other purposes in the health-care system. It should only be introduced if its health gains exceed the gains from the intervention forgone elsewhere.	Genetic test is only reimbursed if the cost per QALY falls below a threshold value which represents the price of the health gain forgone.	• Cost-utility analysis and other methods of health economic evaluation well developed	• Used by some decision makers • Limited sensitivity to other than health outcomes
	Maximise welfare	A new genetic test consumes resources which alternatively would have been spent for other purposes, e.g. health care, education or private consumption. It should only be introduced if its benefits, measured in terms of WTP, exceed the opportunity costs.	Genetic test is only reimbursed if the mean willingness to pay exceeds the test costs (or funding is left to the market so that only those whose WTP exceeds the service costs receive the test).	• CBA to measure WTP established method • Markets to measure WTP practically	• CBA rarely used by decision makers • Markets may cause fairness concerns

| Equitable allocation | Promote equality | Every citizen has equal claims on scarce health-care resources. Problem to determine 'equality of what' – health, health-care spending, access to care according to equal need? | All of the above are of equal priority. If resources are not sufficient to fund all tests, a lottery decides. The decision is based on cost per QALY but gains to individuals in very bad health receive higher weight which improves cost-effectiveness. | • Lotteries and random assignment (like for organs)
• Equity-weights in CUA (which still face methodological difficulties) | • Lotteries ignore too much info to be used in practice
• Rather: allocate equitably according to criteria above |
| | Avoid inequity | As no conclusive concept of equity exists, legal or ethical boundaries define which types of inequality are unacceptable; efforts are made to avoid or overcome these. | Predictive HH test is offered both to males and females even if cost-effectiveness is much worse in females to avoid sex discrimination. | • Methods to measure specific types of (in)equity | • Boundaries to rather than tool for priority setting |

Abbreviations: CBA = cost–benefit analysis; CUA = cost-utility analysis; FDR = first-degree relatives; HD = Huntington's disease; HH = hereditary haemochromatosis; HNPCC = hereditary nonpolyposis colorectal cancer; QALY = quality-adjusted life year; WTP = willingness to pay

Discussion

This study provided an overview of normative criteria for prioritising genetic tests. All of these are faced with particular strengths and limitations: prioritisation based on claims which accrue from medical need appears to have the strongest ethical basis and practical acceptability. However, there is limited methodology and practical experience available with frameworks of measuring and balancing health and intervention needs and costs. Frameworks establishing intervention need, such as the EGAPP framework, are too resource-consuming to be applied to all genetic tests which exist and are applied in decision practice; moreover, they are currently unable to prioritise across different intervention needs.

Benefit maximisation is the standard criterion applied by health economic frameworks and well-developed evaluation methods are available and applied by institutions such as NICE. However, they can be even more resource-consuming than frameworks for evidence assessment. Additionally, different economic schools of thought exist with different associated outcome measures and practical implications, so that an ethically grounded choice of the most appropriate framework needs to be made. Finally, there is ethical criticism to benefit maximising frameworks, because individual claims rather than overall benefit could be considered an appropriate normative basis for prioritising health-care resources.

In addition, treating people equally is a frequently stated principle of fair resource allocation. However, it is a challenging task, because it requires a specification of which dimensions of equality are considered normatively relevant. Rather than a principle on its own, it is likely to be relevant in terms of applying other criteria with a firm normative basis equitably to all patients requesting a genetic test.

The principle of rewarding and promoting social usefulness has a long-standing tradition in the reflection over fair allocation, tracing back to Aristotelian ethics. However, applying this criterion in the prioritisation of genetic tests is unlikely to be acceptable, for example, because it would require intrusive questions to patients.

Overall, claims based on health and intervention need appear to be the strongest normative basis for allocating scarce health-care resources to genetic tests; however, benefit maximisation frameworks are much further developed for addressing problems of resource scarcity.

Limitations

There are many issues in the design and provision of genetics services which are ethically relevant but could not be addressed within this study which focused only on the prioritisation of beneficial genetic tests. These are, for example, how incidental findings should be addressed appropriately, ethical issues with preconception and prenatal screening, and privacy concerns related to information spillovers of genetic tests.

Reasonable people may disagree about which of the four sets of criteria should guide the prioritisation of genetic tests. Moreover, there may be conflicting analyses of the policy implications of common values, for example, because of different interpretations of the criteria or scientific evidence of benefits or economic and social costs (Baily, 2009). In such situations of disagreement about substantive criteria, it has been claimed that decisions should meet criteria of procedural fairness (Daniels and Sabin, 1998). Therefore, prioritisation activities should also account for principles of procedural justice, such as the framework of accountability for reasonableness by Norman Daniels (Daniels and Sabin, 1998) which could not be addressed in this study.

Clearly, the prioritisation of health-care resources is in the remit of those whose resources are prioritised – thus, the payers of health insurance distributions or committees of third-party payers on their behalf. Therefore, any recommendation developed on a European level can only serve as a complementary national and state regulation.

Implications for Further Research

Further research is necessary to arrive at a recommendation of prioritisation criteria or even an algorithm to derive a standardised priority score in conjunction with information sources such as the EuroGentest clinical utility gene cards or the UKGTN gene dossiers. This includes the following steps: first, a normative framework needs to be chosen to identify relevant prioritisation criteria; second, the criteria following from the framework need to be operationalised to allow for empirical assessment; and third, relative weights for the criteria need to be determined, for example, through discrete choice experiments (Severin et al., 2013).

To improve the legitimacy of such weights, the empirical evidence should attempt to capture value judgments of key stakeholders, such as clinicians and patient representatives. Furthermore, given that disagreement may persist, any prioritisation guidance should additionally be developed in a decision process oriented at principles of procedural justice, such as accountability for reasonableness.

Finally, prioritisation of care is interrelated with, but still separate from, prioritisation of applied research. Therefore, research with stakeholder involvement on prioritisation of research would also be desirable.

Implications for Decision Makers

Public health-care budgets are faced with particular resource constraints in the current economic climate. This is likely to lead to situations where not all desirable tests can be funded and priorities have to be set which genetics services to provide – therefore, this activity is generally of high relevance for decision makers.

Fair and reasonable prioritisation of genetic tests is a complex challenge for which no easy solutions exist. Therefore, efforts should be made to choose an appropriate framework for the explicit prioritisation of genetic tests in a normatively and economically reflected manner. Otherwise, there is the risk that limits are set implicitly in an unfair manner. This overview of criteria can be used as a first orientation for reflecting whether current service provision corresponds with reasonable priorities. Such reflection can feed into the development of standard operating procedures, for example, regarding which patients receive higher priority and which are assigned to waiting lists.

Evolving science has led to multiple new genetic tests becoming available; research and practical experience in health-care priority setting can help allocate these medical innovations in a reasonable and fair manner.

References

Adair, A., Hyde-Lay, R., Einsiedel, E. and Caulfield, T., 2009. Technology assessment and resource allocation for predictive genetic testing: a study of the perspectives of Canadian genetic health care providers. *BMC Medical Ethics*, 10, p.6.

Anell, A., 2004. Priority setting for pharmaceuticals. The use of health economic evidence by reimbursement and clinical guidance committees. *European Journal of Health Economics*, 5, pp.28–35.

Arrow, K.J., 1963. Uncertainty and the welfare economics of medical care. *The American Economic Review*, 53, pp.141–9.

Baily, M.A., 2009. Ethics and newborn genetic screening: new technologies, new challenges. In: M.A. Baily and T.H. Murray, eds. *Ethics and newborn genetic screening: new technologies, new challenges*. Baltimore: Johns Hopkins University Press.

Baltussen, R. and Niessen, L., 2006. Priority setting of health interventions: the need for multi-criteria decision analysis. *Cost Effectiveness and Resource Allocation*, 4, p.14.

Boadway, R. and Bruce, N., 1984. *Welfare economics*. Oxford: Basil Blackwell.

Brazier, J., Ratcliffe, J., Salomon, J.A. and Tsuchiya, A., 2007. *Measuring and valuing health benefits for economic evaluation*. Oxford: Oxford University Press.

Broqvist, M., Elgstrand, M.B., Carlsson, P., Eklund, K. and Jakobsson, A., 2011, *National model for transparent prioritisation in Swedish health care*. Revised Version. Linköping: National Center for Priority Setting in Healthcare.

Brouwer, W.B., Culyer, A.J., Van Exel, N.J. and Rutten, F.F., 2008. Welfarism vs. extra-welfarism. *Journal of Health Economics*, 27, pp.325–38.

Carlsson, J., 2012. Nationale und regionale Priorisierung im schwedischen Gesundheitswesen: Erfahrungen aus der Kardiologie [National and regional priority setting in Swedish health care: experiences from cardiology]. *Zeitschrift für Evidenz, Fortbildung und Qualität im Gesundheitswesen*, 106, pp.435–442.

Claxton, K., Briggs, A., Buxton, M.J., Culyer, A.J., McCabe, C., Walker, S. and Sculpher, M.J., 2008. Value based pricing for NHS drugs: an opportunity not to be missed? *British Medical Journal*, 336, pp.251–4.

Cookson, R. and Dolan, P., 2000. Principles of justice in health care rationing. *Journal of Medical Ethics*, 26, pp.323–9.

Culyer, A.J. and Wagstaff, A., 1993. Equity and equality in health and health care. *Journal of Health Economics*, 12, pp.431–57.

Daniels, N. and Sabin, J., 1998. The ethics of accountability in managed care reform. *Health Affairs (Project Hope)*, 17, pp.50–64.

Eisenberg, V.H. and Schenker, J.J., 1997. The moral aspects of prenatal diagnosis. *European Journal of Obstetrics, Gynecology and Reproductive Biology*, 72, pp.35–45.

Garber, A.M., 2004. Cost-effectiveness and evidence evaluation as criteria for coverage policy. *Health Affairs (Project Hope)*, Suppl. Web Exclusives, W4, pp.284–96.

Giacomini, M., Miller, F. and Browman, G., 2003. Confronting the 'gray zones' of technology assessment: evaluating genetic testing services for public insurance coverage in Canada. *International Journal of Technology Assessment in Health Care*, 19, pp.301–16.

Grosse, S.D., Rogowski, W.H., Ross, L.F., Cornel, M.C., Dondorp, W.J. and Khoury, M.J., 2010. Population screening for genetic disorders in the 21st century: evidence, economics, and ethics. *Public Health Genomics*, 13, pp.106–15.

Grosse, S.D., Wordsworth, S. and Payne, K., 2008. Economic methods for valuing the outcomes of genetic testing: beyond cost-effectiveness analysis. *Genetic Medicine*, 10, pp.648–54.

Guindo, L.A., Wagner, M., Baltussen, R., Rindress, D., Van Til, J., Kind, P. and Goetghebeur, M.M., 2012. From efficacy to equity: literature review of decision criteria for resource allocation and healthcare decisionmaking. *Cost Effectiveness and Resource Allocation*, 10, p.9.

Hurley, J., 2000. An overview of the normative economics of the health sector. In: A. Culyer and J.P. Newhouse, eds. *Handbook of health economics*. Philadelphia: Elsevier Science B.V. pp.55–110.

Huster, S., 2011. *Soziale Gesundheitsgerechtigkeit: sparen, umverteilen, vorsorgen? [Social health equity: save, redistribute, provide?]*. Berlin: Wagenbach.

Javaher, P., Kaariainen, H., Kristoffersson, U., Nippert, I., Sequeiros, J., Zimmern, R. and Schmidtke, J., 2008. EuroGentest: DNA-based testing for heritable disorders in Europe. *Community Genetics*, 11(2), pp.75–120.

Johnson, S.R. and Elkins, T.E., 1988. Ethical issues in prenatal diagnosis. *Clinical Obstetrics and Gynecology*, 31, pp.408–17.

Kaye, J., 2008. The regulation of direct-to-consumer genetic tests. *Human Molecular Genetics*, 17, pp.R180–3.

Kenny, N. and Joffres, C., 2008. An ethical analysis of international health priority-setting. *Health Care Analysis*, 16, pp.145–60.

Klonschinski, A. and Lübbe, W., 2011. QALYs und Gerechtigkeit: Ansätze und Probleme einer gesundheitsökonomischen Lösung der Fairnessproblematik [QALYs and fairness: health economic approaches to the fairness issue and their problems]. *Gesundheitswesen*, 73, pp.688–95.

Krawczak, M., Caliebe, A., Croucher, P.J. and Schmidtke, J., 2007. On the testing load incurred by cascade genetic carrier screening for Mendelian disorders: a brief report. *Genetic Testing*, 11, pp.417–19.

Kroese, M., Burton, H., Whittaker, J., Lakshman, R. and Alberg, C., 2010. A framework for the prioritization of investment in the provision of genetic tests. *Public Health Genomics*, 13, pp.538–43.

Marckmann, G., 2009. Priorisierung im Gesundheitswesen: Was können wir aus den internationalen Erfahrungen lernen? [Prioritization in health care: what can we learn from international experience?] *Zeitschrift für Evidenz, Fortbildung und Qualität im Gesundheitswesen*, 103, pp.85–91.

Mardis, E.R., 2010. The $1,000 genome, the $100,000 analysis? *Genome Medicine*, 2, p.84.

McGuire, A.L. and Burke, W., 2008. Raiding the medical commons: an unwelcome side effect of direct-to-consumer personal genome testing. *Journal of the American Medical Association*, 300, pp.2669–71.

Minhas, R., Humphries, S.E., Qureshi, N. and Neil, H.A., 2009. Controversies in familial hypercholesterolaemia: recommendations of the NICE Guideline Development Group for the identification and management of familial hypercholesterolaemia. *Heart*, 95, pp.584–7; discussion pp.587–91.

National Institute for Health and Clinical Excellence, 2008. *Guide to the methods of technology appraisal*. London: NICE.

Otlowski, M., Taylor, S. and Bombard, Y., 2012. Genetic discrimination: international perspectives. *Annual Review of Genomics and Human Genetics*, 13, pp.433–54.

Payne, K., Nicholls, S., McAllister, M., Macleod, R., Donnai, D. and Davies, L.M., 2008. Outcome measurement in clinical genetics services: a systematic review of validated measures. *Value in Health*, 11, pp.497–508.

Persad, G., Wertheimer, A. and Emanuel, E.J., 2009. Principles for allocation of scarce medical interventions. *Lancet*, 373, pp.423–31.

PrioriteringsCentrum, 2008. *Resolving health care's difficult choices. Survey of priority setting in Sweden and an analysis of principles and guidelines on priorities in health care. Rapport 2008:2.* Linköping: National Centre for Priority Setting in Health Care.

Rogowski, W., 2006. Genetic screening by DNA technology. A systematic review of health economic evidence. *International Journal of Technology Assessment in Health Care*, 22, pp.327–337.

Rogowski, W., 2007. Current impact of gene technology on healthcare. A map of economic assessments. *Health Policy*, 80, pp.340–57.

Rogowski, W.H., Grosse, S.D., John, J., Kääriäinen, H., Kent, A., Kristofferson, U. and Schmidtke, J., 2010. Points to consider in assessing and appraising predictive genetic tests. *Journal of Community Genetics*, 1, pp.185–94.

Rogowski, W.H., Grosse, S.D. and Khoury, M.J., 2009. Challenges of translating genetic tests into clinical and public health practice. *Nature Reviews. Genetics*, 10, pp.489–95.

Rogowski, W.H., Hartz, S.C. and John, J.H., 2008. Clearing up the hazy road from bench to bedside: a framework for integrating the fourth hurdle into translational medicine. *BMC Health Services Research*, 8, pp.1–12.

Schmidtke, J. and Cassiman, J.J., 2010. The EuroGentest clinical utility gene cards. *European Journal of Human Genetics*, 18, p.1068.

Schmidtke, J., Pabst, B. and Nippert, I., 2005. DNA-based genetic testing is rising steeply in a national health care system with open access to services: a survey of genetic test use in Germany, 1996–2002. *Genetic Testing*, 9(1), pp.80–4.

Sen, A., 1999. The possibility of social choice. *The American Economic Review*, 89, pp.349–78.

Sequeiros, J., Paneque, M., Guimaraes, B., Rantanen, E., Javaher, P., Nippert, I., Schmidtke, J., Kääriäinen, H., Kristoffersson, U. and Cassiman, J.J., 2012. The wide variation of definitions of genetic testing in international recommendations, guidelines and reports. *Journal of Community Genetics*, 3, pp.113–24.

Severin, F., Schmidtke, J., Muhlbacher, A. and Rogowski, W.H., 2013. Eliciting preferences for priority setting in genetic testing: a pilot study comparing best-worst scaling and discrete-choice experiments. *European Journal of Human Genetics*, 21, pp.1202–8.

Van Doorslaer, E., Koolman, X. and Jones, A.M., 2004. Explaining income-related inequalities in doctor utilisation in Europe. *Health Economics*, 13, pp.629–47.

Wailoo, A., Tsuchiya, A. and McCabe, C., 2009. Weighting must wait: incorporating equity concerns into cost-effectiveness analysis may take longer than expected. *Pharmacoeconomics*, 27, pp.983–9.

Wasson, K., Cook, E.D. and Helzlsouer, K., 2006. Direct-to-consumer online genetic testing and the four principles: an analysis of the ethical issues. *Ethics & Medicine*, 22, pp.83–91.

West, R., 1988. Ethical aspects of genetic disease and genetic counselling. *Journal of Medical Ethics*, 14, pp.194–7.

Williams, A., 1997. Intergenerational equity: an exploration of the 'fair innings' argument. *Health Economics*, 6, pp.117–32.

Chapter 17

Personalised Medicine as Orphan Drugs? Legal and Ethical Questions[1]

Sina Gottwald and Stefan Huster[2]

The development of 'personalised medicine' currently is a widely discussed issue. In particular personalised pharmacotherapy is gaining increasing importance, as a consequence of the developments in the fields of pharmacology and molecular genetics. This requires an examination of the consequences of personalised pharmacotherapy on the German Statutory Health Insurance System (Gesetzliche Krankenversicherung – GKV) and on the quality of patient health care. In this context, a question that arises is the issue of 'orphanisation': if personalised medicinal products could regularly be designated as orphan drugs, that is as medicinal products for rare diseases, it would as a general rule not be necessary to provide proof under the Pharmaceutical Market Restructuring Act (Arzneimittelmarktneuordnungsgesetz – AMNOG) of the additional benefit in the context of the early benefit assessment to be carried out by the German Joint Government Committee (Gemeinsamer Bundesausschuss – G-BA). The decisive aspect for the designation of a medicinal product as an orphan drug is, among others, the prevalence rate of the group of patients whose condition is intended to be treated with the product. In this context, the stratification of patent groups within the framework of personalised pharmacotherapy

1   This chapter was originally published in German in a slightly modified form, under the title 'Personalisierte Medizin als Orphanisierung: rechtliche und ethische Fragen' in: *Ethik in der Medizin* 2013, 25, 259–66. With kind permission of Springer Science+Business Media.

2   This study was conducted in the research network Personalised Medicine in Oncology: An Interdisciplinary Study on Ethical, Medical, Economical and Legal Aspects (Grant project number: 01 GP 1001A-C), which is supported by the German Federal Ministry of Education and Research (Bundesministerium für Bildung und Forschung – BMBF). The authors confirm that they are not subject to conflicts of interests.

has particular significance. An 'orphanisation' such as this would in particular have price-related consequences for the GKV, due to the lack of knowledge regarding a medicinal product's additional benefit; for the patients, the consequences must be considered in a more differentiated manner.

Regulation of Prices for Medicinal Products in the GKV

Due to the continuously increasing spending on medicinal products in the GKV in recent years, which now constitute the second largest group of costs (Wille, 2011, p.35) a multitude of measures has already been taken in the past in order to reduce costs in the area of medicinal product supply. The Pharmaceutical Market Restructuring Act (Arzneimittelmarktneuordnungsgesetz – AMNOG (Deutscher Bundestag, 2010c,, p.1)[3]) supplements these endeavours, specifying as its objective profitability and cost efficiency regarding prices and prescriptions of medicinal products (Deutscher Bundestag, 2010c). An important issue with regard to the price regulation of medicinal products as introduced by the AMNOG is their additional benefit, whereby this principle applies only to a restricted extent to medicinal products for rare diseases (so-called orphan drugs) (for a detailed discussion on reimbursement of personalised medicine see Chapter 15, this volume).

Significance of the Additional Benefit

For medicinal products with new active ingredients,[4] section 35a of the Social Security Code Book 5 (Sozialgesetzbuch – SGB V) always provides for an early benefit assessment by the G-BA. Pursuant to section 35a (1) 2 of the SGB V, this includes, among other aspects, the assessment of the additional benefit, the extent of the additional benefit and its therapeutic significance. An additional benefit is deemed to exist if the benefit, under quantitative and qualitative aspects, is greater than the benefit of the appropriate comparative treatment[5] (section 2 (4) of the Decree on the Assessment of the Benefit

---

3   With regard to AMNOG as an instrument for cost reduction, also see Cassel (2011, pp.15ff.).

4   Pursuant to the definition in section 2 (1) 1 of the AM-NutzenV, these are medicinal products containing active ingredients, the effects of which are not generally known in medical science upon their initial marketing authorisation.

5   The appropriate comparative treatment is the treatment, the benefit of which is compared to the benefit of a medicinal product with new active ingredients in the course of the benefit assessment pursuant to section 35a of the SGB V (section 2 (5) of the AM-NutzenV).

of Medicinal Products (Arzneimittel-Nutzenbewertungsverordnung – AM-NutzenV)). Pursuant to section 2 (3) of the AM-NutzenV, the 'benefit' is the therapeutic effect with relevance for the patient, in particular with regard to the improvement of health or quality of life, the reduction of the duration of the condition, the prolongation of life or the reduction of side effects. For medicinal products with new active ingredients, the pharmaceuticals company must file a dossier with the G-BA when the product is first placed on the market (section 4 (3) No. 1 of the AM-NutzenV), in which proof must be provided of the additional benefit of the medicinal product in comparison to the appropriate comparative treatment. The G-BA must finalise and publish the benefit assessment after three months (section 7 (3) of the AM-NutzenV) and must carry out a hearing; the final resolution regarding the benefit assessment must be taken after a further three month period after the hearing (section 7 (4) of the AM-NutzenV).

The results of this assessment are decisive for the process for the determination of prices for the medicinal product in the GKV: only if an additional benefit can be proven will a reimbursement amount in the form of a discount on the pharmaceutical company's sales price be agreed between this company and the Central Federal Association of Health Insurance Funds (Spitzenverband Bund der Krankenkassen) (section 130b (1) of the SGB V). If an additional benefit cannot be determined, the medicinal product will be classified in the fixed-price group pursuant to section 35 (1) of the SGB V, with medicinal products which are comparable under pharmacological-therapeutic aspects (section 35a (4) 1 of the SGB V). If a medicinal product without proven additional benefit cannot be classified into one of the fixed-price groups, the Spitzenverband Bund der Krankenkassen and the pharmaceutical company, after consultation with the Association of Private Health Insurance Companies (Verband der privaten Krankenversicherung), agree on a reimbursement sum which does not lead to higher treatment costs than the appropriate comparative treatment (section 130b (3) 1 in conjunction with (1) 1 of the SGB V).

Due to the importance of the additional benefit with regard to pricing, it is therefore of considerable significance for the pharmaceutical companies to provide such proof. At the same time, they are faced with the problem that only limited data material is available upon market introduction, on the basis of which proof has to be provided (Heinemann and Lang, 2011, p.150). If the pharmaceutical companies feel that based on the early benefit assessment there is a risk that they may have to accept a price which, in their opinion, is unduly low, this may lead to them refraining from marketing the product in Germany (*ÄrzteZeitung*, 2011a, 2011b, 2011c, 2012a, 2012b; Laschet, 2011; Preusker, 2011).

Special Rules for Orphan Drugs

These problems are alleviated by the statutory exception provisions regarding the obligation to provide proof. Here, the legal classification of the medicinal products for the treatment of rare diseases (orphan drugs) is interesting.[6]

For medicinal products which are authorised under Regulation (European Communities (EC)) No. 141/2000 of the European Parliament and of the Council of 16 Dec. 1999 on orphan medicinal products, proof of the benefits and additional benefits is not required. For such products, proof of the additional benefit is deemed to have been provided pursuant to section 35a (1) 10 of the SGB V through the authorisation for marketing.[7] However, it is nevertheless necessary to provide proof of the extent of the additional benefit assumed in this manner, and of its therapeutic significance,[8] also for orphan drugs.[9] The relevant determination by the G-BA is done on the basis of the authorisation and the studies on which the authorisation is based.[10]

---

6   In addition to the exception for orphan drugs, another exception is provided for in section 35a (1a) of the SGB V, according to which the G-BA is obligated to release the pharmaceutical company upon request from the obligation to present proof pursuant to subsection 1, and to release the medicinal product from the benefit assessment pursuant to subsection 3 if it is to be expected that the GKV will only incur minor expenses for such a medicinal product.

7   This was not taken into account by the Institute for Quality and Profitability in the Health Sector (Institut für Qualität und Wirtschaftlichkeit im Gesundheitswesen – IQWIG) when it, during its first orphan drug assessment under the AMNOG (dossier assessment of 12 December 2011 regarding the active ingredient Pirfenidon), reached the conclusion that the medicinal product had to be classified as 'additional benefit not proven' (IQWIG, 2011, p.23), see to this effect Gieseke and Schmitt-Feuerbach (2012), Schmitt-Feuerbach (2012) and Willhöft and Lietz (2012, pp.19, 21). In its resolution of 15 March 2012, the G-BA correctly did not endorse this opinion, but rather attributed the active ingredient with an unquantifiable additional benefit. With the agreement between the GKV umbrella organisation and the manufacturer regarding a reimbursement sum for Pirfenidon, the first discount for an orphan drug was negotiated in July 2012.

8   See section 35a (1) 2 of the SGB V, chapter 5, section 5 (7) No. 1 through 4 of the Code of Procedure of the G-BA (Verfahrensordnung des G-BA – VerfO-G-BA), as amended on 18 December 2008.

9   Commenting critically in this context: Schickert and Schmitz (2013, pp.128ff.).

10   G-BA in its resolution of 15 March 2012 regarding the assessment of the active ingredient Pirfenidon (Gemeinsamer Bundesausschuss, 2012, p.3). For Pirfenidon, it reached the conclusion that the additional benefit was unquantifiable, because the scientific database currently does not allow this. With regard to the other seven orphan drugs assessed up to now by the G-BA under the AMNOG, the following applies: the G-BA determined that there was an unquantifiable additional benefit for two other orphan drugs (active ingredient Brentuximab vedotin, resolution of 16

An exception to the exception exists in the event of the turnover of the medicinal product in the GKV at pharmacy sales prices including VAT during the last 12 calendar months exceeding a sum of 50 million Euro, section 35a (1) 11 of the SGB V. In this case, the pharmaceutical company, within three months from a corresponding request by the G-BA, must provide documents of proof pursuant to section 35a (1) 3 – for example, also regarding the medicinal benefit and the additional benefit – and in these prove the additional benefit in comparison to the appropriate comparable treatment.[11]

The exception regulation for orphan drugs was introduced into the legislative process by an amendment application filed by the CDU/CSU and FDP parliamentary parties (Deutscher Bundestag, 2010b), and was highly controversial (ACHSE e.V., 2010; *ÄrzteZeitung*, 2010; Deutscher Bundestag, 2010a, pp.4ff.; Rieser, 2010, p.A-1887). The reasons given for the application were that for a medicinal product for the treatment of a rare disease, proof of its effectiveness has been provided through the authorisation for marketing, that this has to be acknowledged as an additional benefit in this area of application, and that it can usually be assumed that there is no therapeutically equivalent alternative for the treatment of a disease (Deutscher Bundestag, 2010b).

'Orphanisation' through Personalised Medicine?

In this context, the development summarised under the headline 'personalised medicine' now is of interest, which also, and in particular, includes the possibilities of a 'personalised pharmacotherapy'. In the treatment of cancer, for instance, the characteristics of the tumour are determined with the help

---

May 2013; active ingredient Bosutinib, resolution of 17 October 2013). In four other cases, the G-BA reached the conclusion that there is a minor additional benefit (active ingredient Tafamidis Meglumin, resolution of 7 June 2012; active ingredient Pasireotid, resolution of 6 December 2012; active ingredient Ruxolitinib, resolution of 7 March 2013; active ingredient Decitabin, resolution of 2 May 2013). With regard to the active ingredient Ivacaftor, the judgment was differentiated: for the treatment of children, a small additional benefit was found, for adolescents and adults, however, a significant additional benefit (resolution of 7 February 2013). With regard to two other orphan drugs (active ingredients Pomalidomid and Ponatinib), the assessment process has not yet been finalised.

11   Here, the question is what the consequences of the fact that the medicinal product has already been authorised, and that the European Commission has already determined the significant benefit of the medicinal product in this context, are for the determination by the G-BA with regard to the benefits or additional benefits of the medicinal product; regarding the issue of the binding effect of the designation as an orphan drug for the G-BA (Schickert and Schmitz, 2013, pp.135ff.).

of biomarkers – such as certain gene sequences or surface proteins – which allow an assessment regarding the effectiveness or tolerability of a specific medicinal active ingredient, with the consequence that the pharmacotherapy in conclusion is only available for a specific sub-set (Pfundner, 2009, pp.182ff.; see also Chapter 14 this volume).[12] The question is whether the prerequisites for the designation of a medicinal product as an orphan drug are fulfilled with this type of stratification and/or creation of sub-sets, and what the consequences would be of such 'orphanisation' (Huster and Gottwald, 2012, pp.449, 453).

Prerequisites for the Designation of a Medicinal Product as an Orphan Drug

Two alternatives exist for the designation of a medicinal product as an orphan drug, both of which include requirements as to the seriousness of the condition and as to the health care situation, and furthermore alternatively provide for a prevalence criterion and/or economic criterion. Pursuant to Art. 3 (1a) Alt. 1 of regulation (EC) No. 141/2000, a medicinal product can be designated as an orphan drug if proof has been provided that it is intended for the diagnosis, prevention or treatment of a life-threatening or chronically debilitating condition affecting not more than five in 10,000 persons in the community when the application is made (Kamann, 2000, p.170; Remmele, 2007).

The second alternative pursuant to Art. 3 (1a) Alt. 2 of this Regulation sets less stringent requirements on the quality of the disease, as under this alternative, in addition to a life-threatening or chronically debilitating condition, serious and chronic conditions suffice. A medicinal product can be considered to be rare pursuant to this alternative if the marketing of the medicinal product in the Community without any incentives is unlikely to generate sufficient return to justify the necessary investment.

Both alternatives furthermore cumulatively require that no satisfactory method of diagnosis, prevention or treatment of the condition in question exists that has been authorised in the Community or, if such method exists, that the medicinal product will be of significant benefit to those affected by that condition.[13]

---

12   Pursuant to a publication by the vfa, 37 authorised medicinal products currently exist in Germany which can be attributed to the area of personalised medicine, see http://www.vfa.de/de/arzneimittel-forschung/datenbanken-zu-arzneimitteln/individualisierte-medizin.html (last updated 2 October 2013; last accessed 18 November 2013).

13   Art. 3 (1b) of Regulation (EC) No. 141/2000.

Designation of Personalised Medicinal Products as Orphan Drugs?

The prerequisite of the degree of seriousness of a condition is usually fulfilled by personalised medicinal products, which are used mainly in the area of oncology, and therefore usually treat a condition which is to be classified as life-threatening. However, the prevalence of the respective condition is problematic. In order to be able to designate a medicinal product as an orphan drug, it will be decisive whether or not the relevant sub-sets can, or have to, be regarded as 'independent' conditions within the meaning of the regulation, or whether the issue has to be considered using the 'generic term' of the disease (Enzmann and Lütz, 2008, pp.500, 506). If the decisive aspect for the prevalence rate were the existence of the stratifying sub-set characteristics, this may lead to an inflation of the status of rare diseases, due to the current and expected future progress in molecular biology (Enzmann and Lütz, 2008, pp.500, 506).

Even though it can be said that differences regarding the degree of seriousness and the stages or places of manifestation of a condition do usually not lead to a differentiated view in the context of the prevalence assessment, and even though this applies even if they make a differentiated treatment necessary (Enzmann and Lütz, 2008, pp.500, 506), there are no significant differences in the condition itself with regard to these criteria, in contrast to the sub-sets created within the framework of personalised medicine. For instance, different degrees of seriousness and stages usually relate to the specific progression of one specific disease. On the other hand, the differentiation on which personalised pharmacotherapy is based is often caused by the disease itself, for instance if the differentiation is linked to the question of whether the number of HER2 proteins has massively increased on the surface of a tumour.[14] If such characteristics of a tumour exist, which can be measured clearly, for instance with the help of biomarkers, and which are characteristic and causal for the effectiveness of a medicinal product, the classification as an independent condition within the meaning of the regulation is logical (Enzmann and Lütz, 2008, pp.500, 506).[15]

---

14 For HER2-positive breast cancer, for instance, the selective treatment with Trastuzumab, depending on the stage of the disease, allows a doubling of survival time, or may even prevent progression of the disease (see Pfundner, 2009, pp.169ff.).

15 However, a recommendation by the European Medicines Agency (EMA) (EMA/COMP/15893/2009) of 2 March 2010 must be taken into consideration, which views critically the 'slicing' of common conditions into sub-sets during the determination of prevalence. An abuse of the Orphan Drug Act is at least to be assumed to exist if the medicinal product is split up in order for it to be designated as an orphan drug, and is then nevertheless applied to several or all sub-sets of the disease (Remmele, 2007). However, for personalised medicine, the latter is specifically not the case. With regard to such 'slicing', see also Cassel and Heigl (2013, pp.10, 20).

Also, the fulfilment of the alternative requirement in Art. 3 (1a) of regulation (EC) No. 141/2000, which requires that, without incentives, it is unlikely that the marketing of the medicinal product would generate sufficient return to justify the necessary investment, does not seem to be far-fetched for personalised medicinal products. Insufficient return in the meaning of this provision in particular typically exists if the medicinal product can actually only be used for the treatment of a small number of patients.

The cumulative requirement that no satisfactory method of treatment of the condition exists that has been authorised in the community will probably usually be typical for oncological treatments. However, as, due to the positive results of the risk–benefit assessment during the authorisation for marketing, all authorised medicinal products are deemed to constitute satisfactory methods in the meaning of Art. 3 (1b) of the regulation, the applicant will have to prove that significant (additional) benefits[16] are to be expected in comparison to all existing authorised medicinal products (Remmele, 2007).[17] Even though this significant benefit must be proven by presenting documents of proof or data,[18] this requirement does not constitute a major obstacle; due to the probably minor or non-existent clinical experience, it is to be assumed that the additional benefit assumed by the applicant actually exists.[19]

Therefore, it can be stated as an interim conclusion that personalised medicinal products will often fulfil the criteria for the designation as orphan medicinal products.

Consequences of an 'Orphanisation'

With regard to the consequences of an 'orphanisation', a differentiation is necessary between the consequences for the GKV and for the patients and insured persons.

Consequences for the GKV

For the GKV, a potential 'orphanisation' through personalised medicine has, above all, price-related consequences (Huster and Gottwald, 2012, pp.449, 454). The negotiations between the Spitzenverband Bund der Krankenkassen and

---

16 Art. 3 (1b) 2nd Alt. of Regulation (EC) No. 141/2000.

17 See A. 3. of the Communication from the Commission on orphan medicinal products (2003/C 178/02).

18 See A. 4. of the Communication from the Commission on orphan medicinal products (2003/C 178/02).

19 A. 4. of the Communication from the Commission on orphan medicinal products (2003/C 178/02).

the pharmaceutical companies regarding the reimbursement sum will then take place without having knowledge with regard to whether the medicinal products actually provide an additional benefit. Insofar, there is the risk that the GKV may incur increased costs without this necessarily leading to an increase in the quality of health care.[20] Even though an additional benefit exists under legal aspects, this does not necessarily need to correspond to the actual facts. In particular, proof of such additional benefits does not become obsolete through the authorisation for marketing, due to the different assessment standards under the Act on Medicinal Products (Arzneimittelgesetz – AMG) and the SGB V. Whilst the assessment in the context of the decision on the authorisation for marketing can be based on surrogate parameters which mostly do not have direct relevance with regard to a patient-oriented benefit, the assessment under the SGB V is made on the basis of patient-relevant end points (Huster, 2011, pp.76, 80; Windeler et al., 2010, p.A-2032–3). This means that the decisive issue in this context is the improvement of the health condition, the shortening of the duration of the condition, the prolongation of survival, the reduction of side effects or an improvement in the quality of life.[21] Furthermore, the authorising authority does not necessarily carry out a comparative assessment of benefits, whilst this is a decisive component of the benefit assessment under the SGB V (Huster, 2011, pp.76, 80). In this context, the legislator also is wrong in basing the justification of the exception rule for orphan drugs on the assumption that no therapeutically equivalent alternative exists for the treatment of such a condition (Deutscher Bundestag, 2010b): for some indications, several orphan drugs with different active ingredients have already been designated.[22]

Consequences for Patients and Insured Persons

Under aspects of patient protection, the fact that an assessment of the (additional) benefit does not take place does not – at least in theory – cause any risks. Only the decision on the authorisation for marketing is responsible for the safety of medicinal products, an assessment which insofar is not made (again) within the framework of the early benefit assessment under the SGB

---

20 Some even are of the opinion that the financial viability of the health care system as a whole may be in danger, see Fricke (2011). On the spending by the GKV for orphan drugs, see Kleinfeld et al. (2013, pp.181ff.).

21 See section 2 (3) of the AM-NutzenV.

22 Based on the list of the Association of Researching Pharmaceutical Manufacturers (Verband der forschenden Pharmahersteller e. V. – vfa) on orphan drugs, last amended on 5 November 2013 (http://www.vfa.de/embed/orphan-drugs-list.pdf; accessed 18 November 2013) almost 30 per cent of the medicinal products designated as orphan drugs are not soloists with regard to the treatment of the relevant indication.

V. However, when taking his/her decision on whether or not to use a medicinal product for the treatment of his/her – often life-threatening – condition, the patient has to do without information on the patient-relevant additional benefit of the medicinal product. Information as to whether the medicinal product will lead to a prolongation of survival or an improvement in the quality of life can usually not be provided to the patient. Furthermore, he/she does not have an information basis for the decision among various medicinal products if more than one medicinal product is designated as an orphan drug for the relevant indication. The assessment of the additional benefit under the SGB V would therefore improve the patient's possibility of reaching a self-determined decision on the application of a medicinal product (Windeler et al., 2010, p.A-2032). On the other hand, the orphan drug rules may increase the incentive for pharmaceutical companies to also develop and introduce into the market in Germany personalised medicine which is effective only for a small sub-set. This would at least create the chance of a patient-relevant improvement of the health care situation for this small group of patients, which otherwise would possibly not exist.[23]

Conclusion

The specified legal issues and developments within the framework of personalised pharmacotherapy all point towards a fundamental problem: the steering of innovations in the health care sector. On the one hand, medicinal innovations are obviously welcome in as far as they improve the quality of health care. Whether or not this is the case can, however, on the other hand not always be assessed unambiguously. As the producers of such innovations at the same time push into the market with all their might, this leads to a dilemma for a publicly-funded health-care system such as the GKV: on the one hand, the insured persons are not to be blocked from access to such innovations, whilst on the other hand a steering must take place in view of the limited resources.

In the long run, the community of insured persons which is based on the principle of mutual solidarity will probably not be able to avoid an open discussion of the price it is willing to pay for which additional benefit. This requires the best possible clarification of the additional benefit and the largest possible level of transparency with regard to the existing results. The regulation on orphan drugs as introduced by the AMNOG therefore has rather counterproductive effects. Should personalised pharmacotherapy in the future

---

23   In this respect, the Alliance for Chronical and Rare Diseases (Allianz chronischer seltener Erkrankungen – ACHSE) supports the exception rules for orphan drugs (see ACHSE e.V., 2010).

try to facilitate market access via this rule, it will probably be necessary to reconsider its reasonability.

References

ACHSE e.V., 2010. Statement on the draft act introduced by the CDU/CSU parliamentary parties regarding the AMNOG (AMNOG BT DS 17/2413) and the amendment applications submitted by CDU/CSU and FDP on this act. http://www.achse-online.de/cms/medienbord/download-dokumente/101008_AMNOG_ACHSE_240910.pdf (accessed 20 March 2014).

ÄrzteZeitung, 2010. Streit um schnelle Nutzenbewertung für Orphan Drugs. *ÄrzteZeitung*, 26 October 2010. http://www.aerztezeitung.de/politik_gesellschaft/arzneimittelpolitik/article/625826/streit-schnelle-nutzenbewertung-orphan-drugs.html?sh=3&h=-657915867 (accessed 20 March 2014).

ÄrzteZeitung, 2011a. (Ver)früh(t)e Nutzenbewertung. *ÄrzteZeitung*, 28 August 2011. http://www.aerztezeitung.de/politik_gesellschaft/arzneimittelpolitik/article/667519/verfruehte-nutzenbewertung.html?sh=1&h=1059925918 (accessed 20 March 2014).

ÄrzteZeitung, 2011b. AMNOG stoppt die zweite Innovation. *ÄrzteZeitung*, 2 September 2011. http://www.aerztezeitung.de/politik_gesellschaft/arzneimittelpolitik/article/668434/amnog-stoppt-zweite-innovation.html?sh=1&h=-1334834879 (accessed 20 March 2014).

ÄrzteZeitung, 2011c. Folge des AMNOG: Rasilamlo® außer Vertrieb. *ÄrzteZeitung*, 25 August 2011. http://www.aerztezeitung.de/praxis_wirtschaft/unternehmen/article/667308/folge-des-amnog-rasilamlo-ausser-vertrieb.html?sh=2&h=-1532392813 (accessed 20 March 2014).

ÄrzteZeitung, 2012a. GKV kompromisslos – Glaxo zieht Retigabin zurück. *ÄrzteZeitung*, 31 May 2012. http://www.aerztezeitung.de/politik_gesellschaft/arzneimittelpolitik/article/814561/gkv-kompromisslos-glaxo-zieht-retigabin-zurueck.html?sh=6&h=1114409503 (accessed 20 March 2014).

ÄrzteZeitung, 2012b. Nutzenbewertung: Den Drohungen folgen jetzt Taten. *ÄrzteZeitung*, 11 May 2012. http://www.aerztezeitung.de/politik_gesellschaft/arzneimittelpolitik/article/813066/nutzenbewertung-drohungen-folgen-taten.html?sh=2&h=-678091188 (accessed 20 March 2014).

Cassel, D., 2011. Arzneimittel-Innovationen im Visier der Kostendämpfungspolitik. *G + G Wissenschaft* 11: 15–24.

Cassel, D. and Heigl, A., 2013. AMNOG in der Umsetzung: Preisregulierung als Innovationsbremse?, *Rechtsdepesche für das Gesundheitswesen*, 10.

Deutscher Bundestag, 2010a. Ausschussdrucks (printed papers of the German parliament) 17(14)0065(8neu).

Deutscher Bundestag, 2010b. Ausschussdrucks (printed papers of the German parliament) 17(14)0067.

Deutscher Bundestag, 2010c. Drucksache (printed papers of the German parliament) 17/2413.

Enzmann, H. and Lütz, J., 2008. Förderung von Arzneimitteln für seltene Leiden durch die Europäische Gemeinschaft. *Bundesgesundheitsbl – Gesundheitsforschung – Gesundheitsschutz* 5: 500–8.

Fricke, A., 2011. Individualisierte Medizin: Hoffnung und Risiko zugleich. *ÄrzteZeitung*, 22 February 2011. http://www.aerztezeitung.de/politik_gesellschaft/arzneimittelpolitik/article/642186/individualisierte-medizin-hoffnung-risiko-zugleich.html?sh=6&h=-1574724143 (accessed 20 March 2014).

Gemeinsamer Bundesausschuss, 2012. Summarising documentation on the amendment of the Directive on Medicinal Products. http://www.g-ba.de/downloads/40–268–1915/2012–03–15_AM-RL-XII_Pirfenidon_ZD.pdf (accessed 20 March 2014).

Gieseke, S. and Schmitt-Feuerbach, B., 2012. Fingerhakeln um den Preis beginnt. *ÄrzteZeitung*, 22 January 2012. http://www.aerztezeitung.de/politik_gesellschaft/arzneimittelpolitik/article/802270/fingerhakeln-preis-beginnt.html?sh=1&h=2126635865 (accessed 20 March 2014).

Heinemann, A.-K. and Lang, C., 2011. Der Begriff des Nutzens in der Frühbewertung nach den AMNOG. *Medizinrecht* 29: 150–3.

Huster, S., 2011. Rechtsfragen der frühen Nutzenbewertung. *Gesundheitsrecht* 2: 76–82.

Huster, S. and Gottwald, S., 2012. Rechtliche Implikationen der personalisierten Medizin. *Gesundheitsrecht* 8: 449–56.

IQWIG, 2011. Pirfenidon. Nutzenbewertung gemäß § 35a SGB V. https://www.iqwig.de/download/A11–18_Pirfenidon_Nutzenbewertung_35a_SGB_V.pdf (accessed 20 March 2014).

Kamann, H.-G., 2000. Die neuen E.G.-Regeln über Arzneimittel für seltene Leiden. Ein Förderungssystem für die sog. Orphan-Präparate aus Solidarität mit den Patienten. *Pharmarecht* 6: 170–4.

Kleinfeld, A., Bensing, C. and Schwarz, R., 2013. Der GKV-Verordnungsmarkt für Orphan Drugs. In: B. Häussler and K.-J. Preuß, eds. *Seltene Helden, Orphan Drugs in Deutschland*. Düsseldorf: Verlagsgruppe Handelsblatt, pp.181–96.

Laschet, H., 2011. AMNOG – Stoppschild für viele neue Wirkstoffe. *ÄrzteZeitung*, 12 October 2011. http://www.aerztezeitung.de/politik_gesellschaft/arzneimittelpolitik/article/673783/amnog-stoppschild-viele-neue-wirkstoffe.html?sh=1&h=312063017 (accessed 20 March 2014).

Pfundner, H., 2009. Personalisierte Medizin als Innovationsstrategie. In: H. Rebscher and S. Kaufmann, eds. *Gesundheitssysteme im Wandel.* Heidelberg: Economica-Verlag, pp.169–91.

Preusker, 2011. Verzicht – der Ausweg für innovative Unternehmen? *ÄrzteZeitung,* 14 September 2011. http://www.aerztezeitung.de/politik_gesellschaft/arznei mittelpolitik/article/669684/verzicht-ausweg-innovative-unternehmen. html?sh=3&h=346306849 (accessed 20 March 2014).

Remmele, C., 2007. Arzneimittel für seltene Leiden ('Orphan Drugs') im E.G.- und US-Recht. Augsburg, Shaker Verlag, Dissertation.

Rieser, S., 2010. Wann soll denn der wirkliche Nutzen festgestellt werden? *Deutsches Ärzteblatt* 40: A1887–A1888.

Schickert, J. and Schmitz, A., 2013. Orphan Drug in der schnellen Nutzenbewertung nach dem § 35a SGB V. In: B. Häussler and K.-J. Preuß, eds. *Seltene Helden, Orphan Drugs in Deutschland.* Düsseldorf: Verlagsgruppe Handelsblatt, pp.115–47.

Schmitt-Feuerbach, B., 2012. Ein Jahr Tauziehen um den Zusatznutzen. *ÄrzteZeitung,* 2 February 2012. http://www.aerztezeitung.de/politik_ gesellschaft/arzneimittelpolitik/article/803275/jahr-tauziehen-zusatznutzen. html?sh=1&h=-1698240275 (accessed 20 March 2014).

Wille, M., 2011. Die wichtigsten Regelungen des Gesetzes zur Neuordnung des Arzneimittelmarktes (AMNOG). *Wege zur Sozialversicherung* 2: 35–42.

Willhöft, C. and Lietz, C., 2012. Die frühe Nutzenbewertung von Orphan Drugs nach § 35a SGB V. *Arzneimittel & Recht* 1: 19–23.

Windeler, J., Koch, K., Lange. S. and Ludwig, W.-D., 2010. Zu guter Letzt ist alles selten. *Deutsches Ärzteblatt* 42: A2034–A2034.

Chapter 18

Personalised Medicine: Priority Setting and Opportunity Costs in European Public Health-Care Systems[1]

Jochen Vollmann[2]

Introduction

Modern medicine now has access to extensive genetic information about humans. The entire human genome was decoded in the international *Human Genome Project* and technical progress in the field of sequencing technologies enables inexpensive analyses of the complete genome of an individual. Clinical medicine is seeking to utilise these insights from molecular genetics research to treat patients more effectively. Knowledge about the individual genes of a patient in the field of medical diagnostics and treatment is being used to develop custom-tailored, individualised treatments (Chin et al., 2011; McDermott et al., 2011; Phimister et al., 2012; Sledge, 2012). Doctors can determine, for example, whether or not a cancer drug will be effective against a specific tumour by determining specific genetic biomarkers in a patient prior to starting treatment. Ineffective treatments can be excluded from the outset, and patients can, therefore, also be spared unnecessary adverse side effects. Furthermore, the pharmaceutical industry contends that considerable health-care costs can be saved by avoiding ineffective treatments (Richter-Kuhlmann, 2012a).

1   Major parts of this article were previously published in German under the title 'Persönlicher – besser – kostengünstiger? Kritische medizinethische Anfragen an die "personalisierte Medizin"' in: *Ethik in der Medizin* 2013, 25, 233–41. With kind permission of Springer Science+Business Media.

2   This study was conducted in the research network Personalised Medicine in Oncology: An Interdisciplinary Study on Ethical, Medical, Economical and Legal Aspects (Grant project number: 01 GP 1001A-C), which is supported by the German Federal Ministry of Education and Research (Bundesministerium für Bildung und Forschung – BMBF).

This concept of personalised medicine is not only often used in oncology, but also raises hopes of successful treatments for other common diseases, such as cardiovascular diseases, type 2 diabetes mellitus and mental disorders. Personalised medicine is frequently used as a synonym for progress and the promise of modern medicine *per se* and is presented in an uncritically positive way in research, business and the media (Collins, 2011; Holsboer, 2011; Schwan, 2013). Public research funding has declared personalised medicine to be a priority both at the European and also at the national level (Bundesministerium für Bildung und Forschung, 2010), and large pharmaceutical and biotechnology companies invest billions of euros in this research. Modern medicine is facing a new 'revolution' (Richter-Kuhlmann, 2012a) due to new scientific insights and the close co-operation of research, clinics and industry (Hüsing, 2010; Collins, 2011; Mirnezami et al., 2012). The treatment concept also appeals to medical laypersons as something that is worthy of support. However, are the hopes associated with personalised medicine well-founded, and are the high investments justified?

The Concept of a Person and 'Personalised Medicine'

The term 'personalised medicine' insinuates a kind of medical care which focuses on the health situation and the particular needs of each individual person. This is incorrect and misleading in two ways. First, the molecular genetic complexity of many illnesses makes the possibility of a treatment custom-tailored to each individual person very improbable, while the extremely high efforts and costs of this approach do not appear feasible in the current health-care system. What the term connotes is, therefore, not *personalised* diagnosis and treatment, but at best, diagnostic and therapeutic approaches which are targeted at specific patient subgroups, for example, groups which have the same tumour biomarkers (*stratified medicine*).

Second, medical care focused on molecular genetic characteristics has nothing to do with medical care oriented on the individual patient. *Individualisation* only takes place at the molecular genetic level, but not at the personal level between doctor and patient. In order to achieve a personal treatment, the person of the patient should be placed at the centre of treatment, and this is exactly what so-called personalised medicine does not do (Hüsing, 2010; Dabrock et al., 2012). A person is not only distinguished by biological traits, but also by individual psychological and social characteristics and needs. Individuals have their own lifestyles, values and preferences (Yurkiewicz, 2010). Law and ethics emphasise the normative implications of the concept of personhood, as evident in ongoing debates about so-called 'personhood' (Mahowald, 1995; Lampe, 1986). As a consequence, the patient in the doctor–patient relationship is entitled to adequate education and information from the doctor and has the individual right to consent to or to refuse a treatment (Kohnen et al., 2012). The patient's self-determined decision must be respected, even if it goes against the doctor's advice and against a medical indication, precisely because we ascribe the person these rights (Vollmann, 2008).

This ethical and anthropological understanding of the 'person' is expressed by many people in their wishes about modern medicine. Patients wish to be perceived by their doctors and by medical institutions as individual persons with questions, wishes and normative preferences. In the citizens' report 'High-Tech Medicine – What Kind of Health Care Do We Want?' of the German Federal Ministry of Education and Research, citizens demand that medical and nursing staff should have better communication skills. Furthermore, alongside the specialist subjects, mental and interpersonal aspects in day-to-day patient care must play an equal role in medical and nursing education and training and in research. The importance of taking time for the patient should be rediscovered in modern medicine (Bundesministerium für Bildung und Forschung 2011; Siegmund-Schultze, 2011; Koch, 2012). This broader cultural understanding of the term 'person' and the wishes of citizens for personal medical care are not considered in so-called personalised medicine. The term sounds appealing, but is misleading. The intention of the inappropriate use of the term 'person', which is conveyed in numerous texts and images in advertising materials, is to achieve a positive image and wide acceptance in society. It is important to debunk this questionable advertising strategy because it abuses the concept of personhood, perceives patients primarily as carriers of molecular genetically determined traits, suggests a genetic determinism for medicine (Tauber and Sarkar, 1993; Kerr and Cunningham-Burley, 2000) and aims at setting specific priorities in research funding. The latter, in particular, requires a transparent and critical discussion, as well as democratic decision-making.

Basic Research and Clinical Application

Additional doubts arise with regard to the statement of the US Food and Drug Administration (FDA) that after a decade of billions of dollars in investments in the *Human Genome Project* and in subsequent genetic analysis studies, the yield has only been a small number of clinical treatments on the basis of genetic biomarkers (Hüsing, 2010; Marshall, 2011). In addition, for the president of the Max Planck Society, the hope of immediately deriving rapid medical progress from the deciphering of the human genome has hardly been fulfilled (Gruss, 2011). The reason for this discrepancy is clear upon closer scientific observation. The clinical applications that have been successful until now are mainly in the field of oncology and are limited to a few tumour types for which the molecular genetic biomarkers are known and for which there is a treatment available. This fortunate constellation is the exception in clinical practice; these new treatments are of no benefit for the majority of patients. The scientific explanation for the slow clinical progress lies in the complexity of tumour biology, where the variability and mutation dynamics of the genetic traits of many tumours complicate the development of targeted therapies. Progress in clinical treatment and practice does not necessarily follow from a brilliant treatment approach that is derived from basic research (Burke and Psaty, 2007; Konstantinopoulos et al., 2009; Browman et al., 2011; Ludwig, 2012). Unfortunately, the international experience during the last decade makes rapid clinical progress for the majority of cancer patients very unlikely.

Medical Research and Industry under Pressure to Succeed

This sobering conclusion is contrary to the euphoria about the promise of personalised medicine. After decades without innovation breakthroughs, many biomedical researchers long for significant therapeutic progress (Hudson, 2009; Collins, 2011; Holsboer, 2011). The pharmaceutical industry is in a similar situation – its patents for the strongest selling drugs (so-called 'blockbusters') are due to expire in the coming years, and many companies do not have any new innovative drugs in their development pipeline (Collier, 2011; Greiner, 2012). Rather, the pharmaceutical and biotechnology industries are under pressure from the markets to reduce their high costs for research and development, since these, given the lack of innovation, do not refinance themselves (Aiolfi, 2011; Hunt et al., 2011; KPMG, 2011; Dhankhar et al., 2012). Compared to the stock price development of other companies, the value of many pharmaceutical companies has declined, while the return on investment from the high expenditures in research and development has been falling for years. As a result, consultants predict tough times ahead for the pharmaceutical industry (*Frankfurter Allgemeine Zeitung*, 2012).

In this difficult economic situation, many pharmaceutical companies are counting on rapid progress in the new field of personalised medicine. However, the high expectations are contrasted by the sluggish progress in the clinical application of personalised medicine (Ludwig, 2012). In practice, there is a danger that insufficiently tested drugs might be introduced too hastily into clinical care. New 'personalised' diagnostics and therapeutics may not have been approved without sufficient proof of their effectiveness. However, validation studies that are required for scientific proof of effectiveness are seldom carried out because these are long-term, complex and costly (Ludwig, 2012). It is commonly argued that the relevant cost and time-consuming proof of effectiveness in personalised medicine does not apply and should be abbreviated to get approval for the drug. However, the effectiveness and benefit of new drugs, even in small patient groups and targeted treatments, must be scientifically proven to ensure the health and welfare of the patients and to avoid unnecessary health costs (Ludwig et al., 2009; Richter-Kuhlmann, 2012a).

For this reason, drugs in the field of personalised treatments must be checked according to normal approval procedures in order to meet scientific and therapeutic standards. Since current clinical research in the field of personalised medicine is primarily financed by the pharmaceutical industry, conflicts of interest are inevitable (Valachis et al., 2012). In order to promote the necessary gain in scientific knowledge in this new field, therefore, we need more clinical research that is publicly funded and is independent from the private sector. This would strengthen serious patient-oriented clinical research that is independent of short-term economic interests (Vollmann et al., 2011). At present, however, universities and other public research organisations in this field are hardly autonomous and independent, so that the content of research activities and research strategies are often heavily influenced by industry (Dreger, 2011).

Priority Setting and Opportunity Costs

The high investment costs in research based on molecular genetic criteria raise the question of opportunity costs. This type of research ultimately provides stratified medical care that only benefits subgroups of patients. Investments in this field have been made for more than a decade and, due to many open research questions, will continue to be made in the future (Rauprich, 2010). Given the limited resources in the health-care sector, a prioritisation decision is required already at the research level regarding the extent of public resources that will flow into particular areas of the health-care system. A research priority in one area limits the remaining research funds for other medical speciality areas. With regard to the promotion and funding of personalised medicine, this difficult normative and political decision is further exacerbated since there are only a relatively small number of patients who may benefit from these very expensive measures. That is why clinical physicians are concerned that other important clinical and health-care areas which might be beneficial for many patients will be neglected through the prioritised promotion of personalised medicine (Browman et al., 2011; Siegmund-Schultze, 2011; Koch, 2012; Ludwig, 2012). Thus far, only a minority of patients have benefited from this expensive, research- and economics-driven project of personalised medicine (Hamburg and Collins, 2010; Browman et al., 2011; Deutscher Ethikrat [German Ethics Council], 2012). Based on previous experience, high profits can be expected from expensive cancer drugs for small patient groups (so-called 'niche busters') and, therefore, this approach continues to appear lucrative for the pharmaceutical industry, without taking into account the health needs of the majority of patients in our health-care system.

Whereas in oncology, at least a small portion of patients have benefited from the innovations of personalised medicine, they have until now brought no benefit for patients in other socially and medically important disease groups. An example is the common disease type 2 diabetes: no molecular genetic descriptions of subgroups, biomarkers, and so on, are superior to the usual preventive, diagnostic and treatment options and they do not improve the health situation of the patients affected (Schulze, 2011). Moreover, screening for type 2 diabetes does not offer any relevant advantages (Simmons et al., 2012). Rather, as our society ages, our nutrition, exercise and lifestyle play an increasingly crucial role in the prevention and treatment of type 2 diabetes (Kurth, 2012; Richter-Kuhlmann, 2012b). For this disease, modern medicine does not primarily require new molecular genetic insights, but rather sociomedical care approaches and intensive public health research to enable and support at-risk and affected people to adopt healthy behaviours as individuals. However, this research is seriously underfunded in our health-care system.

Another example is the increasing importance of mental illness as a public health concern in our society. Mental illness and its treatment and prevention is of great significance for the patients affected, health insurance companies, pension fund insurance companies who bear the cost for rehabilitation, and for the labour market. According to the German Federal Ministry of Labour and Social Affairs, the days missed from work due to mental disorders have increased from 6.6 per cent in 2001 to 13.1 per cent in 2010, which is associated with economic costs of approximately EUR 8–10 billion annually. The most important causes specified are higher demands in the workplace, increased personal responsibility, pressure to be flexible, irregular employment relationships and job insecurity (*Deutsches Ärzteblatt*, 2012). The current care of these patients in our health-care system is under criticism due to excessively long sick-leave times, excessive waiting times for psychiatric and psychotherapy treatment and/or inpatient rehabilitation measures, and too frequent early retirements due to mental disorders. Investments are, therefore, required in research to develop new concepts for social-psychiatric prevention and treatment, for example, enabling effective prevention and early intervention at the workplace and improving the co-operation between, for example, the company doctor, primary care physician, psychiatrist and hospital. This raises the issue whether we, as a society, should respond to the increasing importance of mental illness primarily with high investments in molecular genetic research for 'personalised treatment', or invest at least in equal measure in social psychiatric and mental health research, which is allocated relatively little funding in current research policy.

Therefore, from a medical ethics perspective, the existing preference for molecular genetics medicine in personalised medicine in contrast to other research fields in the publicly funded health-care system needs to be critically examined. In essence, all prioritisation decisions are ethical decisions in which competing values must be weighed (Rauprich, 2010). In doing so, transparency must prevail regarding who decides about what facts, which criteria are used and on which arguments decisions are based. Therefore, it is ethically unacceptable that influential individual interests *de facto* determine medical research priorities and resource allocation in the publicly funded health-care system; but this is exactly what is currently happening under the innocuous label of 'personalised medicine'. Cost–benefit assessments of the individual treatments – now often discussed – are also insufficient, since, on the basis of empirical data, they only allow statements about the medical benefits and the costs of the treatment area under investigation. In practice, the selection of the treatment area for research already frequently represents a setting of priorities within the overall spectrum of possible health-promoting measures without prior reflection on the norms involved. What is required for our health care in the future are transparent and democratically legitimised superordinate medical and research policy prioritisations.

However, our society leaves crucial research policy decisions to internationally active stakeholders from research and industry. Whereas public funds have invested heavily in basic research (for example, the *Human Genome Project*), priority setting in the field of clinical applications is left to the discretion of the international pharmaceutical industry. Universities and other public research organisations in Germany have little influence on content prioritisation in this field because, as I noted above, independent research hardly exists due to the lack of public funding. To be sure, co-operation with the public health authorities is always emphasised in order to co-ordinate health-care and socio-economic priorities. In reality, however, this hardly plays a role. The reason is that international pharmaceutical companies develop diagnostics and drugs for the world market (Hunt et al., 2011; KPMG, 2011; Dhankhar et al., 2012; *Frankfurter Allgemeine Zeitung*, 2013; Schwan, 2013). However, the health-care needs and the financing of the health-care systems differ greatly in the various countries. The currently still largest health-care market in the United States, with its strong private sector orientation and a high proportion of citizens who lack medical insurance, for example, differs greatly from European health-care systems. The demographic trend of Western societies contrasts sharply to that of the economically emerging countries, such as Brazil and India, with their high proportion of young people in the population and a growing, upwardly mobile middle class that finances its medical care privately (Agarwal et al., 2012). In these so-called *emerging markets*, the pharmaceutical industry in 2020 will proportionately make equivalent profits as in the currently largest pharmaceutical market, the United States (KPMG, 2011). These profits will originate from innovative products, including products in the fields of personalised medicine, which are expensive and have to be paid for privately (Griggs, 2009). By contrast, the importance of European health-care markets for the development of new drugs is declining.

Given the different socio-economic and health priorities, which vary from country to country, the research and development investments of the pharmaceutical industry will follow international market opportunities, which are not necessarily congruent with health-care needs in Germany and other European countries. In order to provide optimal health care for our population, it is essential to develop our own strategic research and health-care policy in the public health sector. To achieve this, those responsible for health and research policy must recognise the existing problems and put them forward for public debate. However, past experience with a public discussion about setting priorities and rationing in the health-care system in Germany gives little cause for optimism. A wealthy, shrinking and ageing society cannot muster the strength to carry out a reform or to design its own public health system. Thus, society should not complain when global stakeholders set priorities under the lofty-sounding label of personalised medicine – priorities that do not correspond to society's own health-care needs.

Conclusion

Genetic biomarker-based personalised medicine does not contribute to a more personal treatment of individual patients, in contrast to patient – or person-centred – medical care. Subgroups of patients, for example, in oncology, may have medical advantages from the present progress in personalised medicine, but it is unlikely that this will be the case for the overall majority of patients. The promise of less expensive health care through personalised medicine lacks any empirical evidence. Rather, based on past experience, an increase of costs is more likely.

A public debate is needed on priority setting in medical research and treatment and about how societies and public health systems can influence the development of the research agenda regarding future health-care priorities.

References

Agarwal, S., d'Almeida, J. and Francis, T., 2012. Capturing the Brazilian pharma opportunity. Global pharma companies are missing a chance to serve

Brazil's increasingly prosperous and growing middle class. *McKinsey Quarterly*, March, pp.1–4.

Aiolfi, S., 2011. Die Pharmaforschung ist zu teuer. Investoren zeigen sich irritiert über einen offensichtlichen Mangel an Effizienz [Pharmaceutical research is too expensive. Investors are irritated about an apparent lack of efficiency]. *Neue Zürcher Zeitung*, 31 December.

Browman, G., Hébert, P.C. and Coutts, J., 2011. Personalized medicine: a windfall for science, but what about patients? *Canadian Medical Association Journal*, 183(18), p.E1277.

Bundesministerium für Bildung und Forschung, 2010. *Ideen. Innovation. Wachstum – Hightech-Strategie 2020 für Deutschland [Ideas. Innovation. Growth – high-tech strategy 2020 for Germany]*. Berlin: Bundesministerium für Bildung und Forschung.

Bundesministerium für Bildung und Forschung, 2011. *Bürgerreport: Hightech-Medizin – Welche Gesundheit wollen wir? [Citizens report: high-tech medicine – what health do we want?]*. Berlin: Bundesministerium für Bildung und Forschung.

Burke, W. and Psaty, B.M., 2007. Personalized medicine in the era of genomics. *Journal of the American Medical Association*, 298, pp.1682–4.

Chin, L., Andersen, J.N. and Futreal, P.A., 2011. Cancer genomics: from discovery science to personalized medicine. *Nature Medicine*, 17, pp.297–303.

Collier, R., 2011. Bye, bye blockbusters, hello niche busters. *Canadian Medical Association Journal*, 183, pp.E697–8.

Collins, F.S., 2011. *Meine Gene – mein Leben [My genes – my life]*. Heidelberg: Spektrum Akademischer Verlag.

Dabrock, P., Braun, M. and Ried, J., 2012. Individualisierte Medizin: Ethische und gesellschaftliche Herausforderungen [Individualised medicine: ethical and societal challenges]. *Forum*, 27, pp.209–13.

Deutscher Ethikrat [German Ethics Council], 2012. *Pressemitteilungen: Ethikrat rückt den Patienten in den Fokus der personalisierten Medizin [Press release: ethics Council puts the patient in the focus of peronalised medicine]*. Berlin: Deutscher Ethikrat.

Deutsches Ärzteblatt, 2012. Krankschreibungen: Mehr Fehltage wegen psychischer Erkrankungen [Sick leave: more days of absence due to mental disorders]. *Deutsches Ärzteblatt*, 109, p.A-948.

Dhankhar, A., Evers, M. and Møller, M., 2012. *Escaping the sword of Damocles: toward a new future for pharmaceutical R&D*. Chicago: McKinsey & Company.

Dreger, P., 2011. Brief: Priorisierung in der Forschung [Letter: prioritization of research]. *Deutsches Ärzteblatt*, 108, p.A-2286.

Frankfurter Allgemeine Zeitung, 2012. Im Gespräch: Thomas Strüngmann, Unternehmer und Investor in der Pharmabranche [Interview: Thomas Strüngmann, entrepreneur and investor in the pharmaceutical industry]. *Frankfurter Allgemeine Zeitung*, 10 April, p.15.

Frankfurter Allgemeine Zeitung, 2013. Sanofi schmerzt Patentauslauf. Gewinn des Pharmakonzerns könnte 2013 sinken [Sanofi hurt by patent expiry. Profits of the pharmaceutical company could fall in 2013]. *Frankfurter Allgemeine Zeitung*, 8 February, p.16.

Greiner, W., 2012. Ökonomische Herausforderungen der individualisierten Medizin [Economic challenges of individualised medicine]. *Forum*, 27, pp.203–8.

Griggs, J.J., 2009. Personalized medicine: a perk of privilege? *Clinical Pharmacology & Therapeutics*, 86, pp.21–3.

Gruss, P., 2011. Der Faktor Mensch [The human factor]. *MaxPlanckForschung*, 1, pp.6–7.

Hamburg, M.A. and Collins, F.S., 2010. The path to personalized medicine. *New England Journal of Medicine*, 363(4), pp.301–4.

Holsboer, F., 2011. *Biologie für die Seele: Mein Weg zur personalisierten Medizin* [*Biology for the soul: my path to personalised medicine*]. München: dtv.

Hudson, T.J., 2009. Personalized medicine: a transformative approach is needed. *Canadian Medical Association Journal*, 180, pp.911–13.

Hunt, V., Manson, N. and Morgan, P., 2011. A wake-up call for big pharma: pharmaceuticals & medical products practice. *McKinsey Quarterly*, December, pp.1–6.

Hüsing, B., 2010. Individualisierte Medizin – Potenziale und Handlungsbedarf [Individualised medicine – potential and action]. *Zeitschrift für Evidenz, Fortbildung und Qualität im Gesundheitswesen*, 104, pp.727–31.

Kerr, A. and Cunningham-Burley, S., 2000. On ambivalence and risk: reflexive modernity and the new human genetics. *Sociology*, 34, pp.283–304.

Koch, M., 2012. Arzt-Patienten-Beziehung: In falsches Fahrwasser geraten [Doctor–patient relationship: having run into the wrong channel]. *Deutsches Ärzteblatt*, 109, p.A-20.

Kohnen, T., Schildmann, J. and Vollmann, J., 2012. Patients' self-determination in 'personalized medicine': the case of whole genome sequencing and tissue banking in oncology. Individualized medicine between hype and hope. In: P. Dabrock, M. Braun and J. Ried, eds. *Individualized medicine between hype and hope: exploring ethical and societal challenges for healthcare*. Zürich: Lit Verlag. pp.97–110.

Konstantinopoulos, P.A., Karamouzis, M.V. and Papavassiliou, A.G., 2009. Educational and social-ethical issues in the pursuit of molecular medicine. *Molecular Medicine*, 15, pp.60–3.

KPMG, 2011. *Pharmaceuticals: future pharma. Five strategies to accelerate the transformation of the pharmaceutical industry by 2020*. London: KPMG.

Kurth, B-M., 2012. Erste Ergebnisse aus der 'Studie zur Gesundheit Erwachsener in Deutschland' (DEGS) [First results of the 'Study on Adult Health in Germany' (DEGS)]. *Bundesgesundheitsblatt*, 55, pp.980–90.

Lampe, E.-J., 1986. Persönlichkeit, Persönlichkeitssphäre, Persönlichkeitsrecht [Personality, privacy, personal rights. In: E-J. Lampe, ed. *Persönlichkeit, Familie, Eigentum: Grundrechte aus der Sicht der Sozial- und Verhaltenswissenschaften* [*Personality, family, property: fundamental rights from the perspective of social and behavioural sciences*]. Opladen: Westdeutscher Verlag. pp.73–102.

Ludwig, W.-D., 2012. Möglichkeiten und Grenzen der stratifizierenden Medizin am Beispiel von prädiktiven Biomarkern und 'zielgerichteten' medikamentösen Therapien in der Onkologie [Possibilities and limitations of stratifying medicine using the example of predictive biomarkers and 'targeted' drug therapies in oncology]. *Zeitschrift für Evidenz, Fortbildung und Qualität im Gesundheitswesen*, 122, pp.11–22.

Ludwig, W.-D., Fetscher, S. and Schildmann, J., 2009. Teure Innovationen in der Onkologie – für alle? Überlegungen zu Voraussetzungen für eine rationale Pharmakotherapie und ethische Herausforderungen [Expensive innovation in oncology – for all? Considering conditions for rational pharmacotherapy and ethical challenges]. *Der Onkologe*, 15, pp.1004–14.

Mahowald, M., 1995. Person. In: W.T. Reich, ed. *Encyclopedia of Bioethics*. New York: Macmillan. pp.1934–40

Marshall, E., 2011. Waiting for the revolution. *Science*, 331, pp.526–9.

McDermott, U., Downing, J.R. and Stratton, M.R., 2011. Genomics and the continuum of cancer care. *New England Journal of Medicine*, 364, pp.340–50.

Mirnezami, R., Nicholson, J. and Darzi, A., 2012. Preparing for precision medicine. *New England Journal of Medicine*, 366, pp.489–91.

Phimister, E.G., Feero, G.W. and Guttmacher, A.E., 2012. Realizing genomic medicine. *New England Journal of Medicine*, 366, pp.757–9.

Rauprich, O., 2010. Rationierung unter den Bedingungen der Endlichkeit im Gesundheitswesen [Rationing under the conditions of finiteness in health care]. In: G. Thomas, M. Höfner and S. Schaede, eds. *Endliches Leben Interdisziplinäre Zugänge zum Phänomen der Krankheit* [*Finite life interdisciplinary approaches to the phenomenon of disease*]. Tübingen: Mohr Siebeck. pp.229–56.

Richter-Kuhlmann, E., 2012a. Pränataldiagnostik: Paradigmenwechsel [Prenatal diagnosis: a paradigm shift]. *Deutsches Ärzteblatt*, 109, p.A-1306.

Richter-Kuhlmann, E., 2012b. Gesundheitssurvey des Robert-Koch-Instituts: Zivilisationskrankheiten nehmen zu [Health survey by the Robert Koch Institute: lifestyle diseases are increasing]. *Deutsches Ärzteblatt*, 109, pp.C-1171–2.

Schulze, M., 2011. *Programme of the international symposium: predictive genetic testing, risk communication and risk perception: value of genetics. Information for diabetes risk prediction*. Berlin: Robert Koch Institut.

Schwan, S., 2013. Die Dividendenhoffnungen bleiben intakt [The dividend hopes remain intact]. *Frankfurter Allgemeine Zeitung*, 14 January, p.22.

Siegmund-Schultze, N., 2011. Versorgung von Krebspatienten: Menschliche Zuwendung aufwerten [Care of cancer patients; enhance human affection]. *Deutsches Ärzteblatt*, 108, p.A-932.

Simmons, R.K., Echouffo-Tcheugui, J.B., Sharp, S.J., Sargeant, L.A., Williams, K.M., Prevost, A.T., Kinmonth, A.L., Wareham, N.J. and Griffin, S.J., 2012. Screening for type 2 diabetes and population mortality over 10 years (ADDITION-Cambridge): a cluster-randomised controlled trial. *Lancet*, 380, pp.1741–8.

Sledge, G.W., 2012. The challenge and promise of the genomic era. *Journal of Clinical Oncology*, 30, pp.203–9.

Tauber, A.I. and Sarkar, S., 1993. The ideology of the human genome project. *Journal of the Royal Society of Medicine*, 86, pp.537–40.

Valachis, A., Polyzos, N.P., Nearchou, A., Lind, P. and Mauri, D., 2012. Financial relationships in economic analyses of targeted therapies in oncology. *Journal of Clinical Oncology*, 30, pp.1316–20.

Vollmann, J., 2008. *Patientenselbstbestimmung und Selbstbestimmungsfähigkeit: Beiträge zur klinischen Ethik* [*Patient self-determination and self-determination ability: contributions to clinical ethics*]. Stuttgart: Kohlhammer.

Vollmann, J., Schildmann, J. and Kohnen, T., 2011. Onkologie: Sehr gut recherchiert [Oncology: very well-researched]. *Deutsches Ärzteblatt*, 108, p.A-2341.

Yurkiewicz, S., 2010. The prospects for personalized medicine. *Hastings Center Report*, 40, pp.14–18.

PART IV
Personalised Medicine in Oncology: Recommendations for Future Development

Chapter 19

'Personalised Medicine': Multidisciplinary Perspectives and Interdisciplinary Recommendations on a Framework for Future Research and Practice

Jan Schildmann, Miriam Böttcher, Maria Gabriel, Arnold Ganser,
Sina Gottwald, Franz Hessel, Stefan Huster, Rebecca Jahn, Anja Neumann,
Michael Noweski, Matthias Port, Laura Pouryamout, Verena Sandow,
Felicitas Thol, Sebastian Wäscher, Anke Walendzik,
Jürgen Wasem and Jochen Vollmann[1]

Introduction

'Personalised medicine' (PM) has raised great hopes and expectations among researchers, patients, health-care providers and politicians in past years. Although the term 'person' in PM suggests an approach of medicine which takes into account psychosocial and value aspects of the patient as human being, most articles refer to PM as strategies limited to biological features of individuals which are used to stratify patient groups for the purposes of prevention, diagnosis and treatment of disease.

This approach to medicine has gained considerable success in recent years, especially for some patient groups in oncology. However, current research also indicates that targeted treatment seems realistic only for a minority of patients in the near future. Among the reasons for this are the multitude of genetic variations

1   The authors form part of the collaborative research network 'Personalised Medicine in Oncology: An Interdisciplinary Study on Ethical, Medical, Economical and Legal Aspects' (Grant project number: 01 GP 1001A-C), which is supported by the German Federal Ministry of Education and Research (Bundesministerium für Bildung und Forschung – BMBF).

associated with a disease, the interplay between environment and genetic make-up, and mechanisms of resistance as they can be observed in patients receiving targeted treatment. Other challenges regarding the implementation of PM cover the scarcity of high-quality valid and reliable biomarker tests and a lack of education and professional expertise which enables health-care providers to interpret the relevance of data which are currently generated by high-output gene sequencing technologies regarding possible associations between biomarkers and diseases.

In addition to the medical-technical challenges mentioned above, the further development and implementation of PM also raises a number of ethical issues. Questions about the rights to information and self-determination of those participating in biobank research and those, such as relatives, possibly affected by biobank research are examples. From a social-ethics perspective, there has to be a balance in financing the various sectors of health care. On the one hand, targeted treatment is needed to improve the quantity and quality of life in cancer patients. On the other hand, the implementation of PM requires enormous resources in medical-technical foundations, as well as education and further prerequisites for implementing PM in times when money in health care is scarce. After all, there are opportunity costs associated with the spending of resources in PM, for example, limitations on spending the money in other areas of medicine such as psychosocial support of patients. Furthermore and relevant from an economic perspective, it is a matter of current methodological debate how one can determine the costs and benefits of the often complex PM interventions and how to compare the (cost-)effectiveness with other approaches in medicine. Last but not least, there are several issues still to be solved from a legal perspective: regulation of biobanks, approval of new kinds of pharmaceutical products and reimbursement of additional testing are three urgent tasks with regards to the implementation of PM interventions within a public health-care system.

During four years between 2011 and 2014, the authors, researchers from the fields of medical ethics, medicine, health economics and law, have collaborated in the research network 'Personalised Medicine in Oncology: an Interdisciplinary Study on Ethical, Medical, Economical and Legal Aspects', which has been funded by the German Federal Ministry of Education and Research (FK 01GP 1001A-C). In this chapter, the experts in the different fields summarise selected findings of the work conducted in different work packages with a focus on the relevance of the findings for the future development of PM. In the first section, Matthias Port and colleagues provide an up-to-date account of scientific foundations as well as challenges from a medical perspective. The following section reports on findings from the joint work of researchers in health economics and medicine conducted by Laura Pouryamout and colleagues on methodological challenges associated with cost–benefit analysis of PM interventions. Referring to considerations in the field of economics, Michael Noweski and colleagues explain in a third part how to encourage the industry to invest in innovative and cost-effective solutions in PM. The two final sections provide an outlook on future development and regulation of PM from a legal (Sina Gottwald and Stefan Huster) and ethical (Jan Schildmann and colleagues) perspective. The chapter will conclude with summarising joint recommendations of all participants of the research project.

Scientific Foundations and Challenges: A Medical Perspective[2]

There has been a tremendous increase in our knowledge of tumour biology (Hanahan and Weinberg, 2011) in the last decade. Major advances in technologies, such as high-throughput DNA sequencing, have led to insights into tumour signalling pathways that modulate cell growth and differentiation, cell death or metastasis formation. The discoveries in the area of tumour biology have already resulted in new therapeutic strategies, as shown for the advances in treatment of melanoma. After decades of almost no progress in the treatment of metastatic melanoma and 10 years after the discovery that B-Raf proto-oncogene (BRAF) mutation is present in 40 per cent of melanomas, studies on the inhibition of mutated BRAF have shown a dramatic benefit for personalised therapy in this disease (Flaherty et al., 2010). This is a prime example showing that these new findings need to be evaluated in well-conducted clinical trials. Understanding the biology of tumours has to take into account the heterogeneity (Gerlinger et al., 2012) and escape strategies of tumours to counteract targeted therapies. In order to address the clinical problems in the context of PM requires more than just inhibiting mutated gene products; it needs a profound knowledge of major and minor signalling pathways which have to be selectively inhibited to prevent tumour cell escape. This profound knowledge is also required to avoid unwanted adverse effects in organ systems distant from the tumour. According to the technical progress in medicine, genetic information on individuals and knowledge about related health consequences are growing steadily. The use of biomarker-based or molecular genetic tests for diagnosis, especially in malignant diseases, leads to information about the potential success concerning treatment options and may optimise therapy.

The implementation of PM is associated with several challenges. There are already, for example, more than 20 mutations and genes known to play a role in the development and prognosis of acute myeloid leukaemia (AML). The integration of these and other mutations still to be detected as well as classic

---

2   The work presented in this section has been conducted by Matthias Port, Miriam Böttcher, Maria Gabriel, Felicitas Thol and Arnold Ganser.

prognostic markers, such as age, performance status, cytogenetics, response to induction therapy or quantification of residual disease, is a great challenge for future research (Damm et al., 2011). It is uncommon and almost impossible to evaluate the benefit of implementing prognostic markers in prospective studies. Although this might increase the evidence, especially in rare diseases or even more when defining further subgroups, it takes years to collect material in biobanks to evaluate the impact of these parameters. Since new mutations were detected during the course or after the end of many of the trials, these analyses cannot be but retrospective. In order to circumvent these limitations, part of the studies were used to generate hypotheses, while others served to verify or disprove them.

Gain of knowledge in diseases with smaller and smaller genetically defined subgroups will depend on international collaboration and exchange of individual patient datasets in order to obtain insights into the interdependencies of molecular findings. The danger of identifying individual patients even when using pseudonymised datasets also has to be taken into account, as well as the tremendous challenges of defining common and sufficiently detailed patient datasets and describing or evaluating complex disease courses. In order to optimise treatment, it might be necessary to continually evaluate patients even after marketing authorisation. To meet this need and because of the high complexity in the field of cancer treatment and individualisation, it might be necessary to refer the patient to specialists for the optimal treatment management. This would be one step further to enable medicine to match patient and treatment at its best and to minimise medical harm. For this purpose, scientific findings from retrospective studies, including meta-analyses and integration of the World Health Organization (WHO) disease classification, should be gathered with the aim of making testing mandatory in cases in which optimised treatment decisions can reliably be based on the findings of biomarkers.

To summarise: PM, with an increase of knowledge in the biology of patients and their diseases, is about to change our way of treatment. The successful integration of the scientific findings into new treatment strategies remains a constant challenge and needs to be evaluated in well-designed controlled trials.

Benefit and Costs of Personalised Medicine: The Case Example of Acute Myeloid Leukaemia[3]

In addition to dealing with the medical challenges of implementing the concept of PM described above, interdisciplinary analysis of benefits and costs of

---

3 The work presented in this section has been conducted by Laura Pouryamout, Anja Neumann, Matthias Port, Arnold Ganser and Jürgen Wasem.

different strategies for diagnosis and treatment is an important step to inform the different stakeholders about the contribution of PM in practice. In the following, we describe the factors which need to be taken into account when performing an analysis of benefits and costs of PM interventions using the case of stratification of patient groups with AML.

AML is a malignant disease of the haematopoietic system, which may lead to death within a few weeks if left untreated. The basis of treatment is chemotherapy. A further therapy option is the method of allogeneic stem cell transplantation. Known prognostic factors are the patient's age, leukocyte count, cytogenetic and previous haemato-oncological diseases, and, most important, response to induction chemotherapy. AML is a disease in which molecular genetic studies play an important role. Therefore, methods of PM seem to be appropriate – by determination of molecular genetic markers – for a further risk classification of patients with AML, as they may give information about the prognosis of the disease. This, in turn, may influence the decision with regard to the optimal treatment strategy depending on the risk classification.

The identification of markers by molecular genetic testing allows further risk classification of AML patients previously classified as intermediate risk into a high- and low-risk type due to the existence of certain genetic markers or marker combinations. AML patients with a normal karyotype, who are classified as low-risk type due to the molecular genetic testing (for example, in the presence of the marker-mutated nucleophosmin-1 (NPM1)), seem to have a better prognosis in terms of overall survival and recurrence-free survival. By contrast, the presence of the marker fms-related tyrosine kinase 3 (FLT3-ITD) positive is an indicator of a rather poor prognosis (Schlenk and Döhner, 2009). We included data from over 1,400 to 1,900 patients in a meta-analysis conducted as part of the project, looking especially at three frequent mutations: mutations of FLT3-ITD, NPM1 and the CEBPA gene (encoding the CCAAT/enhancer binding protein-alpha). A clear negative impact both on overall survival (OS) and disease-free survival (DFS) was seen for FLT3-ITD, while positive prognostic impact of both NPM1 and CEBPA mutations could be demonstrated (Port et al., 2014).

In terms of a health economic analysis, the cost–benefit ratio of PM in AML, both the cost of molecular genetic tests and of related therapeutic decisions, which are based on the molecular genetic studies, are of importance. Based only on cytogenetic diagnostics, all AML patients with normal karyotype were classified as medium risk. The treatment decision after cytogenetic diagnostics with regard to stem cell transplantation was mainly triggered due to the additional prognostic factors mentioned above, for example, the patient's response to induction therapy or age. The risk classification based on the molecular genetic testing performed additionally implies that patients of the 'medium risk group' can be further subdivided into a group of patients with high-risk or low-risk.

Concerning treatment, there is a focus on stem cell transplantation in the high-risk group, whereas patients in the low-risk group only receive chemotherapy. The transplantation of patients within the high-risk group involves initially high costs. However, treatment of these patients with chemotherapy alone is associated with a high risk of recurrence, reduced overall survival and a potential decision for stem cell transplantation after relapse. Therefore, costs occur for initial treatment as well as for relapse therapy. A classification of patients in the low-risk group due to a favourable combination of biomarkers leads to an abandonment of stem cell therapy in many cases, which is associated with lower side-effects as well as possibly lower cost. Finally, the cost of molecular genetic analyses, which have to be done in addition to the already expensive cytogenetic analyses, has to be taken into account. To what extent this example of PM, in other words, the treatment decision supported by molecular genetic information, may be cost-effective in relation to the treatment decision without this additional information is currently being analysed.

From a health economics perspective, the use of methods of PM, such as the biomarker-based or molecular genetic tests described above, and related adaption of therapy are considered as an economic challenge (Greiner, 2012). The financing especially will pose substantial challenges for the German health-care system. Since not all innovative methods can be financed, the methods which show an additional benefit for the patient and should be financed by the publicly financed health-care system have to be analysed. In terms of these circumstances, cost-effectiveness analyses are becoming increasingly important due to the fact that they enable a comparison of cost and effects even in terms of patient-related outcomes, for example, overall survival of different competitive technologies. The financial feasibility and the patients' benefit are limited by the fact that many innovative methods are tailored for smaller patient groups suffering from severe diseases, especially in the field of oncology.

The overall goal in terms of PM should be to avoid inefficiency and unnecessary risks (Maio, 2012). In the following section, we will provide an outlook on factors which can support the development of PM interventions from a health economic perspective.

Promoting the Development of Personalised Medicine: A View from Health Economics[4]

Seen from the perspectives of industrial economics and welfare policy, it should be noted that new therapeutic options with additional benefits will only be

---

4 The work presented in this section has been conducted by Michael Noweski, Franz Hessel, Anke Walendzik, Rebecca Jahn and Jürgen Wasem.

available if the companies develop new products, such as in the case of PM drugs with associated pre-tests. We assume that, under conditions of market competition, research-orientated pharmaceutical companies only invest in the development of products which are profitable to market, but not necessarily targeting the most prevalent medical needs of the patients. Keeping in mind the current financial pressure, governments could successfully improve the situation by supporting companies to develop PM technologies which are profitable for manufacturers and clinically beneficial for patients without imposing an unjustified additional budget impact on health-care payers. To achieve this, legislators have to improve the preconditions of research, market approval and reimbursement, as well as to implement adequate evaluation structures. At the same time, authorities must assure that the burden for the payers keeps in a reasonable relationship to the benefit generated by new drugs.

The product development of personalised drug therapy is influenced by the research policies of the industrialised countries, because private and public research is closely intertwined. The development projects of the pharmaceutical companies benefit from the results of the 'Human Genome Project' and technologies that have been developed in publicly funded research institutions (Wiechers et al., 2013). Fourteen per cent of the new chemical entities that were approved by the US Food and Drug Administration (FDA) in the period from 1990 to 2007 were discovered by public laboratories (Stevens et al., 2011). University hospitals are important partners of the industry not only in the clinical phase. The importance of this interdependency is rising because universities and other public research institutions are increasingly using external funding from industrial sponsors. On the other hand, companies benefit from access to subjects and patient records. The influence of the government on this research area is considerable in all developed countries. There are at least two approaches to make the conditions for investments in new products with additional clinical benefit more attractive:

1. the improvement of data availability; and
2. the strengthening of research translation.

The research system should generate and provide more information on potential and validated biomarkers to improve the availability of data. It should also generate and provide more specific clinical data by retrospective studies, as mentioned above in this chapter. The matching of both data streams should be more effective. Governments are already funding organisations and projects and more initiatives are being formed to share data. An example of networking is the 'EurocanPlatform', an alliance of cancer institutions and organisations, which is funded by the European Union (Tsimberidou et al., 2013). In compliance with the necessary confidentiality of the patient's personal data, the legislator should create a favourable regulatory environment to attract volunteers for research, to establish biobanks and to create large datasets with treatment data. The availability of data must be accompanied by adequate strategies and appropriate study designs to generate convincing clinical, patient-relevant evidence for new test-drug combinations.

Research funding should place further emphasis on the translation of the results of basic research to product development and market access. There is already a strong awareness of the problem among stakeholders. There are meaningful projects, for example, the funding programme 'Clinical and Translational Science Awards', launched by the National Institutes of Health in the United States in 2006, and specialised units in research institutes were strengthened over the last few years. However, the translation often has to cope with extremely large amounts of data. Further investments in data processing centres and appropriate software are needed. Bioinformatics as a new scientific discipline needs further support.

The marketing approval of test-drug combinations is more complex for the companies than that of drugs without pre-test, because an additional, in many cases separate, process is required for the test. It has been possible for some years in the United States for the approval of drug and test to fall apart over time. The American system has the advantage, however, that both components will be reviewed within the FDA, allowing the co-ordination of procedures, at least in principle. In Europe, the process routes are institutionally separated. The industry benefits from the fact that the approval process of the tests is less strict and delays are very unusual. The requirements, however, were increased in small steps in the past and will be significantly raised by a proposed amendment of the EU *In Vitro* Directive, the European regulatory framework for *in vitro* diagnostics, in the near future. Consequently, the probability of delays in the approval process of tests will increase. The solution would be an integrated authorisation procedure for test and drug. While the FDA establishes organisational preconditions to achieve, the European Medicines Agency (EMA) in Europe lacks the jurisdiction for approving the tests. A transfer of these competencies to the EMA seems advisable.

Improvement opportunities also exist with regard to reimbursement. A drug needs sufficient reimbursement by private and public payers to be profitable. Insurers in many health systems assess the medical benefits and/or the cost efficiency of a new product before including it in the scope of service. The amount of refund depends on the results of this evaluation. The procedures and requirements vary between the welfare states. They vary between different regions, different kinds of health-care payers and product groups. Seen from the position of the manufacturers, a reduction of the confusing diversity would be desirable. A network of national Health Technology Assessment (HTA) organisations has been constituted in Europe, developing proposals for alignment

(Borlum Kristensen, 2012). However, recommendations have to be based on current organisational realities, taking into consideration that structural changes are only achievable through systemic reforms and reimbursement decisions are within the jurisdiction of EU member states. There are two ways to improve the investment conditions of the industry within this regulatory framework:

1. an attractive amount of reimbursement for innovative products with additional benefit and sufficient cost-effectiveness; and
2. predictable and fast decision-making whether the product will be reimbursed and for what price.

The amount of reimbursement should be based on the value of the drug from society's perspective. It should reward innovations that are useful for the overall health-care system with a premium price (value-based pricing). Both medical and economic advantages concerning comparable products or therapies can be considered. Medical benefit is understood here in terms of a lower rate of non-responders, fewer side effects and new therapeutic options for hitherto poorly treatable patient groups. Economic benefits from the perspective of insurers can be lower treatment costs, for example, caused by non-responders avoiding treatment, and also a more productive workforce. What criteria are applied in a specific case depends on the national assessment procedures and regulations.

In addition to these incentives, the way of decision-making is crucial for the manufacturer affected. The reimbursement decision-making process is often lengthy and exhausting (Fischer, 2012). Every month of waiting for the manufacturer increases the cost of capital. Companies need transparency, reliability and predictability. It is important, especially in the context of value-based pricing, that the judgements, no matter whether they are based on early benefit assessment or cost–benefit assessment, are not arbitrary. The stakeholders should take advantage of the potentials linked with joint scoping processes.

There is a strong consensus in Germany that the pre-tests of drug therapy should be performed only by accredited laboratories. Therefore, the reimbursement of the testing consists of the remuneration of hospitals or physicians in their own practices. They buy the test kits and perform the testing themselves, or they send the samples to special providers where the analysis takes place. The inclusion of testing in the remuneration systems of public insurance is the responsibility of the so-called 'common self-government' of associations of providers and insurance funds. There may be disagreements and delays, particularly in the case of tests that are not stated on the label of the drug as being a compulsory companion diagnostic. Single evaluations have lasted up to six years (Stock and Sydow, 2013). Although the legislative may influence the relevant organisations only indirectly, it should use its power to embed new billing numbers in the remuneration schemes. A recent example of such an initiative taken by the German government was a change in law which mandated the responsible committee ('Evaluation Committee') to decide by March 2013 which new procedures of telemedicine will be included in the remuneration of medical practitioners of ambulatory care.

In contrast to the drugs, there is no central price negotiation for the test kits. A 'fourth hurdle' of evaluation concerning medical and economic additional benefit compared to products or procedures previously available (Rogowski, 2013) does not exist and there is also no benefit assessment as a reference for pricing. The relevant organisations define the amount of remuneration for the testing to a certain extent, referring to the price of the test kit claimed by the manufacturers. Thus, the statutory health insurance does not send out any signal of price sensitivity. A better option may be an 'early benefit assessment' as practiced in the case of drugs, known as 'AMNOG evaluation', named after the implementing law Arzneimittelmarktneuordnungsgesetz – AMNOG ('Act on the Reform of the Market for Medicinal Products'). Such a rapid evaluation process could shed light on the additional benefit of the test. A deadline for decision of six months should be set to sustain a favourable investment climate. Longer waiting times would not be manageable for small companies. Quite a few start-ups have only one single product. Even vital start-ups could become insolvent if they had to face a longer period without sales. It is part of the responsibility of the government to avoid regulatory disproportionalities. Furthermore, the public bodies involved should inform the industry what kind of data is required to justify the inclusion of testing in the remuneration. Such guidance does not yet exist. Designing a regulatory framework for PM will be detailed in the next section showing the situation in Germany from a jurisprudential perspective.

Personalised Medicine and the Legal Considerations: An Analysis based on Current German Law[5]

Considering the legal aspects of PM carries some specific difficulties and limitations. Among these difficulties is, above all, the fact that PM does not raise any completely new legal questions and that these questions relate to a variety of areas of law; we are, therefore, from the legal point of view, dealing with a cross-section issue (Huster and Gottwald, 2011). Furthermore, legal analysis typically reacts to problems regarding the application of existing rules to known facts. However, the further development of PM can hardly be predicted, therefore, it is uncertain to which facts the law will have to react. Finally, the development

---

5   The work presented in this section has been conducted by Sina Gottwald and Stefan Huster.

which is summarised under the term 'personalised medicine' is a multifaceted matter. The production of individualised protheses raises different legal questions compared to predictive genetic diagnostics, which, in turn, lead to different legal problems compared to a therapy based on a stratification using bio-markers, as this is the focus of this section. Therefore, there will not be a uniform legal problem relating to PM in general, but rather a bundle of various legal issues.

We will focus the legal analysis in the following on the collection of genetic (and clinical) data relevant for PM and on consequences which PM may have for the system of the German statutory health insurance funds.

The Collection of Genetic Data and Legal Regulation Requirements

The collection of data for research purposes in so-called biobanks in Germany – in contrast to many other countries – has not, up to now, been made subject to special statutory regulations (Antonow, 2006; Söns, 2008; Deutscher Ethikrat, 2010).

The collection of human genetic information for treatment purposes, however, has already been regulated in the Act on Genetic Diagnostics (Gendiagnostikgesetz – GenDG). In as far as PM has to rely on such human genetic examinations, it remains to be seen whether the rules provided for in the GenDG and in other applicable norms require adaptation. Should processes from PM develop into medical standards, the requirements with regard to the provision of genetic information and advice for the patients will become more demanding. This may also have consequences for the ongoing training of physicians and for the remuneration of the relevant services. Due to their cross-border character, 'direct-to-consumer tests' will only be open to a very limited extent to regulation by the German legal system.

From this perspective, an extension of genetic diagnostics, furthermore, poses more fundamental questions. The massive extension of predictive genetic diagnostics may lead, for instance, to an individualisation of health responsibility, or even to a 'health obligation' relating to the genetic risks detected (Damm, 2011). Furthermore, it cannot be excluded that knowledge of disease risks may, in the long-term, undermine the acceptance of the solidarity-based safeguarding of such risks in the context of a collective health fund system.

In addition to this, the health fund system, as well as the definition of the term 'disease' as used for the regulation of this system, may be faced with new challenges should predictive genetic diagnostics be able to determine with a high probability the future materialisation of disease risks. For such 'healthy sick people', the question will be whether they have a claim against the health fund system to be provided with prophylactic treatment. This already addresses the consequences which PM may have for the system of the German statutory health insurance fund (Gesetzliche Krankenversicherung – GKV).

Personalised Medicine and Possible Consequences for the System of the German Statutory Health Insurance Fund

Medicinal measures must always prove their (additional) benefit in order to be incorporated into the catalogue of services of the GKV. In this context, health insurance law has aligned this benefit assessment strictly along the principles of evidence-based medicine (EBM). With regard to PM, the demand is also that the requirements of EBM must be fulfilled (Schillinger, 2011; Windeler, 2012; Grafin von Hardenberg and Wilman, 2013; Windeler and Lange, 2013). The stratification of patient groups and the ever-shrinking subgroup of patients for whom the application of the relevant personalised therapy is an option may have the consequence that evidence can no longer be obtained through the application to as large a group and as large a number of cases as possible as required by EBM. This would require significant revisions of the laws with regard to the proof of benefits required in order to prevent new therapies of PM being included in the catalogue of services without valid proof of benefits having been provided (Eberbach, 2011).

A similar problem occurs regarding the determination of prices for personalised medicinal products. In the procedure of early benefit assessment and negotiation of reimbursement sums introduced in 2011, the legislative provided for a privilege for medicinal products for the treatment of rare diseases by assuming that their additional benefit has been proven upon their authorisation for marketing under pharmaceutical law. Should the stratification of the patient population have the consequence that personalised medicinal products are generally classified as orphan drugs, this provision would have to be reconsidered (Huster and Gottwald, 2013a).

These medicinal products lead to another regulatory problem, insofar as their authorisation for marketing requires, or at least recommends, accompanying tests. As outlined already in the section on health economic aspects in Germany, medicinal products are eligible for prescription for the account of the health insurance fund upon their authorisation, but this does not apply to the same extent to tests as 'companion diagnostics'. Even assuming that, due to their direct link to the medicinal product, they do not require a special authorisation decision by the Joint Federal Committee (Gemeinsamer Bundesausschuss – G-BA) for incorporation into the services of contract physicians, the reimbursement of their costs depends on their inclusion into the uniform assessment standard (Einheitlicher Bewertungsmaßstab). It would have to be considered whether application rights for the diagnostics manufacturers and decision obligations for the uniform evaluation committee (Einheitlicher Bewertungsausschuss) should be provided for in order to prevent the blocking of the use of the authorised medicinal product due to lack of payment for the tests (Huster and Gottwald, 2013b).

Finally, the stratification of patient populations may also lead to the consideration to refuse to provide a subgroup of patients with a treatment which has very unlikely or minor benefits. If alternative treatments do not exist and if the disease is life-threatening, this refusal of treatment would constitute a violation of the requirements developed by the German federal constitutional court (Bundesverfassungsgericht) in its decisions regarding the service obligations of the statutory health insurance fund. Insofar as this is so, stratification would have limitations under constitutional law (Beschluss des BVerfG, 2005).

Benefits and Harms of Personalised Medicine and the Respect for Patient Autonomy: An Ethical Analysis in Light of Evidentiary Uncertainty[6]

Numerous issues of ethical relevance have been raised in the preceding sections concerning medical, health economic and legal aspects of PM. Examples are the value judgements relevant to determine benefit, cost and harm of PM, ethical issues relevant to private–public partnerships and possible conflict of interests, the protection of privacy in light of the aggregation of large amounts of biological and clinical data, professional competency in times of PM, and issues relevant from an allocation ethics perspective when it comes to investments in research and products regarding PM by public institutions.

The subsequent analysis from an ethics perspective starts from the premise that while important innovative diagnostic and treatment strategies in the context of PM have doubtless been developed, it is, at the moment, far from clear whether PM will be a justified dominant model for research and clinical practice in the future. Based on the current scientific evidence and the challenges pointed out in the medical section, we suggest rather that an ethical analysis should be guided by considerations which take into account the continuation of success of PM in some fields of medicine as well as failure in other fields. Against this background and taking up selected challenges which have been pointed out already in the sections above, we will focus our analysis on three aspects: first, the debate about evidentiary standards for PM and inherent value judgements, second, the importance of unbiased information for research participants and patients, and third, ethical issues relevant to decisions about the resources spent on the research and practice of PM.

---

6   The work presented in this section has been conducted by Jan Schildmann, Sebastian Wäscher, Verena Sandow and Jochen Vollmann.

Standards for Evidence-Based (Personalised) Medicine and Value Judgements

Based on the possibility of translating biological concepts, identified in the context of PM, into clinical practice, it has been argued that the usual cascade of phase 1–3 trials requested to prove the benefit of a new substances may not be necessary to prove the benefit of PM interventions (Mandrekar and Sargent, 2009; Kaplan et al., 2013; Sleijfer et al., 2013). One rationale for this claim is that, in light of the multitude of markers which have been detected to be associated with diseases and the limited number of resources which are available for clinical trials to test PM interventions, it will simply not be possible to prove the benefit of PM interventions according to the established criteria of EBM, as they have been described, for example, by Windeler and Lange in this book (Chapter 13). It has also been pointed out that the decreasing number of patients with a specific marker requires changes in trial design. This is because it will not be possible to get a sufficiently high number of patients into trials due to small populations characterised by a certain marker. In contrast to the various suggestions to change research methodology for PM interventions, there are also a considerable number of statements by researchers and other stakeholders suggesting that it is only by adhering to established standards of evidence-based medicine that the benefit of PM can be proven. In order to bolster their cautious stance, critics refer to the findings of more recent research studies within the context of PM which have pointed out considerable heterogeneity regarding genetic mutation at different sites of the cancer (Browman, 2012; Ludwig, 2012). Furthermore, critics argue that if PM is effective, the smaller numbers should not be a problem, taking into account a sufficient size of effect.

The sketch above only describes some of the current points of controversy concerning the question of acceptable evidentiary levels. What evidence is needed to accept PM interventions as being of more benefit than harm? The answers to this question differ depending whether they come from the perspective of a clinician, a natural science researcher, a representative of the pharmaceutical industry or a body which is responsible for making decisions about the funding of approved substances. Empirical research and methodological analysis may inform judgements on evidence. However, at the end and without exception, there will be also a normative component when making judgements about the evidentiary level (Browman et al., 2014). Factors relevant here are our views on the required level of efficiency of research designed to translate biological developments into clinical practice or the clinical utility which we wish to have shown (and the different ways in which we define such a clinical utility). From a medical ethics perspective, there are several things which seem important with regard to advancement in this debate. First, we require an exploration of empirical challenges relevant to the methodology of PM, including suggestions and arguments for alternative approaches to determine the benefit and harm of a concrete PM (for suggestions in this respect, see Chapter 3, this volume). Second, it is of utmost importance to identify the often cryptonormative value judgements associated with the differing accounts regarding the (in-) appropriateness of the research methodology of PM. Last but not least, and relevant from a procedural ethics perspective, it is necessary to determine legitimate bodies who make decisions about the level of evidence necessary to define benefit or harm of PM.

Patient Autonomy and the Need for Unbiased Information

Informing patients and research participants about PM interventions is associated with several ethical challenges. In the context of PM and informational self-determination, the issues of reporting back results of genomic analysis, information about the future use of tissue samples and aspects of privacy have been analysed in numerous ethical analyses (Secko et al., 2009; Kohnen et al., 2013). While these issues are doubtless important from an ethical perspective, we would like to add two less frequently discussed aspects which, in our view, are highly relevant from a practical point of view.

The first issue which follows from the analysis on evidentiary uncertainty above is the question on ethically appropriate information about this uncertainty in the context of clinical research. Take the example of a patient diagnosed with AML who is offered participation in a trial in which patients will be treated based on the analysis of different biomarkers.[7] As has been shown in the medical section, there is evidence for biomarkers associated with better and worse prognosis. However, this evidence stems from retrospective genome-wide association studies (GWAS) and it is far from clear whether a more aggressive treatment in patients with a more risky genetic make-up will lead to better results. It is also unclear whether patients with a less favourable genetic make-up could profit even more from a more aggressive treatment such as stem cell transplantation.

A second aspect relevant for informed decision-making from the side of the patient can be framed as the complexity of genetic information and appropriate ways of communicating such information. Both the risks associated with certain biomarkers and those associated with biobank research are complex. Against such a background, we need to explore ways which facilitate the understanding of such information so that patients and/or research participants can make informed decisions. To get back to the example of the patient with AML who is offered participation in a trial including stratification according to biomarkers.

---

7   The case analysis of a patient with acute myeloid leukaemia has been published in a more detailed version in Kohnen et al. (2013).

In practice, this patient, shortly after having received the bad news of a life-threatening disease, receives a package with written information, whereas time for detailed discussions necessary to understand the information is limited in the clinical research context. Patients who consent to participate in the clinical research usually consent also to the use of data for other research which at the time is not known in detail. From a medical ethics perspective and with a focus on patient autonomy, it has to be questioned whether such an approach takes the principle of patient self-determination seriously enough. After all, it is unlikely that patients having received the diagnosis of a life-threatening disease are in a position to make far-reaching decisions, such as the use of data in future research. Against this background, we suggested a more process-orientated approach to information and consent which focuses on the question at which point in time may patients be in a good position to make a decision (Kohnen et al., 2013). Furthermore, and in light of the evidentiary uncertainty underlying current clinical research strategies in the context of PM, it seems necessary to explore what information on this aspect of PM should be conveyed to patients in which way. Given unavoidable value judgements guiding decisions about research design and treatment recommendation, such considerations are important to empower patients to make decisions which are in line with their priorities and attitudes.

Financing PM and Opportunity Costs from an Allocation Ethics Perspective

The high investment costs in research based on molecular genetic criteria raise the question of opportunity costs. Given the limited resources in the health-care sector, a prioritisation decision is already required at the research level regarding the extent of public resources that should flow into particular areas of the health-care system (Vollmann, 2012). A research priority in one area limits the remaining research funds for other medical speciality areas. With regard to the promotion and funding of PM, this difficult normative and political decision is further exacerbated since only a relatively small number of patients benefit here from these very expensive measures. That is why clinical physicians are concerned that other important clinical and health-care areas benefiting many patients will be neglected through the prioritised promotion of PM (Browman et al., 2011; Ludwig, 2012, Wäscher et al., 2013) Thus far, only a minority of patients have benefited from this expensive, research- and economics-driven project of PM (Browman et al., 2011). From a medical ethics perspective, the existing preference for molecular genetics medicine in PM, in contrast to other research fields in the publicly funded health-care system, needs to be critically examined. In essence, all prioritisation decisions are ethical decisions in which competing values must be weighed (Vollmann, 2015). In doing so, transparency must prevail regarding who decides about what facts, which criteria are used and on which arguments decisions are based. Therefore, it is ethically unacceptable that influential individual interests *de facto* determine medical research priorities and resource allocation in the publicly funded health-care system; but this is exactly what is currently happening under the innocuous label of 'PM'. Cost–benefit assessments of the individual treatments – now often discussed – are also insufficient, since they only allow statements about the medical benefits and the costs of the treatment area under investigation on the basis of empirical data. Frequently, the selection of the treatment area for research in practice already represents a setting of priorities within the overall spectrum of possible health-promoting measures without prior reflexion about the norms involved. Transparent and democratically legitimised superordinate medical and research policy prioritisations are required for our health care in the future (for a discussion from a health economist perspective, see Chapter 16, this volume).

Joint Summarising Recommendations for Future Development of the Research and Practice of 'Personalised Medicine'

As shown in the analysis above, there can be little doubt that PM already plays and will in the future play a role with regard to research and practice in medicine. However, it is also obvious that, for the moment, it is difficult to estimate the impact of this approach on medicine. Based on the multidisciplinary analysis, which includes different emphases and diverging views by the collaborating researchers, we jointly recommend the following measures and strategies.

Evidence and Professional Competency

There is currently considerable uncertainty regarding the clinical relevance of data gathered in the context of PM research. Strategies to determine the benefit and harm of PM interventions for patients are, therefore, of utmost importance. In additional to technological solutions, this may also include new research designs which, in turn, need to be critically discussed with regard to strengths and weaknesses compared with established standards of EBM. Last but not least, physicians and, where appropriate, other health-care providers need to acquire the necessary knowledge and medical and professional skills (for example, interpretation and communication of genetic risks) to apply PM in clinical practice.

Information, Management and Protection of Data

The collection and storage of a large amount of biological and clinical data is a prerequisite to determine the benefit and harm of PM interventions.

The enhancement of technologies to systemise, exchange and analyse the data with regard to their relevance in clinical practice is crucial. At the same time, protection of data of patients and/or research participants must have primacy in any concept of biobank and related data storage. Potential research participants should be informed appropriately given the increasing possibilities to link genetic data with individuals and the possible harm associated with such events for the participating individuals and their biological relatives. Given the complexity of such an information process, models and tools which facilitate the understanding of complex information should be developed.

Approval and Reimbursement, Setting of Priorities

The combination of tests and treatment (companion diagnostics) is characteristic for PM. However, the regulation regarding approval and reimbursement of such interventions in public health systems is insufficiently implemented at the moment and should be adapted. Given the high investments necessary for PM interventions, a transparent approach towards approval and reimbursement is required. On the other hand, the problem of opportunity costs associated with this approach have to be analysed and discussed in the light of the high investments necessary to implement PM within the public health-care system. These settings of public priorities in research and clinical practice are ethical decisions which have to be made public and decided by democratic legitimised bodies.

References

Antonow, K., 2006. *Der rechtliche Rahmen der Zulässigkeit von Biobanken zu Forschungszwecken [The legal framework of the admissibility of biobanks for research purposes]*. Düsseldorfer Rechtswissenschaftliche Schriften Band 40. Baden-Baden: Nomos.

Beschluss des BVerfG, 2005. 1 BvR 347/98. *Entscheidungen des Bundesverfassungsgerichts*, 115, p.25.

Borlum Kristensen, F., 2012. Development of European HTA: from vision to EUnetHTA. *Michael Quarterly*, 9(2), pp.147–56.

Browman, G., 2012. Special series on comparative effectiveness research: challenges to real-world solutions to quality improvement in personalized medicine. *Journal of Clinical Oncology*, 30(34), pp.4188–91.

Browman, G., Vollmann, J., Virani, A. and Schildmann, J., 2014. Improving the quality of 'personalized medicine' research and practice – through an ethical lens. *Personalized Medicine*, 11(4), pp.413–23.

Browman G., Hébert P.C., Coutts J., Stanbrook M.B., Flegel K. and MacDonald N.E., 2011. Personalized medicine: a windfall for science, but what about patients? *CMAJ*, 183(18), p.E1277.

Damm, F., Heuser, M., Morgan, M., Wagner, K., Görlich, K., Grosshennig, A., Hamwi, I., Thol, F., Surdziel, E., Fiedler, W., Lübbert, M., Kanz, L., Reuter, C., Heil, G., Delwel, R., Löwenberg, B., Valk, P.J., Krauter, J. and Ganser, A., 2011. Integrative prognostic risk score in acute myeloid leukemia with normal karyotype. *Blood*, 117(17), pp.4561–8.

Damm, R., 2011. Personalisierte Medizin und Patientenrechte – Medizinische Optionen und medizinrechtliche Bewertung [Personalised medicine and patients' rights – medical options and medical legal evaluation]. *Medizinrecht*, 29(1), pp.7–17.

Deutscher Ethikrat, 2010. *Humanbiobanken für die Forschung* [*Human biobanks for research*]. Berlin: Druckerei Hermann Schlesener KG.

Eberbach, W.H., 2011. Juristische Aspekte einer individualisierten Medizin [Legal aspects of individualised medicine]. *Medizinrecht*, 29(12), pp.757–70.

Fischer, B., 2012. 'Deutschland ist ein Top-Standort [Germany is a top location]'. Interview with Birgit Fischer, CEO, vfa. VC-Magazin, 6, Sonderbeilage Personalisierte Medizin [Special supplement on personalised medicine], pp.14–15.

Flaherty, K.T., Puzanov, I., Kim, K.B., Ribas, A., McArthur, G.A., Sosman, J.A., O'Dwyer, P.J., Lee, R.J., Grippo, J.F., Nolop, K. and Chapman, P.B., 2010. Inhibition of mutated, activated BRAF in metastatic melanoma. *New England Journal of Medicine*, 363(9), pp.809–19.

Gerlinger, M., Rowan, A.J., Horswell, S., Larkin, J., Endesfelder, D., Gronroos, E., Martinez, P., Matthews, N., Stewart, A., Tarpey, P., Varela, I., Phillimore, B., Begum, S., McDonald, N.Q., Butler, A., Jones, D., Raine, K., Latimer, C., Santos, C.R., Nohadani, M., Eklund, A.C., Spencer-Dene, B., Clark, G., Pickering, L., Stamp, G., Gore, M., Szallasi, Z., Downward, J., Futreal, P.A. and Swanton, C., 2012. Intratumor heterogeneity and branched evolution revealed by multiregion sequencing. *New England Journal of Medicine*, 366(10), pp.883–92.

Gräfin von Hardenberg, S. and Wilman, N., 2013. Individualisierte Medizin als Exklusiv-Medizin? [Individualised medicine as exclusive medicine?] *Medizinrecht*, 31(2), pp.77–82.

Greiner, W., 2012. Wirtschaftliche Potenziale individualisierter Medizin [The economic potential of individualised medicine]. *Gesundheit und Gesellschaft Wissenschaft*, 12(1), pp.20–6.

Hanahan, D. and Weinberg, R.A., 2011. Hallmarks of cancer: the next generation. *Cell*, 144(5), pp.646–74.

Huster, S. and Gottwald, S., 2011. Rechtliche Implikationen der personalisierten Medizin [Legal implications of personalised medicine]. *GesundheitsRecht*, pp.449–56.

Huster, S. and Gottwald, S., 2013a. Personalisierte Medizin als Orphanisierung: rechtliche und ethische Fragen [Personalised medicine as orphanisation: legal and ethical questions]. *Ethik in der Medizin*, 25(3), pp.259–66.

Huster, S. and Gottwald, S., 2013b. *Die Vergütung genetischer Diagnostik in der Gesetzlichen Krankenversicherung [The remuneration of genetic testing in statutory health insurance]*. Baden-Baden: Nomos.

Kaplan, R., Maughan, T., Crook, A., Fisher, D., Wilson, R., Brown, L. and Parmar, M., 2013. Evaluating many treatments and biomarkers in oncology: a new design. *Journal of Clinical Oncology*, 31(36), pp.4562–8.

Kohnen, T., Schildmann, J. and Vollmann, J., 2013. Patients' self-determination in 'personalised medicine': the case of whole genome sequencing and tissue banking in oncology. In: M. Braun and P. Dabrock, eds. *'Individualised medicine' between hype und hope*. Münster: LIT. pp.97–110.

Ludwig, W.D., 2012. Possibilities and limitations of stratified medicine based on biomarkers and targeted therapies in oncology. *Zeitschrift für Evidenz, Fortbildung und Qualität im Gesundheitswesen*, 106(1), pp.11–22.

Maio, G., 2012. Chancen und Grenzen der personalisierten Medizin – eine ethische Betrachtung [Opportunities and limitations of personalised medicine – an ethical consideration]. *Gesundheit und Gesellschaft Wissenschaft*, 12(1), pp.15–19.

Mandrekar, S. and Sargent, D., 2009. Genomic advances and their impact on clinical trial design. *Genome Medicine*, 1(7), p.69.

Port, M., Böttcher, M., Thol, F., Ganser, A., Schlenk, R., Wasem, J., Neumann, A. and Pouryamout, L., 2014. Prognostic significance of FLT3 internal tandem duplication, nucleophosmin 1, and CEBPA gene mutations for acute myeloid leukemia patients with normal karyotype and younger than 60 years: a systematic review and meta-analysis. *Annals of Hematology*, 93(8), pp.1279–86.

Rogowski, W., 2013. An economic theory of the fourth hurdle. *Health Economics*, 22(5), pp.600–10.

Schillinger, G., 2011. Pille nach Maß – Heilung für jeden? [Pills to measure – healing for everything?] *Gesundheit und Gesellschaft*, 11, pp.22–6.

Schlenk, R.F. and Döhner, K., 2009. Impact of new prognostic markers in treatment decisions in acute myeloid leukemia. *Current Opinion in Hematology*, 16, pp.98–104.

Secko, D., Preto, N., Niemeyer, S. and Burgess, M., 2009. Informed consent in biobank research: a deliberative approach to the debate. *Social Science and Medicine*, 68(4), pp.781–9.

Sleijfer, S., Bogaerts, J. and Siu, L., 2013. Designing transformative clinical trials in the cancer genome era. *Journal of Clinical Oncology*, 31(15), pp.1834–41.

Söns, U., 2008. *Biobanken im Spannungsfeld von Persönlichkeitsrecht und Forschungsfreiheit* [*Biobanks in the area of conflict between personal rights and freedom of research*]. Hamburg: Dr. Kovac Verlag.

Stevens, A.J., Jensen, J.J., Wyller, K., Kilgore, P.C., Chatterjee, S. and Rohrbaugh, M.L., 2011. The role of public-sector research in the discovery of drugs and vaccines. *New England Journal of Medicine*, 364(6), pp.535–41.

Stock, G. and Sydow, S., 2013. Personalisierte Medizin. Paradigmenwechsel in der Arzneimittelforschung und –therapie [Personalised medicine. Paradigm shift in drug research and therapy]. *Bundesgesundheitsblatt – Gesundheitsforschung – Gesundheitsschutz*, 56(11), pp.1495–501.

Tsimberidou, A.M., Ringborg, U. and Schilsky, R.L., 2013. *Strategies to overcome clinical, regulatory, and financial challenges in the implementation of personalized medicine.* American Society of Clinical Oncology Educational Book 49, pp.118–25.

Vollmann, J., 2012. Ein trügerisches Versprechen [A deceptive promise]. *Frankfurter Allgemeine Zeitung*, 105, p.10.

Vollmann, J., 2015 (in print). Personalised medicine: priority setting and opportunity costs in different social rooms. In: R. ter Meulen and R. Huxtable, eds. *The voices and rooms of European bioethics*. Routledge.

Wäscher, S., Schildmann, J., Brall, C. and Vollmann, J., 2013. Personalisierte Medizin in der Onkologie. Erste Ergebnisse einer qualitativen Interviewstudie zu Wahrnehmungen und Bewertungen onkologisch tätiger Ärzte [Personalised medicine in oncology. First results of a qualitative interview study of perceptions and evaluations of oncology-based physicians]. *Ethik in der Medizin*, 25, pp.205–14.

Wiechers, I.R., Perin, N.C. and Cook-Deegan, R., 2013. The emergence of commercial genomics: analysis of the rise of a biotechnology subsector during the human genome project, 1990 to 2004. *Genome Medicine*, 5(9), p.83.

Windeler, J., 2012. Individualisierte Medizin – unser (Un)Verständnis [Individualised medicine – our (mis)understanding]. *Zeitschrift für Evidenz, Fortbildung und Qualität im Gesundheitswesen*, 106, pp.5–10.

Windeler, J. and Lange, S., 2013. Nutzenbewertung personalisierter Interventionen: Methodische Herausforderungen und Lösungsansätze. *Ethik in der Medizin*, 25(3), pp.173–82.

Index

Page numbers in **bold** refer to figures and tables.

3 20